Cataract Surgery and Intraocular Lenses

Cataract Surgery and Intraocular Lenses

Lucio Buratto, MD
Centro Ambrosiano Oftalmico
Milan, Italy

Stephen F. Brint, MD, FACS
Associate Clinical Professor of Ophthalmology
Tulane University School of Medicine
New Orleans, Louisiana

Domenico Boccuzzi, MD, PhD
Clinica Mediterranea
Naples, Italy

CRC Press
Taylor & Francis Group
Boca Raton London New York

CRC Press is an imprint of the
Taylor & Francis Group, an **informa** business

Illustrations courtesy of Massimiliano Crespi and Lucio Buratto.

First published in 2014 by SLACK Incorporated

Published 2024 by CRC Press
2385 NW Executive Center Drive, Suite 320, Boca Raton FL 33431

and by CRC Press
4 Park Square, Milton Park, Abingdon, Oxon, OX14 4RN

CRC Press is an imprint of Taylor & Francis Group, LLC

Library of Congress Cataloging-in-Publication Data
Buratto, Lucio, author.
Cataract surgery and intraocular lenses / Lucio Buratto, Stephen F. Brint, Domenico Boccuzzi.
p. ; cm.
Includes bibliographical references and index.
ISBN 978-1-61711-604-9
I. Brint, Stephen F., 1946- author. II. Boccuzzi, Domenico, author. III. Title.
[DNLM: 1. Cataract Extraction. 2. Lenses, Intraocular. WW 260]
RE451
617.7'42059--dc23
2013050996

ISBN: 9781617116049 (hbk)
ISBN: 9781003522874 (ebk)

DOI: 10.1201/9781003522874

Dedication

To Vittorio Picardo, a dear friend and highly esteemed colleague.

Lucio Buratto, MD

I have been so fortunate to have great teachers and friends who have helped me though the management of the inevitable complications of cataract surgery and have made me a better surgeon.

Stephen F. Brint, MD, FACS

To my daughter, Lorenza, and my wife, Tiziana, the constants in my life.

Domenico Boccuzzi, MD, PhD

Contents

Dedication v
Acknowledgments ix
About the Authors xi
Contributing Authors xiii
Foreword by Vittorio Picardo, MD xv

Section I 1

Chapter 1 The History of Intraocular Lenses 3
Lucio Buratto, MD; Stephen F. Brint, MD, FACS; and Domenico Boccuzzi, MD, PhD

Chapter 2 The Materials 7
Lucio Buratto, MD; Stephen F. Brint, MD, FACS; and Domenico Boccuzzi, MD, PhD

Chapter 3 Rigid Intraocular Lenses of the Past 15
Lucio Buratto, MD; Stephen F. Brint, MD, FACS; and Domenico Boccuzzi, MD, PhD

Chapter 4 Soft Intraocular Lenses of the Past 17
Lucio Buratto, MD; Stephen F. Brint, MD, FACS; and Domenico Boccuzzi, MD, PhD

Chapter 5 Currently Used Lenses 23
Lucio Buratto, MD; Stephen F. Brint, MD, FACS; and Domenico Boccuzzi, MD, PhD

Chapter 6 Monofocal Intraocular Lenses 27
Lucio Buratto, MD; Stephen F. Brint, MD, FACS; and Domenico Boccuzzi, MD, PhD

Chapter 7 Toric Intraocular Lenses 39
Lucio Buratto, MD; Stephen F. Brint, MD, FACS; and Domenico Boccuzzi, MD, PhD

Chapter 8 Multifocal Intraocular Lenses 53
Lucio Buratto, MD; Stephen F. Brint, MD, FACS; and Domenico Boccuzzi, MD, PhD

Chapter 9 Accommodative Intraocular Lenses 73
Lucio Buratto, MD; Stephen F. Brint, MD, FACS; and Domenico Boccuzzi, MD, PhD

Chapter 10 Mix and Match 79
Lucio Buratto, MD; Stephen F. Brint, MD, FACS; and Domenico Boccuzzi, MD, PhD

Chapter 11 Refractive Cataract Surgery 83
Lucio Buratto, MD; Stephen F. Brint, MD, FACS; and Domenico Boccuzzi, MD, PhD

Chapter 12 Intraocular Lens Exchange 91
Lucio Buratto, MD; Stephen F. Brint, MD, FACS; and Domenico Boccuzzi, MD, PhD

Chapter 13 Correction of Astigmatism 95
Lucio Buratto, MD; Stephen F. Brint, MD, FACS; and Domenico Boccuzzi, MD, PhD

Chapter 14 Vision Quality 99
Lucio Buratto, MD; Stephen F. Brint, MD, FACS; and Domenico Boccuzzi, MD, PhD

Chapter 15 Viscoelastic Substances 119
Lucio Buratto, MD; Stephen F. Brint, MD, FACS; and Domenico Boccuzzi, MD, PhD

Chapter 16 Instruments Used for Intraocular Lens Insertion 125
Lucio Buratto, MD; Stephen F. Brint, MD, FACS; and Domenico Boccuzzi, MD, PhD

Chapter 17 Injectors and Implantation of Foldable Intraocular Lenses 135
Lucio Buratto, MD; Stephen F. Brint, MD, FACS; and Domenico Boccuzzi, MD, PhD

Chapter 18 Implantation of an Intraocular Lens With Capsular Rupture 155
Lucio Buratto, MD; Stephen F. Brint, MD, FACS; and Domenico Boccuzzi, MD, PhD

Chapter 19 Tear or Damage of the Intraocular Lens 161
Lucio Buratto, MD; Stephen F. Brint, MD, FACS; and Domenico Boccuzzi, MD, PhD

Chapter 20 Irrigation/Aspiration Post Implantation 163
Lucio Buratto, MD; Stephen F. Brint, MD, FACS; and Domenico Boccuzzi, MD, PhD

Chapter 21 Closure of the Incision 167
Lucio Buratto, MD; Stephen F. Brint, MD, FACS; and Domenico Boccuzzi, MD, PhD

Chapter 22 Drugs and Fluids for Intraocular Use 171
Lucio Buratto, MD; Stephen F. Brint, MD, FACS; and Domenico Boccuzzi, MD, PhD

Section II 175

Chapter 23 Latest Generation Multifocal Intraocular Lenses and Emerging Accommodative Intraocular Lenses 177
Jorge L. Alió, MD, PhD, FEBO; Felipe Soria, MD; and Ghassan Zein, MD, PhD, FRCS (Ophth) UK

Chapter 24 Avoiding and Managing Patient Dissatisfaction After Intraocular Lens Implantation After Cataract Surgery 189
Johann A. Kruger, MMed Ophth, FCS (SA) Ophth, FRCS Ed Ophth

Financial Disclosures 193

Index 195

Acknowledgments

The publication of a book is an extremely difficult and exhausting procedure and it involves an incredible amount of work. The completion of such an enterprise would not be possible without the smooth-running organization and the assistance of my reliable team of collaborators.

I would like to thank a number of them personally: Domenico Boccuzzi, Luigi Caretti, Mario Romano, Laura Sacchi, and Rosalia Sorce for their invaluable contribution to the production of this series of books on cataract surgery. Heartfelt thanks also to Massimiliano Crespi, the artist who produced the magnificent drawings and particularly for his unique ability to transfer the author's thoughts and ideas onto paper; my warmest thanks also to Salvatore Ferrandes who was in charge of the iconographic and clinical aspects of the publications.

I would like to thank the staff of Medicongress, in particular Monica Gingardi, for their excellent organizational and operational skills.

Sincere thanks to my dear friend Vittorio Picardo for his revision of the final version of the text.

Thanks are also due to SLACK Incorporated, my American publisher of the English versions, and their first-class work in promoting the international distribution of the publications.

Last but not least, I would like to thank my dear friend and superb coauthor, Steve Brint, for his huge work and invaluable contribution.

Lucio Buratto, MD

About the Authors

Lucio Buratto, MD is a leading international expert in cataract and myopia surgery, and a pioneer in the ocular techniques of intraocular lens (IOL) implantation, in the phacoemulsification procedure for the cataract, in the laser techniques for myopia, astigmatism and hyperopia. In 1978, Dr. Buratto began using the Kelman phacoemulsification technique, and in 1979 he started using posterior chamber intraocular lenses. Since 1980, he has organized and presided over 48 updating congresses on the surgery of cataract and glaucoma and on laser therapy, organized 54 practical courses for the teaching of eye surgery, and taken part as spokesman and teacher in more than 400 courses and congresses.

In 1989, Dr. Buratto became the world's first surgeon to use excimer laser intrastromal keratomileusis, and concurrently began to treat low myopia using PRK techniques. In 1995, he was appointed as Monitor of the United States Food and Drug Administration. In 1996, Dr. Buratto became the world's first surgeon to use a new technique called Down-Up LASIK, which improved the LASIK procedure for the correction of myopia; he holds a United States patent for this technique.

For teaching purposes, Dr. Buratto has performed surgical operations during live surgery sessions for more than 200 international and Italian congresses, performed surgery during satellite broadcasts to 54 countries on 4 different continents, and designed and produced 143 instruments for ocular surgery. In 2004, he was a speaker at the Binkhorst Medal Lecture during the XXII Annual Meeting of the European Society of Cataract and Refractive Surgeons (ESCRS) in Paris, and was the first European surgeon to use the new intralase laser for refractive surgery. In 2011, Dr. Buratto was the first West European surgeon to use the femtosecond laser for cataract surgery.

Dr. Buratto has published over 125 scientific publications and 59 monographs (of which 24 are on cataract surgery, 5 are on glaucoma surgery, and 11 are on myopia). His recent works include, *Phakic IOLs: State of the Art*, *LASIK: The Evolution of Refractive Surgery*, and *PRK: The Past, Present, and Future of Surface Ablation.*

Stephen F. Brint, MD, FACS was the first physician in the United States to perform the LASIK procedure in June 1991, after working with Dr. Lucio Buratto in Milan to perfect the technique. He was the medical monitor of the first US FDA LASIK study and has been a lead investigator for both the Alcon Custom Cornea LASIK procedure as well as the Medical Monitor for all of the US FDA Wavelight Allegretto Wavefront Optimized and Custom Studies. He graduated from Tulane University School of Medicine, New Orleans, Louisiana and completed his residency there as well in 1977, continuing to serve as Associate Clinical Professor of Ophthalmology. In addition to his vast LASIK experience of more than 30,000 LASIK procedures, many with the Intralase All Laser LASIK technique, he is a renowned cataract/lens surgeon, having participated in the FDA clinical trials of the new IOLs, including ReSTOR and ReZOOM, and toric IOLs.

He is board certified by the American Board of Ophthalmology and a Fellow of the American College of Surgeons. He has been recognized as "The Best Doctor in New Orleans" by *New Orleans Magazine* for the past 10 years and has been selected by his peers for the 2000–2012 editions of *The Best Doctors in America.* Dr. Brint is a leading cataract surgeon and instructor and the author of the 3 definitive textbooks on LASIK and cataract surgery, including the most recent, *Custom LASIK.*

Dr. Brint performs surgery and lectures around the world, including Europe, Russia, China, Japan, Australia, Singapore, Africa, and South America.

Dr. Brint has a passion for education and research, and most recently he has been involved with the refinement of the intraoperative aberrometer for selecting IOL power and femtosecond laser-assisted cataract surgery.

Domenico Boccuzzi, MD, PhD is a clinician who specialized in ophthalmology in 2006. He was awarded a Research Doctorate in Molecular Imaging, with his thesis on the IROG method for recording nystagmus in patients affected by congenital nystagmus and subjected to surgery. He lives in Naples and works in the city's Clinica Mediterranea. He is specialized in surgery of the anterior segment and has a particular interest in the development of new technologies for ophthalmology and the implantation of innovative IOLs. Since 2008, he has been a humanitarian volunteer at the Comboni Centre in Sogakope in Ghana.

Contributing Authors

Jorge L. Alió, MD, PhD, FEBO (Chapter 23)
Professor and Chairman
Miguel Hernandez University
Medical Director
Vissum Corporation
Alicante, Spain

Johann A. Kruger, MMed Ophth, FCS (SA) Ophth, FRCS Ed Ophth (Chapter 24)
Tygervalley Eye and Laser Centre
Cape Town, South Africa

Felipe Soria, MD (Chapter 23)
Fellow
Cataract and Refractive Surgery
Vissum Corporation
Alicante, Spain

Ghassan Zein, MD, PhD, FRCS (Ophth) UK (Chapter 23)
Fellow
Harvard Medical School
Boston, Massachusetts
Consultant
Refractive Surgery, Cornea, and Uveitis
Ahmadi Hospital
Al Ahmadi, Kuwait

Foreword

Sir Harold Ridley followed his genial intuition and decided to insert an artificial crystalline lens inside the human eye operated for cataract removal; this type of surgery, at the outset simply a therapeutic procedure to resolve a pathological affliction of the crystalline, would rapidly develop into a rehabilitative technique for improving sight.

The technique started life in the 1950s, and since then it has grabbed the attention of researchers, scientists, and manufacturing companies. The field has developed to such a degree that during the second half of the 20th century, in parallel with the evolution of the surgical techniques, now partially performed with laser technology, the companies produced intraocular lenses (IOLs) with increasingly physiological characteristics—an important and necessary achievement.

This book written by Lucio Buratto, Stephen F. Brint, and Domenico Boccuzzi gives a detailed overview on IOLs and completes the new series of books on cataract surgery. They decided to dedicate one of the books to this specific subject because the choice of the IOL to be implanted is an essential feature in the patient's functional result, with the quality and quantity of sight recovered.

In today's surgical universe, biometric errors are no longer acceptable; the surgeon is duty-bound to be fully aware of the wide range of IOLs available for implantation. The lenses are no longer split into hydrophilic and hydrophobic; aspherical, toric, multifocal, accommodative, etc, are also now available.

When the patient consults an eye specialist, he or she will always have researched his or her condition "thanks" to the Internet and will ask very specific questions about the surgery and the available therapeutic options. The eye specialist must be able to answer all of the questions and clearly explain the pros and cons associated with the implantation of each type of artificial crystalline lens.

This knowledge is also one of the foundations of good a surgical outcome; it is essential that the surgeon selects the most appropriate IOL for the needs of the specific patient, in other words, the surgical procedure must be personalized.

Consequently, the surgeon can be defined as a craftsperson who works with his or her hands; however, his or her professional and manual approach cannot be detached from attentive, correct, and global cultural information, factors that will allow him or her to confidently use his or her knowledge and experience to satisfy the doubts and queries voiced by the patient and advise the patient on the real outcome possibilities of his or her surgery.

This book is the third in the cataract series of 5 books published by Dr. Buratto. Dr. Boccuzzi was the perfect coauthor in this project. The publication combines the experience of the Maestro with the passion and enthusiasm of a young surgeon; it unites the latest information on the most advanced functional diagnostic technology and the use of the latest surgical devices, with the top clinical and technical experience of one of the world's leading surgeons, spiced with a healthy dose of self-criticism.

This book is a wonderful monography, full of information that is easy to read and comprehend. It could be described as a "quality gold star" addition to the other 4 books in the series.

Vittorio Picardo, MD
Head
Ophthalmological Department
Casa di Cura "Nuova Itor"
Rome, Italy

Section I

1

The History of Intraocular Lenses

Lucio Buratto, MD; Stephen F. Brint, MD, FACS; and Domenico Boccuzzi, MD, PhD

In order to fully understand the technological evolution of cataract surgery over the past 50 years, we need to compare current surgical procedures and visual recovery times with those reported half a century ago. A look at the history of cataract surgery clearly shows that its evolution is an outcome of the vision of a few inspired pioneers who had great passion for their profession.

When phacoemulsification was first developed by Charles Kelman, it faced strong opposition and hence took time in being accepted by the majority of eye surgeons (Figure 1-1).

It was only with the introduction of intraocular lenses (IOLs), and to a greater degree with the advent of foldable IOLs, that the technique was accepted and used on a much larger scale.

In the same way, the evolution of the IOL itself was influenced by ongoing technological progress with phacoemulsification devices and phacoemulsification techniques. This progress led to the development of lenses that could be inserted through increasingly smaller incisions. Today we are able to perform cataract surgery in a few minutes, with visual rehabilitation, and we owe it exclusively to a small number of surgeons who firmly believed in these technological innovations. Charles Kelman was unquestionably the most brilliant mind behind this enormous change.

However, to fully understand the current status of IOLs, it is essential to take a step back in time to more than 60 years ago.

In 1949, Sir Harold Ridley invented the first IOL (Figure 1-2). These lenses had little in common with IOLs used today. They were not easy to implant and were associated with many complications. When he was working with the Royal Air Force, treating people injured during World War II, Ridley noticed that when splinters of acrylic plastic from shattered aircraft windscreens penetrated the eyes of injured pilots, they were not rejected by the eye; consequently, he suggested using artificial lenses made up of this material to correct aphakia following removal of the lens. He actually got the idea when a student who was assisting him in cataract surgery innocently asked him why an artificial lens was not inserted to replace the focusing natural lens that had been removed from the eye.

Ridley performed his first surgery on November 29, 1949 at St. Thomas' Hospital; he implanted for the first time an artificial acrylic polymethylmethacrylate (PMMA) IOL in a human eye. The surgery was performed with extracapsular technique on the left eye of a 45-year-old woman with unilateral cataracts. Not sure of the stability of the lens, he removed it in a second surgery on February 8, 1950, when the eye appeared inactive.[1]

The first IOL was produced by the company Rayner in Brighton & Hove, East Sussex, UK. Currently, this company continues to produce and supply the latest generation of IOLs.

In 1952, the first IOL (a Ridley-Rayner lens) was implanted at the Wills Eye Hospital, Philadelphia, PA. Over the following years, Ridley continued developing his idea of cataract surgery with IOL implantation; he was a pioneer for this type of surgery, despite strong opposition from the entire medical community at that time. He worked tirelessly to reduce complications and improve the technique. Working closely with one of his disciples, Peter Choyce, he eventually enjoyed the support of the scientific community for the technique, and the IOL was finally approved as "safe and effective" and was

Buratto L, Brint SF, Boccuzzi D.
Cataract Surgery and Intraocular Lenses (pp 3-6).

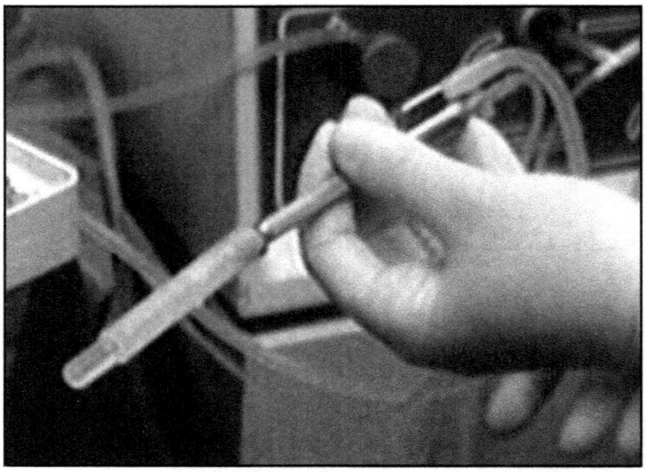

Figure 1-1. The I/A handpiece of the old Cavitron/Kelman phacoemulsifier machine.

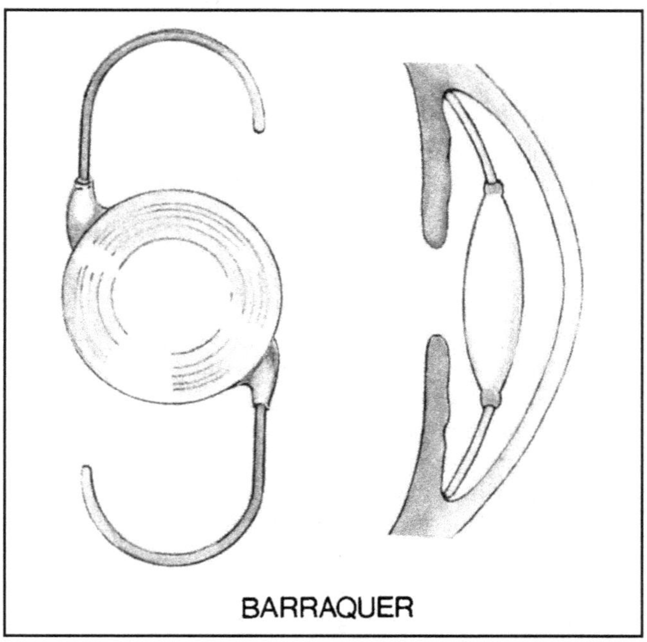

Figure 1-3. The IOL designed by Joaquin Barraquer with J-shaped loops.[3]

permitted by the Food and Drug Administration (FDA) in 1981 for human use in the United States. These first lenses (Choyce Mark VIII and Choyce Mark IX anterior chamber lenses) approved by the FDA were also produced by Rayner. Currently, cataract surgery with lens removal followed by implantation of an artificial lens is the most commonly performed surgical procedure. The first lenses implanted had low reliability, and this type of surgery was associated with a

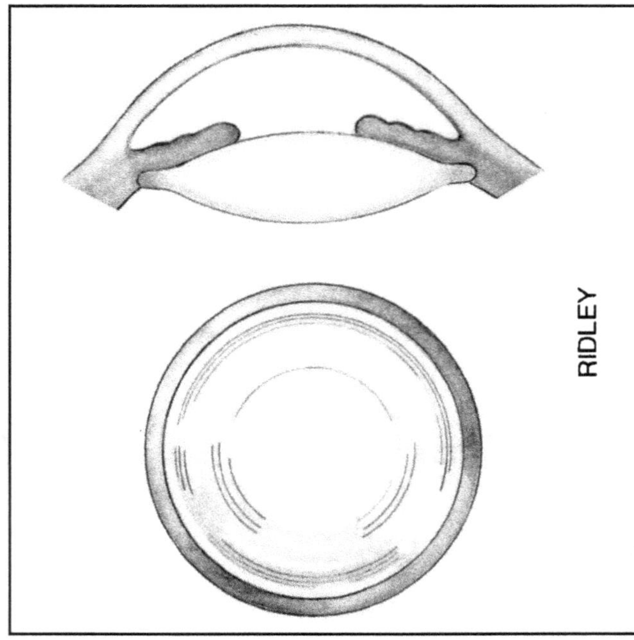

Figure 1-2. The IOL implanted by Ridley, made of plastic.[2]

high number of complications: the haptics of nylon tended to dissolve and this created destabilization of the lens.

It is reported that during the 1950s, 2 surgical techniques were developed in the UK: one for implanting the IOLs and one for removing them! At the end of the 1960s, Cornelius Binkhorst developed an IOL with 4 loops, which greatly reduced the number of complications associated with the implantation technique. Some surgeons began implanting it in the United States using both intracapsular and extracapsular techniques—T. Hamdi, N. Jaffe, H. Byron, and H. Hirschman to name but a few.

However, phacoemulsification was still not accepted by the majority of eye surgeons. Actually, in the mid-1970s, under the pressure of America's "old school" ophthalmic surgeons, who were losing patients to surgeons who performed the innovative ultrasound technique, the government decided that phacoemulsification would not be reimbursed as it was classified as an "experimental" technique.

It was only after a campaign by Dick Kratz and other pioneering colleagues that some years later the government accepted phacoemulsification simply as a variation of the extracapsular technique for removal of the cataract. This was a big achievement as lack of reimbursement had led to interruption in research and development for technical innovations in cataract surgery.

In 1977, Steven Shearing of Las Vegas, Nevada, implanted the first IOL developed for the posterior chamber (p-IOL) (draft from a design by J. Barraquer) (Figure 1-3) with foldable J-shaped loops (Figure 1-4). This was a big stimulus for extracapsular cataract surgery, but did little to

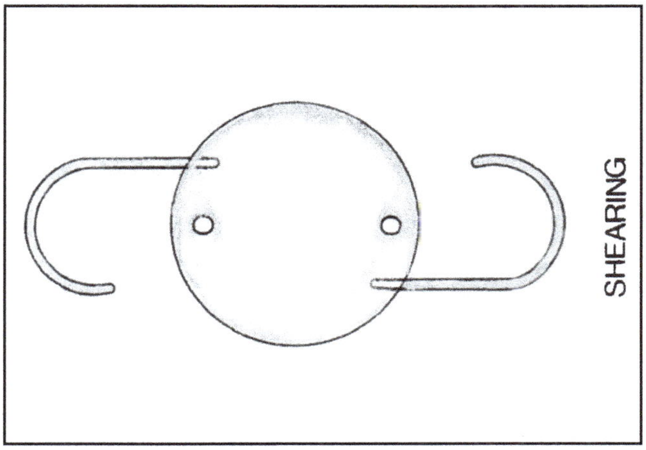

Figure 1-4. The first prototype of the Shearing IOL, Model 101. This photo is a close-up of the lens–loop junctions and the hand-shaped loops (Shearing mod 101).[4]

increase interest in phacoemulsification, a technique that was still being shunned by 90% of American surgeons and approximately 98% of surgeons in the rest of the world.

A turning point came in the 1980s. In 1980, Franz Fankhauser and Daniele Aron Rosa invented the neodymium:yttrium-aluminum-garnet (Nd:YAG) laser, which was able to open the opacified posterior capsule in a noninvasive manner. At the same time, David Miller and Robert Stegmann introduced Healon, the first viscoelastic substance (VES), which greatly improved the safety and operative simplicity of the cataract removal procedure. A couple of years later, Thomas Mazzocco introduced the first foldable silicone lenses that could be implanted through a 3-mm incision, necessary for phacoemulsification, and allowed the procedure to be recognized for what it was in essence: a true stroke of genius (Figure 1-5)! However, initially, the introduction of foldable IOLs was not free from complications, partly because of the design of the lens and partly because the material used in production caused an intense reaction in some eyes. Nevertheless, this development marked a turning point. The complications were greatly reduced following the development of 3-piece acrylic lenses with polypropylene (Prolene) haptic loops.

Sir Harold Ridley showed that the eye could tolerate an artificial lens. Charles Kelman, on the other hand, demonstrated the ability to remove the nucleus and cortex through a small incision. Steve Shearing and Bill Simcoe realized the ideal position for the IOL, and finally, Thomas Mazzocco showed that IOLs could be folded and inserted through small incisions. We must thank these pioneers, as today it is possible to perform cataract removal procedures with mini-invasive techniques and rapid recovery times. In Italy, Lucio Buratto deserves credit for the advancement of the phacoemulsification technique and implantation procedure for a p-IOL.

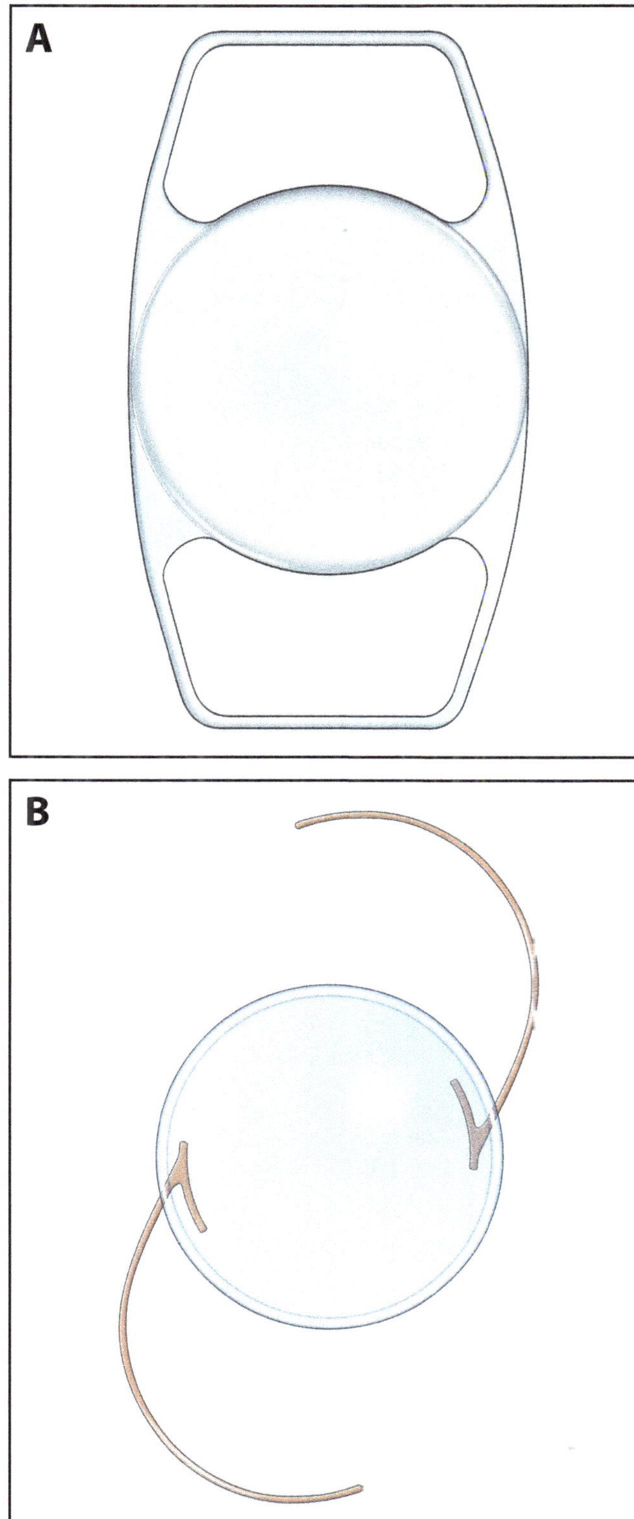

Figure 1-5. The first foldable lenses produced by STAAR Surgical Company for insertion into the posterior chamber. (A) Model AA4004. (B) Model AQ 2010V.[5]

References

1. Williams HP. Sir Harold Ridley's vision. *Br J Ophtalmol.* 2001;85:1022-1023.
2. Apple DJ. Sir Harold Ridley. *Cataract Refract Surg Today.* 2004; March:27-29.
3. Sinskey RM. A history of modern cataract surgery. *Cataract Refract Surg Today.* 2006;July:23-25.
4. Shearing SP. Recreating the posterior chamber lens. *Cataract Refract Surg Today.* 2004;March:30-31.
5. Mazzocco TR. Creating a foldable lens. *Cataract Refract Surg Today.* 2004;March:31-32.

Suggested Readings

Byron HM. Flashback. *Cataract Refract Surg Today.* 2005;August:22-23.

Chang DF. A historical look back: honoring those with the right stuff. *Cataract Refract Surg Today.* 2004;March:22.

Kelman CD. The genesis of phacoemulsification. *Cataract Refract Surg Today.* 2004;March:25-26.

Kratz RP. Cataract surgery and IOLs. *Cataract Refract Surg Today.* 2006;January:32-33.

2

The Materials

Lucio Buratto, MD; Stephen F. Brint, MD, FACS; and Domenico Boccuzzi, MD, PhD

The Optics

The development of the cataract procedure with the advent of phacoemulsification and subsequently with implantation of intraocular lenses (IOLs) is one of the most important achievements of modern medicine; phacoemulsification made it possible to remove the cataract through small incisions with consequent rapid visual and physical rehabilitation for the patient.

The p-IOLs, first the rigid models and then the soft lenses, permit optimal visual rehabilitation with excellent optical qualities. The main chemical constituents of the currently available IOLs can be divided into 2 groups: acrylate/methacrylate polymers and silicone elastomers. Polymethylmethacrylate (PMMA), hydrogel, poly(2-hydroxyethyl methacrylate) (poly-HEMA), and the various co-polymers used in the production of foldable acrylic IOLs all belong to the same group (acrylate and methacrylate); it is a chemical group attached to the main chain of the standard polymer to produce the different properties found. The acrylic used to produce IOLs is an ester of acrylic or methacrylic acids. Two forms are available: rigid and flexible. The rigid acrylic–PMMA is a polymer of methacrylate; it is stiff, is hydrophobic, and promotes cell adhesion to its surface. Its refractive index is between 1.49 and 1.50, and the specific density is 1.19 g/cm^3. It is rigid at room temperature and becomes flexible at a temperature of 105°C. It is an amorphous, transparent, colorless, and water-repellent substance. It transmits 92% of the incident light. Its contact angle is 70 degrees, and its water-absorption index is 0.25%. Incorporating chromophores in the material means that the lens can be produced in a precise color.

The optical portions of PMMA can be produced by 2 methods: grinding and molding.

Grinding

Grinding (or modeling at the lathe) is a method that creates a thinner IOL from much thicker blocks of PMMA. Two techniques can be used with this method: in the first option, the block of PMMA rotates in a support and is cut with a fixed blade; in the second option, the blade rotates around a block of PMMA fixed on a support. The lens is then polished to produce a smooth surface.

Molding

The procedure can be performed in 2 ways:

1. **Injection molding:** In this method, the PMMA is heated until it liquefies (at approximately 160°C to 200°C). The liquid PMMA is then pressure injected into the mold (approximately 140 kg/cm^2). When cooled, the mold is opened and the surface of the lens is polished to achieve the smooth final result.
2. **Compression molding:** In this method, a steel mold filled with PMMA is compressed under pressure of 500 kg/cm^2. The mold is then heated to 20°C and the pressure increased to 2600 kg/cm^2. The pressure is then returned to normal values and the mold cooled with air.

This recently introduced method allows the manufacturing processes to be more repeatable.

Buratto L, Brint SF, Boccuzzi D.
Cataract Surgery and Intraocular Lenses (pp 7-13).

Surface Treatment of Polymethylmethacrylate Intraocular Lenses

The "surface treatments" modify the properties of PMMA IOLs, for example, the balance between the hydrophilic and hydrophobic qualities. The surface can be modified by coating with a deposit and finally by addition of a new molecule (grafting).

- **Surface treatment:** The surface properties are modified principally by chemical reactions, by heating, or under the effects of electromagnetic radiation (bombardment with ionizing radiation or luminous rays; exposure to cold plasma under low pressure). These methods are used to create new chemical functions on the surface of the implant; they can also be used to attach new molecules or to alter surface characteristics such as roughness, durability, or the ability to slide.
- **Coating:** This technique coats the lens surface with a specific material that creates specific properties on the surface. This process is called *dunking* or *soaking*. The PMMA IOL is dipped into the coating solution; however, the solution does not bind chemically with the IOL. The mechanical properties of each individual material remain unchanged. One of the most popular products used to coat a PMMA IOL is clear fluorocarbonate–Teflon AF. Amorphous Teflon is clear and can be dissolved in fluorinated solvents or liquid fluorocarbonates. The properties of these coatings allow the application of very thin layers on substrates, making them completely hydrophobic. Teflon-coated lenses reduce the formation of synechiae between the iris and the implant; Teflon-coated IOLs have lower reactivity and greater biocompatibility. Less cell deposits were detected on IOLs coated with Teflon compared with those without the Teflon coating. Less intraocular trauma is induced with the PMMA Teflon-coated IOL compared with uncoated lenses, and there is less cell loss.
- **Binding or grafting:** Grafting involves the creation of a covalent bond between different types of molecules on the lens surface to produce different properties and improve biocompatibility with ocular tissues.

Despite its excellent optical and physical-chemical properties, PMMA is not totally inert. Surface treatments improve the characteristics of the lens, increasing its biocompatibility with ocular tissues and reducing the incidence and severity of inflammation following implantation.

Heparin-Coated Lenses

The surface of the lenses can be modified by attaching heparin to the surface with covalent bonds through a series of chemical reactions; the high chemical stability of heparin on the surface of the IOL reduces the adhesion of other molecules or pathogenic agents.

The nonstick deterrent properties of heparin-coated IOLs include bacteria such as *Streptococcus*, *Staphylococcus*, and *Pseudomonas aeruginosa*. These lenses must be handled very carefully as the heparin-coated surface risks being damaged by the neodymium:yttrium-aluminum-garnet (Nd:YAG) laser and the surgical instruments.

Intraocular Lenses With a Passivated Surface (A Surface That Has Been Made Chemically Inert)

This treatment aims to create a layer of fluorocarbonate that is chemically bound to the external surface of the lens, reducing its surface energy. Surface passivation of the lens attempts to reduce or eliminate biological reactions of inflammatory origin when the lens is implanted and to reduce surface irregularities. Many studies have reported conflicting results regarding the efficacy of this type of treatment. Koch et al did not observe any major differences between treated and untreated PMMA lenses.[1]

They demonstrated that the lenses with a passivated surface were able to activate the complement cascade, generating the same levels of C3a and C5a as found with normal PMMA lenses.[2]

However, Balyeat et al, in studies on feline eyes, reported a lower incidence of endothelial damage and lower cellular adhesion on the lens with a passivated surface as opposed to untreated PMMA IOLs.[3] However, this procedure is no longer used as surgeons have not found any real improvement in biocompatibility with the treated lenses.

Polymethylmethacrylate Intraocular Lenses Treated With Plasma

This process of fluoridation of the lens surface was introduced in 1990. This method is used to improve biocompatibility of the lens surface by reducing the surface energy of PMMA lenses. The term *plasma* refers to an ionized and electrically neutral gas. It is created artificially by compressing the gas in a closed, high-frequency electromagnetic field inside a polymerizable or nonpolymerizable reactor under low pressure. The gas used is CF4, CF3H, or CF3Cl. There is a chemical change produced on the surface of the polymer; the fluoride ions or the CF2 or CF3 groups are replaced with hydrogen. This layer is less than 0.01-mm thick. Studies reported that, compared with untreated lenses, treated lenses increased the surface hydrophilic properties and there was also an improvement in the angle of contact between the lens and water. Moreover, the granulocytes in contact with treated IOLs were less active, as demonstrated by the percentage of superoxide produced by these cells.

Substances Used to Produce Intraocular Lenses

Silicone

The first silicone IOLs for use in cataract surgery were introduced in 1984. Silicone is a polymer of polyorganosiloxane that is used in the elastomeric form (polydimethylsiloxane [PDMS]) for biomedical applications. The elastomers are polymers that can be subjected to significant reversible deformations. Their properties vary on the basis of additives used, cross-linking, and the catalyst. However, these substances are rarely used as components of medical-quality silicone elastomers because of their poor biocompatibility. The only additives incorporated in silicone IOLs are ultraviolet (UV) chromophores and the phenyl groups. The new generation of silicone-based substances used in the production of IOLs had higher refractive indices, and thus were thinner and easier to handle.

The Physical Properties of Silicone

PDMS was the first elastomer used to produce IOL optics. Its low refractive index (1.412 at 25°C) was responsible for the thickness of IOLs as compared to modern lenses of the same power. Due to their thickness, these lenses were also difficult to fold. A second generation of silicone elastomers was developed using a copolymer—diphenyl and dimethylsiloxane (a copolymer of 2 molecules, namely diphenylsiloxane and dimethylsiloxane). This had a higher refractive index (1.464). Silicone polymers have been developed with even higher refractive indices, but these compounds are not suitable for producing IOLs.

Generally speaking, the silicone lenses produced today have a high refractive index and are extremely easy to fold; their intraocular unfolding is extremely rapid, almost explosive, and difficult to control. Moreover, silicone IOLs are extremely difficult to manipulate when they are wet as the silicone becomes very slippery. Silicone IOLs must not be used in patients who have undergone vitrectomy with the use of silicone oil as a tamponade, or in patients who may require this procedure at a later time, particularly, in those patients who have an open posterior capsule. This is because the exposure of the IOL to silicone oil causes the formation of a silicone interface that is practically impossible to remove. This may interfere with the surgeon's view of the retina and considerably reduce the patient's visual acuity. This phenomenon is not seen with acrylic IOLs, which are therefore strongly recommended in patients having undergone a vitrectomy with PDMS used as a tamponade, or in those patients for whom it may be necessary in the future[4] (Figure 2-1).

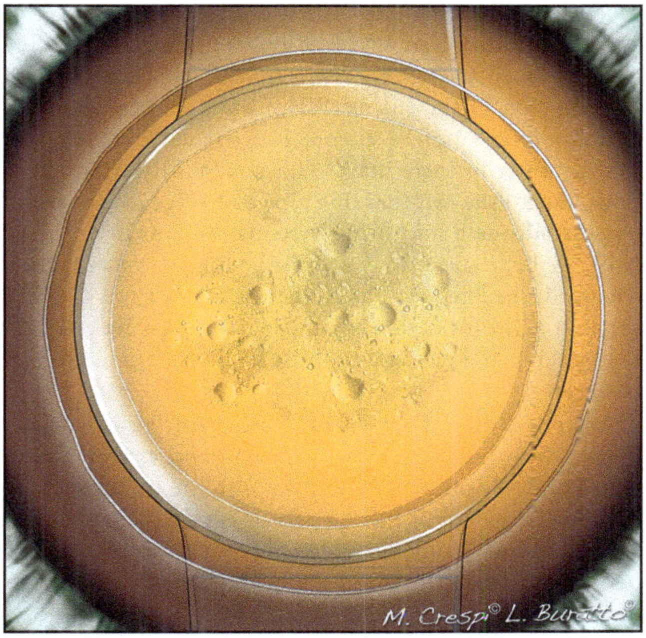

Figure 2-1. An example of the silicone interface on a silicone IOL.

Production of Silicone Intraocular Lenses

Injection molding is the most common method used to manufacture silicone IOLs. Melted silicone is injected into the mold under high pressure; it is then allowed to cool and harden.

The "molding flash" is a rough line along the edge of the lens, seen with electron microscopy; this irregularity is located at the junction point of the 2 sides of the lens and can reduce biocompatibility. This is one of the main disadvantages of this technique.

Occasionally there are irregularities on the surface of silicone IOLs. In addition to the molding flash, small abnormalities can be found at the junction between the optic and the haptic.

As with PMMA IOLs, silicone lenses can undergo surface treatments. To improve the hydrophilic properties of the lens, the PDMS can be exposed to oxygen plasma. The folding process used with silicone IOLs can temporarily compromise the surface of the lens, forming small indentations or folds; however, these are no longer visible after 10 minutes, even when the lens is examined under the electron microscope. Silicone IOLs are not indicated for implantation in the sulcus due to the high probability of decentration. A 1-piece silicone IOL in the capsular sulcus may decenter or there may be horizontal distortion of the optic, due to the fact that this type of 1-piece lens does not possess adequate anchoring systems. Treatment with the Nd:YAG laser must be performed with extreme caution when silicone lenses are used; the use of high energy levels can lead to the formation of pigment spots that are visible at the slit lamp and may compromise the surface and integrity of the lens.

Silicone IOLs can be divided into 3 categories: 1-piece, 3-piece with polypropylene (Prolene) haptics, and 3-piece with PMMA haptics. Silicone IOLs with Prolene haptics are not used frequently as this material is extremely flexible and can easily lose its memory; frequently the haptics remain permanently distorted during implantation. The flexibility of the Prolene haptics is responsible for the forward movement of the lens's optic during contraction of the bag and may also be responsible for cases of pupillary capture.

PMMA haptics are much more resistant than Prolene haptics; this is the correct combination of materials for good stability of the lens in the capsular bag.

Soft Acrylic Intraocular Lenses

Hydrogel and acrylates have joined silicone in the production of foldable lenses.

Hydrogel is a specific compound called poly-HEMA; in reality, this includes a huge group of polymers and poly-HEMA is just one of the compounds. Hydrogel IOLs have 20% maximum water content.

Soft acrylic IOLs are divided into different categories, despite being produced using the same chemical. The groups include the rigid hydrophobic PMMA and the soft hydrophilic hydrogel poly-HEMA lenses.

The vitreal transition temperature (VTT) is a characteristic of acrylic materials and indicates the temperature threshold at which the acrylic material changes from a material that is rigid into a material with greater flexibility. The VTT of PMMA is 110°C; above this temperature PMMA becomes flexible and soft. Methacrylates have a much higher VTT than the acrylates. Appropriate use and selection of acrylates and methacrylates can produce a polymer with an intermediate VTT.

Viteous Transition Temperature

The temperature of vitreous transition is normally indicated with the symbol T_g and represents the value of the temperature below which an amorphous material behaves like a vitreous solid. T_g is the temperature below which the movements of contortion and rotation of segments of molecules of 40 to 50 atoms and translational movements of the entire molecule are frozen and there is energy sufficient only for the vibrations of the atoms around the positions of equilibrium and for the movement of a few atoms belonging to the main chain or the side groups. Analyzing the process implicated in greater detail, in practice, the VTT regulates the second-order transition phase called *vitreous transition* by creating a totally or partially amorphous phase. Classical examples are glass and plastics. It is then possible to supercool the material to T_g, which leads to the formation of a solid vitreous structure. Actually, the VTT marks the threshold between the vitreous amorphous state and the plastic amorphous state (this is a thick liquid state with high viscosity).

The vitreous transition is a kinetic and not a thermodynamic transition; there is no change in the spatial arrangement of the atoms/molecules that is found in the transition between the solid crystalline state and the liquid state. Inorganic or mineral vitreous substances, such as silicate, have a specific T_g value. Thermoplastic polymers have an additional T_g at a lower temperature; below this value, the substances become rigid and fragile and tend to shatter. Moreover, at temperatures higher than T_g, the polymers will become elastic and can be subjected to plastic deformations without fracturing. This property can be exploited in technological situations. The common reference values of vitreous transition are actually mean values and depend on the temperature gradient of cooling; for polymers, they also depend on the distribution of mean molecular weights. Moreover, any additives in the preparation also influence the T_g (Table 2-1). Some pure substances with a low molecular weight may also be associated with a specific VTT, below which their structure is classified as amorphous. For example, water has a $T_g = -173°$ C, and with rapid cooling of water to T_g to prevent the organization of water into a orderly crystalline structure, amorphous ice is obtained.

Common methods used to determine the temperature of vitreous transition are differential scanning calorimetry and dynamic mechanical analysis (Figures 2-2 through 2-4).

TABLE 2-1

VITREOUS TRANSITION TEMPERATURE OF THE MAIN MATERIALS

MATERIAL	T_g (°C)
Polyethylene (LDPE)	–125 (also –30)
Polypropylene (atactic)	–20
Polyvinyl acetate (PVAc)	28
Polyethylene terephthalate (PET)	79
Polyvinyl alcohol (PVA)	85
Polyvinyl chloride (PVC)	81
Polystyrene	95
Polypropylene (isotactic)	0
Polymethylmethacrylate (atactic)	105
Polycarbonate	150
Tellurite	279
Fluoroaluminate	400
Silicate	1175

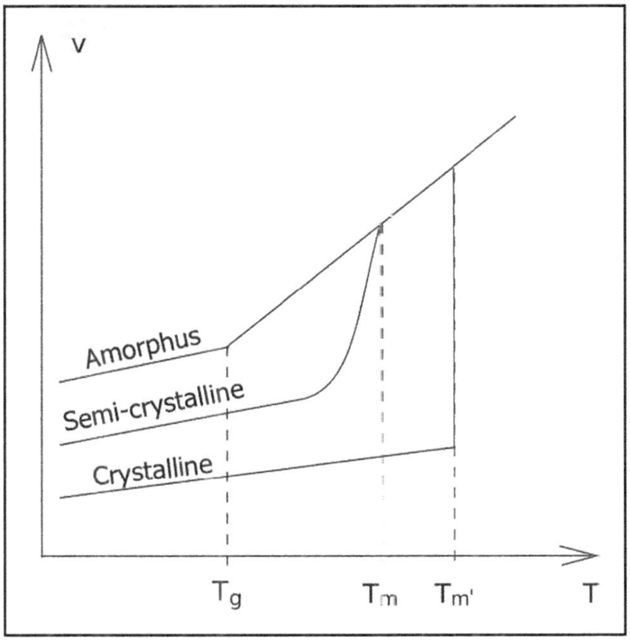

Figure 2-2. Variation of the specific volume with temperature relative to an amorphous semicrystalline and crystalline material. The fusion temperature (T_m and T_m1%) and the VTT (Tg) are indicated. (Reprinted with permission from wikipedia: http://it.wikipedia.org/wiki/Temperatura_di_transizione_vetrosa.)

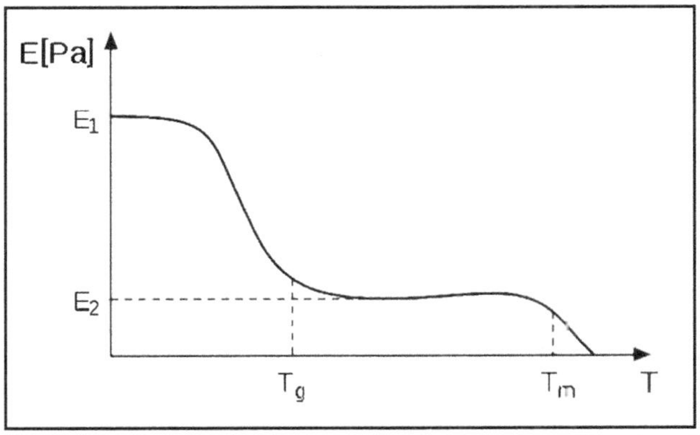

Figure 2-3. VTT in a diagram elastic–temperature. (Reprinted with permission from wikipedia: http://it.wikipedia.org/wiki/Temperatura_di_transizione_vetrosa.)

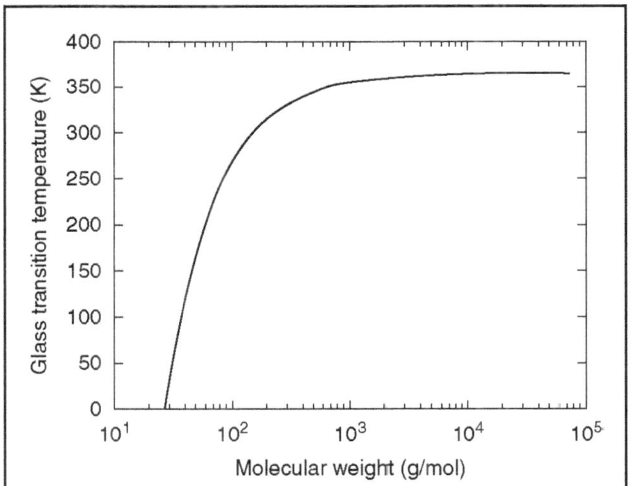

Figure 2-4. Flory–Fox curve representing the variation of VTT with the molecular weight. (Reprinted with permission from wikipedia http://it.wikipedia.org/wiki/Temperatura_di_transizione_vetrosa.)

An appropriate combination of acrylic materials with high refractive indices and a VTT at room temperature allow the creation of copolymers that are ideal for the production of soft acrylic IOLs, while preserving the optical properties of PMMA. A wide range of combinations are possible and these form different copolymers with different refractive indices, compositions, folding and unfolding properties, and surface characteristics.

Poly-HEMA and related compounds are hydrophilic due to the –OH groups of the structures.

The presence of a hydroxyl group allows a rigid lens to absorb water molecules that soften the lens when it is immersed in an aqueous medium, making it more flexible.

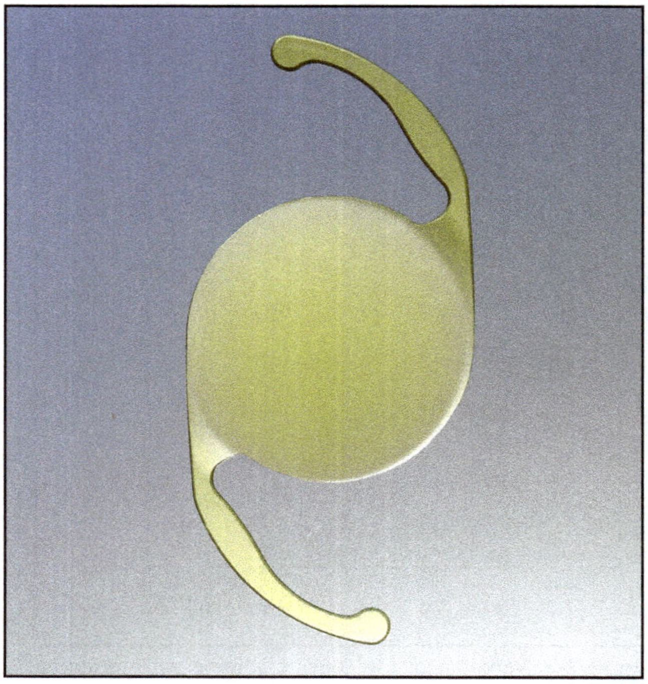

Figure 2-5. Hydrophobic acrylic IOL (Alcon AcrySof Natural) with an incorporated yellow chromophore.

Hydrogel Lenses

The first modern hydrogel lenses were one piece with a biconvex structure and biscuit/cookie-shaped haptics. They were produced in poly-HEMA, which was the most common hydrogel available and had a water content of 38%. The hydrophilic properties of these lenses led to lower cell adhesion in comparison to PMMA lenses; they preserved excellent optic properties and offered visual acuity comparable to lenses of PMMA. They also had greater resistance to YAG-laser treatment. One limitation of this material was that UV filters could not be incorporated into its structure.

The first IOL of poly-HEMA for implantation in the posterior chamber was designed and developed by Graham Barrett and implanted in 1983 in Perth, Australia. The original models of hydrogel lenses were associated with 2 major disadvantages: a greater incidence of posterior capsule opacification (PCO) and a high incidence of dislocation of the lens into the vitreous when the posterior capsule was opened with the YAG laser. The incidence of PCO, with the formation of numerous Elschnig pearls, was not exclusively due to problems with the lens design; the chemical–physical properties of poly-HEMA also contributed to it. Actually, the formation of Elschnig pearls in the capsular bag was due to a difference in osmotic pressure. Fluids and nutrients can pass through the IOL, giving rise to posterior opacities.

The second complication associated with this type of lens was posterior dislocation into the vitreous following treatment with the YAG laser. The high incidence of this complication drove some surgeons to suggest surgical aspiration of the Elschnig pearls, rather than risk dislocation of the lens with the capsulotomy. However, the lens is easily removed, as there is no fusion between the anterior and the posterior capsules. The problems associated with decentration, posterior dislocation, and pigment dispersion led to the production of a new category of poly-HEMA lenses with a new design that would avoid the above-mentioned complications. This new lens had a 6-mm optic with C-shaped haptics. This design allowed fusion between the anterior and posterior capsules and good centration of the lens in the bag.

Soft acrylic lenses are available as hydrophilic or hydrophobic on the basis of hydroxy radicals present or absent in the chemical structure of the lens. These lenses can be folded at room temperature. Their chemical structure derives from the synthesis of 3-dimensional chains formed by the union of an ester of acrylic acid and an ester or 2 of methacrylic acid. A primer (a polymerizer) and a UV filter are added to the lens material. In addition to having a higher refractive index as opposed to PMMA IOLs, and particularly as compared to silicone IOLs, hydrogel lenses have excellent optical characteristics with the added advantage of being foldable.

Once these lenses have been folded and inserted into the eye, they return to their original shape and size, due to the 3-dimensional structure of the chemical chains. Moreover, compared to silicone IOLs, the unfolding process is much slower and more easily controlled. Special attention must be paid during loading and implantation of soft acrylic lenses because the optic is fairly delicate and inappropriate handling can leave permanent marks on the surface.

Hydrophobic Acrylic Lenses

Hydrophobic acrylic lenses consist of a copolymer of acrylate and methacrylate. The properties of flexibility and resistance result from the correct combination of these materials. These lenses are light and relatively inert. Their chemical physical properties ensure that these lenses can be folded at room temperature (VTT is approximately 13°C); they also have a high refractive index (1.44 to 1.55) compared to silicone (1.41 to 1.46) and PMMA (1.49). Consequently, these lenses are extremely thin. The growing popularity of hydrophobic IOLs is due to good mechanical stability, good uveal biocompatibility, and a low incidence of PCO. If vitreoretinal surgery is needed with the use of silicone oil, there is low adhesion without creating problems at the silicone–lens interface (Figure 2-5).

Hydrophilic Acrylic Lenses

Hydrophilic acrylic IOLs are produced from a mixture of poly-HEMA and a hydrophilic acrylic monomer. There are different types of hydrophilic acrylic IOLs available depending on the type of copolymer added and the water content. The quantity of water absorbed generally varies between 18% and 38% and is expressed as the percentage weight of hydrated gel. The hydrophilic surface provides

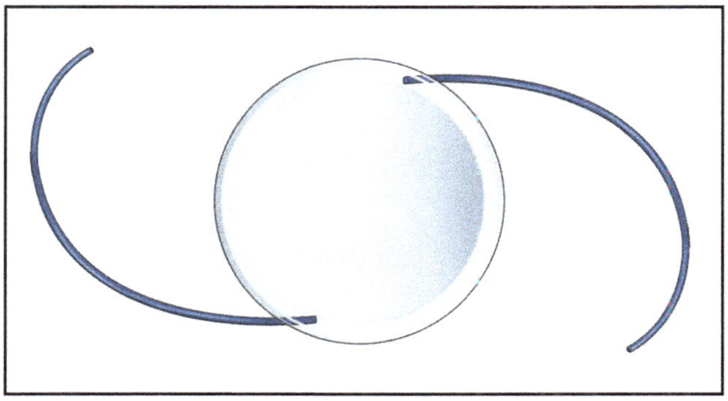

Figure 2-6. Three-piece hydrophilic acrylic IOL, Model Hydromax (Carl Zeiss Meditec).

excellent characteristics of biocompatibility. Due to their soft flexible surface, there is very little or no alteration of the surface of these types of IOLs during the handling and folding procedures required for insertion. The low surface energy and the hydrophilic properties are the main reasons for their good uveal biocompatibility; the same applies to their low potential for endothelial damage with accidental contact (Figure 2-6).

Nevertheless, hydrophilic lenses have poor capsular biocompatibility (there are studies that demonstrate high cell proliferation on the anterior and posterior surfaces with hydrophilic lenses) compared to other materials, causing cell proliferation on the lens, contraction of the anterior capsule, and PCO following implantation (Figure 2-7). They have good resistance to the YAG laser, and with vitreoretinal surgery, this material has a low degree of adherence to silicone oil.

The Haptics

The haptics of acrylic IOLs can be produced in a variety of materials and shapes.

- Polyamide (Nylon): This synthetic material consists of long molecular chains, with an amide group attached at regular intervals. Due to fragmentation by hydrolysis, the use of nylon in the haptics is now obsolete.
- Polypropylene (Prolene): This is a synthetic polymer with high elasticity and resistance to traction. Despite the fact that it is chemoattractive and chemoadhesive for microbial agents, Prolene continues to be a good material for the haptics because of its memory and resistance to biodegradation.
- PMMA is a polymer of methacrylate, as mentioned earlier, which has a very important role, along with Prolene, in the construction of haptics, due to its chemical–physical properties.
- Polyimide is a synthetic material containing a benzyl ring and an imino group. It can be heat sterilized and has high resistance to heat.

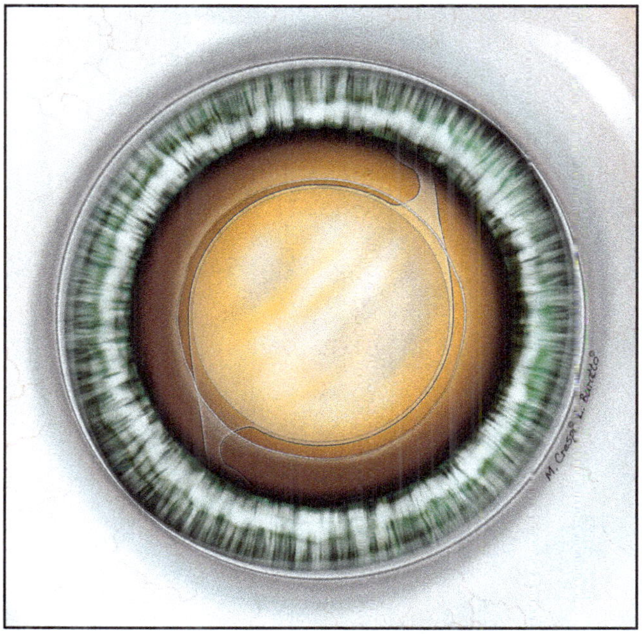

Figure 2-7. Hydrophilic acrylic IOL showing the low capsular biocompatibility and the posterior capsular fibrosis.

References

1. Koch DD, Samuelson SW, Dimonie V. Surface analysis of surface-passivated intraocular lenses. *J Cataract Refract Surg.* 1991;17(2):131-138.
2. Kochunian HH, Maxwell WA, Gupta A. Complement activation by surface modified poly(methyl methacrylate) intraocular lenses. *J Cataract Refract Surg.* 1991;17(2):139-142.
3. Balyeat HD, Nordquist RE, Lerner MP, Gupta A. Comparison of endothelial damage produced by control and surface modified poly(methyl methacrylate) intraocular lenses. *J Cataract Refract Surg.* 1989;15(5):491-494.
4. Khawly JA, Lambert RJ, Jaffe GJ. Intraocular lens changes after short- and long-term exposure to intraocular silicone oil. An in vivo study. *Ophthalmology.* 1998;105(7):1227-1233.

Suggested Readings

Dhaliwal RS, Mandira M. Update on intraocular lenses. In: Garg A, ed. *Advances in Ophthalmology* 2. New Delhi, India: Jaypee; 2005: Chapter 5.

Sachedev MS, Venkatesh P. Phaco intraocular lenses. In: *Phacoemulsification, Laser Cataract Surgery and Foldable IOLs.* New Delhi, India: Jaypee: Chapter 31.

3

Rigid Intraocular Lenses of the Past

Lucio Buratto, MD; Stephen F. Brint, MD, FACS; and Domenico Boccuzzi, MD, PhD

Extracapsular cataract extraction involved implantation of a rigid polymethylmethacrylate intraocular lens (PMMA IOL). Some had large optics (diameter up to 9 mm) and large overall diameters (14 mm) including haptics. This technique did not offer adequate support for the IOL; consequently, it was assumed that the use of lenses with larger optics would avoid the problems of lens decentration. The development of the capsulorrhexis technique allowed implantation of the lens in the bag with greater stability of the IOL; however, it was immediately apparent that this type of lens was very difficult to manage during insertion in the capsular bag, and surgeons realized that optics and lenses of such large sizes were unnecessary. Implantation of the IOL in the capsular bag provided the best results in

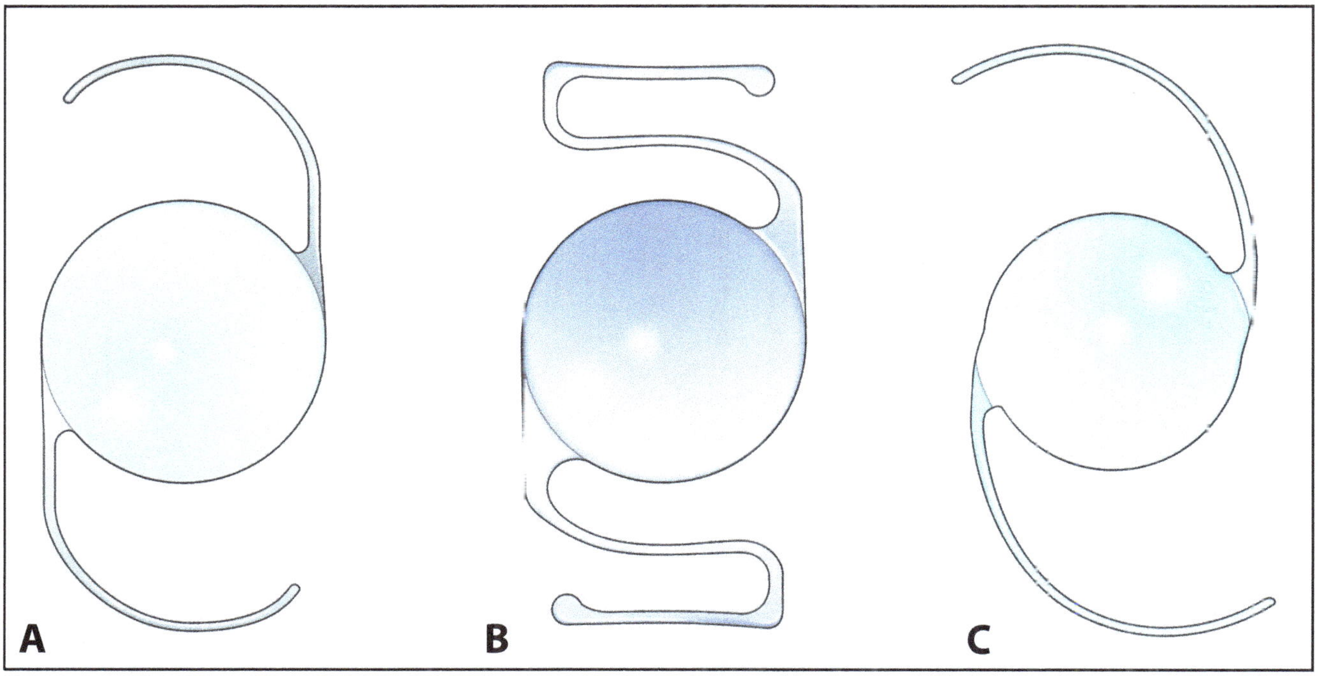

Figure 3-1. Rigid Hexavision IOL of PMMA for implantation in the (A) posterior chamber, (B) anterior chamber, and (C) through small incision.

Buratto L, Brint SF, Boccuzzi D.
Cataract Surgery and Intraocular Lenses (pp 15-16).

terms of lens stability and visual quality. It was therefore essential to develop new types of rigid IOLs.

Newer 1-piece PMMA lenses were round or oval. IOLs with round optics had a diameter of 5.0, 5.25, or 5.5 mm; the diameter of IOLs with the oval optic was predominantly 5.0 or 6.0 mm. The overall length of these lenses was 11.5 and 12.5 mm (ie, approximately corresponding to the diameter of the capsular bag). For implantation, the corneal incision had to be enlarged to correspond to the diameter of the optic of the lens, even though some surgeons believed that it was possible to implant the lenses with incisions that were 0.5 mm smaller than the overall diameter (Figure 3-1).

Suggested Reading

Sachdev MS, Venkatesh P. Phaco intraocular lenses. In: *Phacoemulsification, Laser Cataract Surgery and Foldable IOLs.* New Delhi, India: Jaypee; 1998: Chapter 31.

4

Soft Intraocular Lenses of the Past

Lucio Buratto, MD; Stephen F. Brint, MD, FACS; and Domenico Boccuzzi, MD, PhD

The potential of introducing an intraocular lens (IOL) through a smaller incision, while allowing a lens optic of 6.0 mm, was an important turning point in the field of cataract surgery, for a number of reasons:

- The postoperative inflammatory process is directly proportional to the size of the incision.
- Numerous studies have demonstrated that there are significant differences in the results with a small incision compared to a larger one, at least during the first postoperative month.
- Large incisions also create greater astigmatism as the incision weakens the meridian involved.
- The size of the incision also has an important impact on postoperative vision quality. It is now known that large incisions induce higher-order aberration, for example, trefoil, responsible for deterioration in vision quality.
- Finally, large incisions require numerous sutures, and these can also lead to increased astigmatism.

Silicone Lenses

Even though Kelman introduced the phaco technique with incisions of approximately 3 mm in the early 1970s, the surgical procedure could only be completed with an enlargement of the incision to 6 to 8 mm to allow the introduction of the IOL.

In the early 1980s, Dr. Thomas Mazzocco recognized that in cases of severe myopia, when implantation of an IOL was not indicated, the surgical procedure terminated with removal of the cataract through the 3-mm phaco incision. Dr. Mazzocco found that the postoperative recovery with the small incision was more rapid in these situations. This gave him the idea to insert an IOL through a small incision, without having to enlarge the incision. The idea of using 2 hemi-lenses introduced through the small phaco incision and assembled inside the eye was associated with technical problems and toxicity of the glues. Moreover, 2 hemi-lenses instead of a single piece could lead to problems with visual quality. The second idea was also unsuccessful. It involved creating a small lenticule of 3-mm diameter; this was attached to a diaphragm of black plastic that would create an opaque zone measuring 6 mm with a transparent zone of diameter 3 mm in the center (Figure 4-1).

The only option was to develop a lens using a material that could be folded prior to insertion in the eye through a 3-mm incision. In the early 1980s, there were other medical–surgical devices in soft materials (silicone) that were used predominantly to correct problems caused by ocular trauma.

The experience of Dr. E. Epstein from Johannesburg, South Africa, in the implantation of silicone devices, combined with the idea of Dr. Mazzocco and STAAR Surgical, led to the development of the first foldable silicone lenses (Figure 4-2).

In 1984, the Food and Drug Administration (FDA) approved the use of silicone lenses for implantation; they were produced in 2 models: 3-piece with polyimide loops and 1-piece of silicone. The lens could be folded at its center and could be introduced through the small incisions used for the phacoemulsification procedure. The first lenses were associated with problems of decentration associated with deformation of the haptics induced by the capsular bag.

Buratto L, Brint SF, Boccuzzi D.
Cataract Surgery and Intraocular Lenses (pp 17-22).

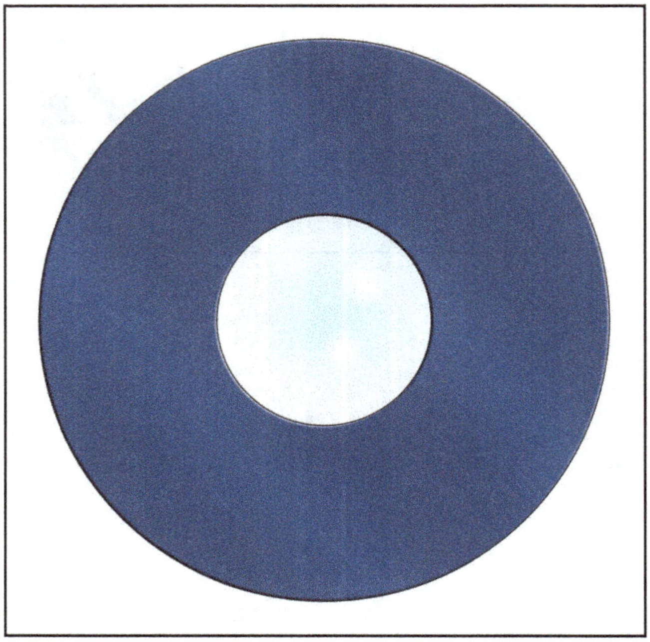

Figure 4-1. Design of the project of Thomas Mazzocco. The idea was to create a 3-mm diameter lenticule to which the surgeon could attach a dark plastic collar after the insertion of the 2 pieces in the anterior chamber.

Creating haptics of greater thickness and rigidity solved this problem.

Soft Hydrophilic Acrylic Lenses

The ORC Memory Lens (Mentor) was one of the most commonly used soft hydrophilic acrylic lenses. This type of lens consisted of polymers with heat-mechanical properties: it was a combination of 2-hydroxyethyl methacrylate (HEMA) and methacrylate (the monomer in PMMA) cross-linked with ethylene glycol dimethacrylate (EGDMA). Ultraviolet (UV) chromophores were integrated in its structure as 4-methacryloxy 2-hydroxy benzophenone (MOBP). The material was then hydrated to 20%. This type of lens had to be stored, folded, at a temperature of 8°C before use. When injected into the eye, it unfolded slowly to return to its original shape after around 10 to 15 minutes at body temperature. Within 1 hour, the lens reacquired its optical properties, and within 24 hours, all of the folds disappeared. The Prolene loops of the prefolded IOL assumed their definitive shape and position as soon as the lens was implanted.

This new technology attempted to eliminate the need for dedicated injectors or surgical instruments known as "holder and folder." The prefolded lens could use the existing small phaco incision.

The Memory Lens was available in 2 models: one with flat haptics (biscuit loops) and a second model with a classical 3-piece design complete with Prolene haptics (Figure 4-3).

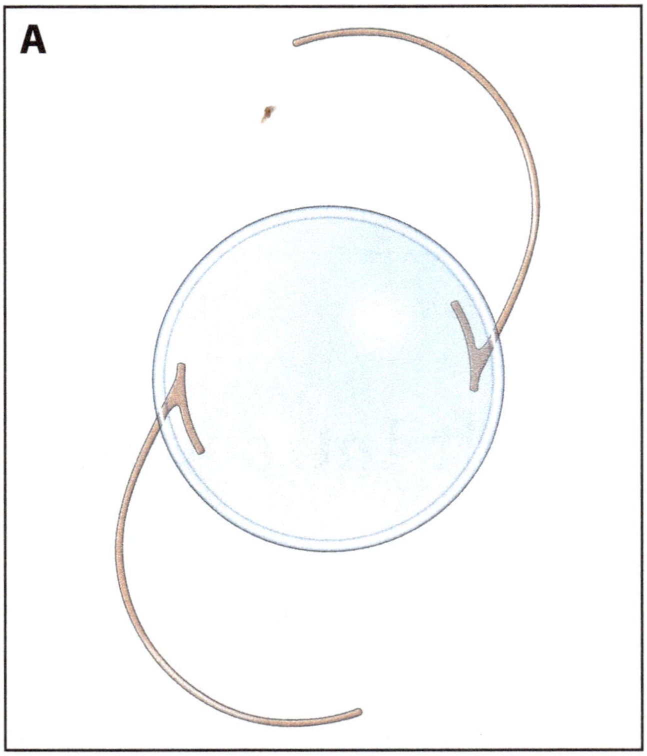

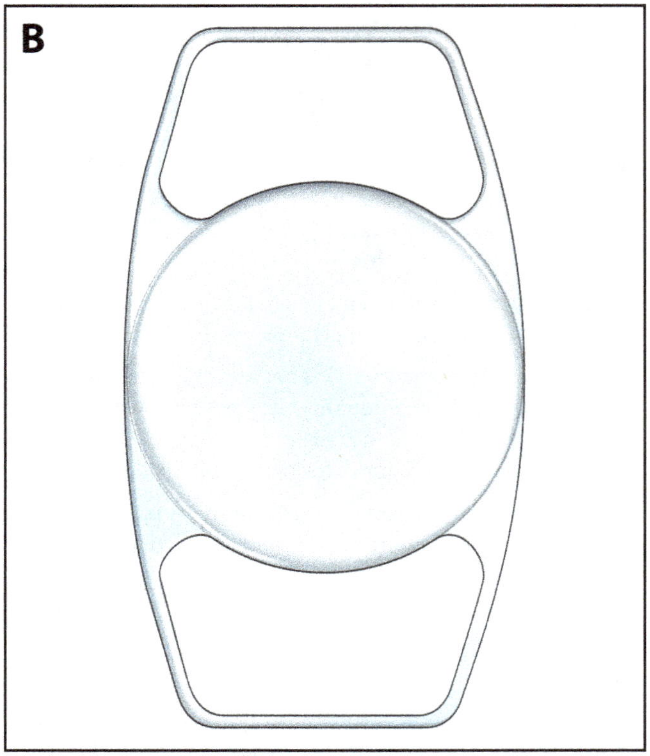

Figure 4-2. The first foldable lenses produced by STAAR Surgical Company for implantation in the posterior chamber. (A) Model AA4004. (B) AQ2010V.

The optic size was 6.0 mm in both. The overall length was 10.5 mm in the former and 13.0 mm in the latter. These lenses were available in powers between 10 and 30 D.

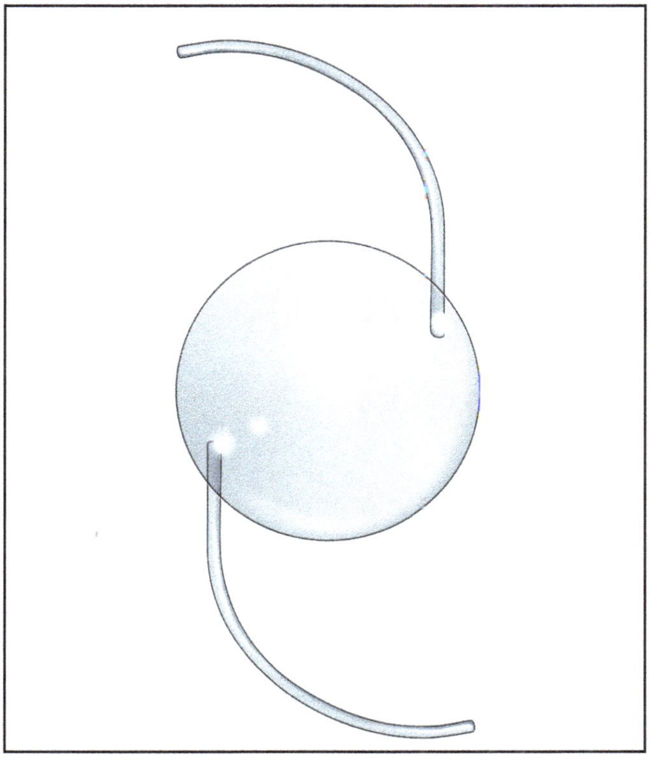

Figure 4-3. ORC Memory Lens. The Memory Lens is produced in poly-HEMA-acrylic (MMA) with a moderate water content and polypropylene loops.

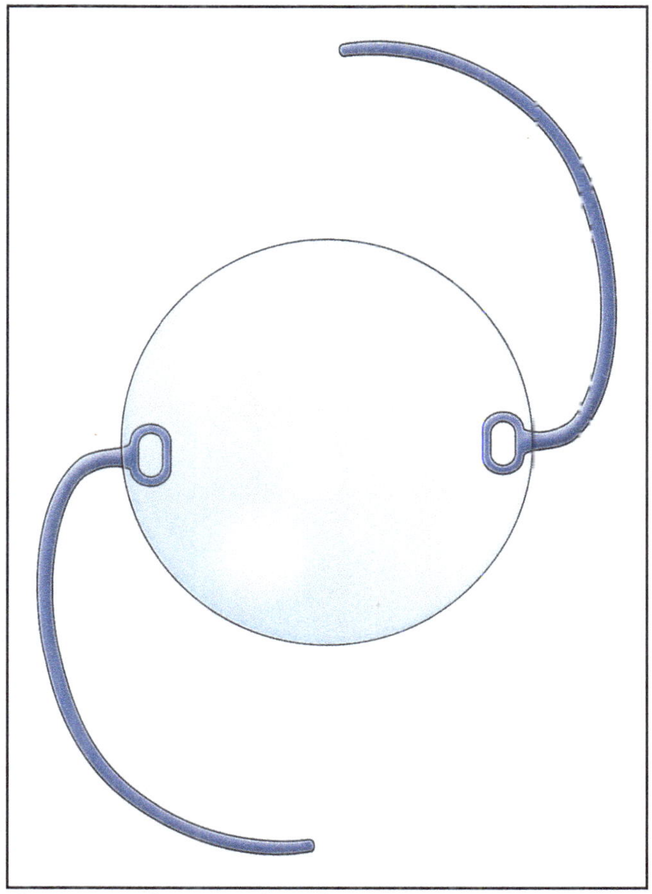

Figure 4-4. The AMO PhacoFlex II SI30NB. This is a second-generation PhacoFlex silicone IOL produced by AMO. This silicone lens with polypropylene loops has a refractive index of 1.46; it is thinner than its predecessor and is also easier to insert in the eye.

Soft Hydrophobic Acrylic Lenses

In 1994, the first foldable hydrophobic acrylic lens was introduced in the United States: the AcrySof. This lens had an optic diameter of 6.0 mm and an overall diameter of 13.0 mm. The C-shaped loops were produced of PMMA and formed an angle of 10 degrees with the optic. Folding and unfolding of the lens was (and still is) possible at room temperature, though higher temperatures are occasionally used as some surgeons (though not all) feel that this makes insertion easier.

This lens, or the material used to produce it, possesses 2 important characteristics: a high refractive index of 1.55, a factor that allows the creation of a very thin lens (0.3 mm) without altering the diameter of the optic and PMMA haptics that allow optimal centration in the bag.

AMO PhacoFlex

Allergan Medical Optics (AMO) introduced 2 generations of foldable lenses in the mid-1990s.[1] The first lens, known as the SLM1, was rapidly removed from the market. It had a silicone optic and a refractive index of 1.41. This lens was very thin at the center (just 1.42 mm); consequently, it was not difficult to fold but strong forceps were required for its introduction into the eye, and these did not enter easily through a small incision suitable for phaco. The second generation of AMO lenses (PhacoFlex II, Epoch, SI30NB) (Figure 4-4) did not have this problem because they were produced in a silicone elastomer that had a refractive index of 1.46. These lenses have a central thickness of 0.9 mm, an optic diameter of 6.0 mm, and a maximum diameter of the haptics of 13.0 mm. The Prolene haptics were a modified C-shaped loop and could be inserted through small incisions. AMO no longer produces the PhacoFlex II lens.

At the end of the 1990s, AMO introduced the first multifocal silicone lens, the AMO Array, in an attempt to produce optimal distance vision and good intermediate vision (Figure 4-5). This was possible by the creation of a series of concentric zones with an addition of +3.5 D with respect to the distance power. This lens was introduced in 1999 and was commercially available until 2004 when it was replaced by the ReZoom. The Array had blue-core PMMA haptics of 10-degree angle and a maximum diameter of 13.0 mm.

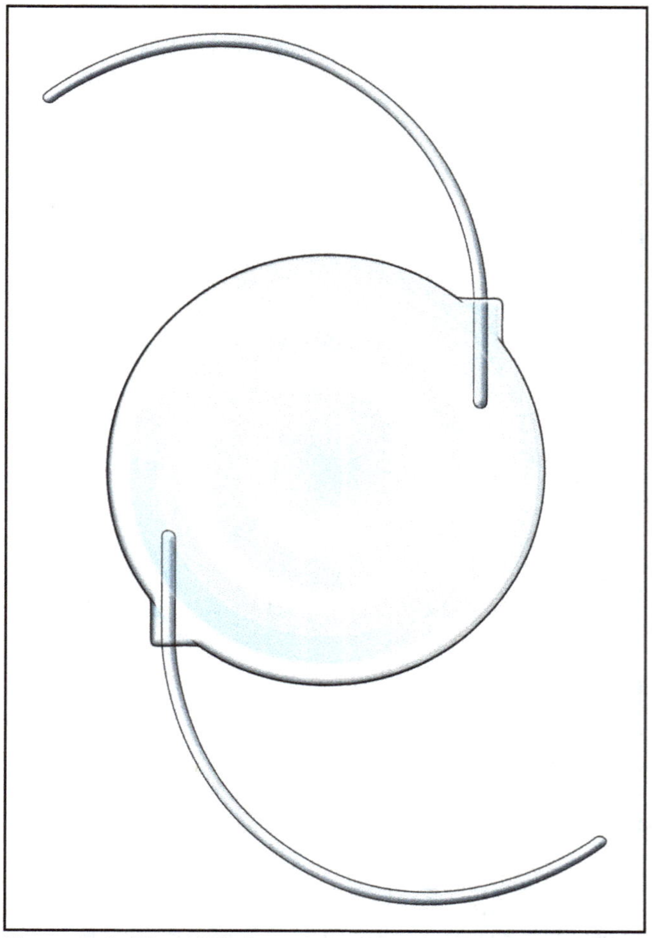

Figure 4-5. The AMO Array lens, SA40N refractive multifocal silicone IOL, which was on the market between 1999 and 2004; it was eventually replaced by the ReZoom lens. This is a refractive lens with optic zones with PMMA loops with blue core.

The lens was foldable and could be inserted through incisions of 3.2 mm. The disadvantages associated with this type of lens were its reduced contrast sensitivity, haloes perceived around light sources, and reduced near vision in subjects with poor pupil movement (because the IOL is refractive and therefore pupil dependent). Moreover, cases of opacification of this type of lens, resulting in explantation of the lens, have been described in the literature.[2] The haloes around light sources are the result of the splitting of light in different foci: 50% distance, 37% near, and 13% intermediate. Papers published in 2005 reported the success as being independence from spectacles in 54.5% of cases; this was extremely interesting as the literature at that time reported independence from spectacles as between 26% and 47% of cases implanted with other lenses. These percentages cannot be compared to current statistics in which independence from spectacles with multifocal lenses is considerably higher. The AMO Array SA40N lens is no longer being produced.[3]

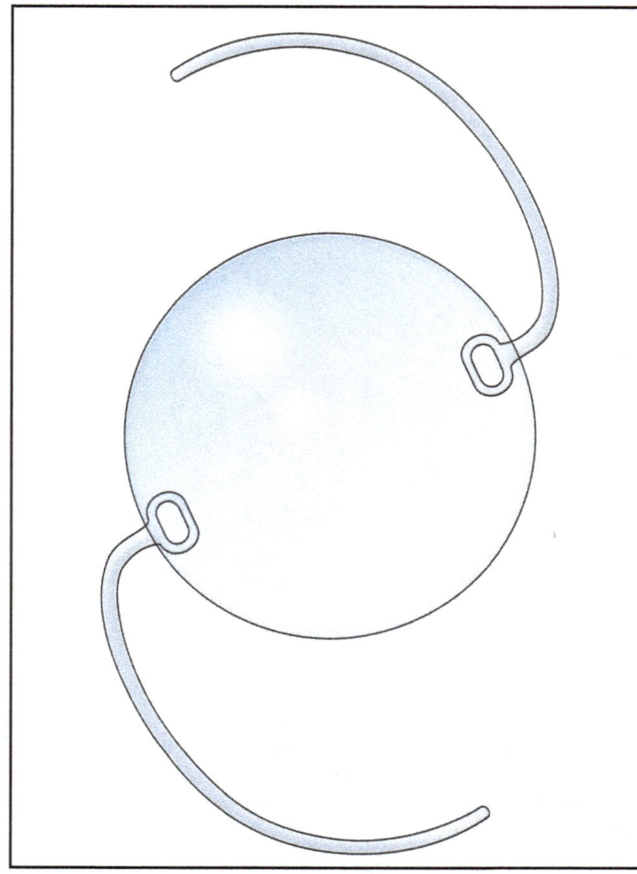

Figure 4-6. The Pharmacia CeeOn lens. This is a foldable lens with a silicone optic and PMMA haptics. This lens possessed the advantages of the memory form of PMMA and the theoretical disadvantages of the silicone elastomers.

Pharmacia CeeOn Foldable Lens

The IOL produced by Pharmacia CeeOn was a foldable lens with a silicone optic and PMMA haptics. This lens had the advantages of the memory form of PMMA and the theoretical disadvantages of the silicone elastomers (compared to the more recently developed foldable lenses). Moreover, there was poor compatibility between the YAG and silicone (Figure 4-6).

Storz Hydroview Lens

The Storz Hydroview Lens was a foldable hydrogel lens produced by Storz Ophthalmic. The hydrated optic of this lens was a copolymer of HEMA and 6-hydroxy-hexyl-methacrylate (HOHEXMA). The compound 1,6-hexane-diol dimethacrylate (HDDM) was added as a cross-linker to create dimensional stability. Moreover, a UV filter–benzotriazole was added. The blue-core PMMA loops were cross-linked with EGDMA and polymerized with the body

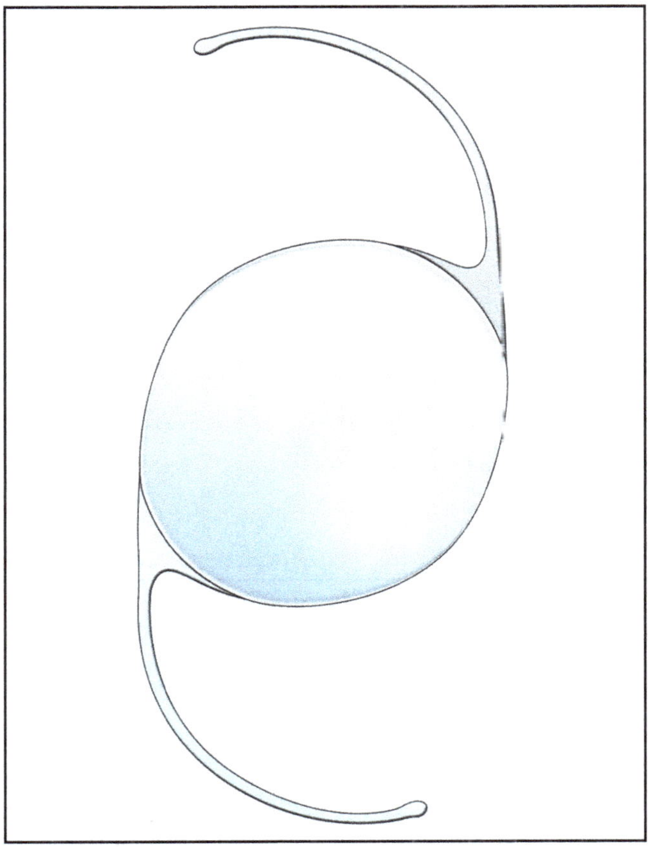

Figure 4-7. The Storz Hydroview Lens. This is a foldable lens of hydrogel produced by Storz Ophthalmic. The material used to produce the lens is called xerogel, or zero water hydrogel.

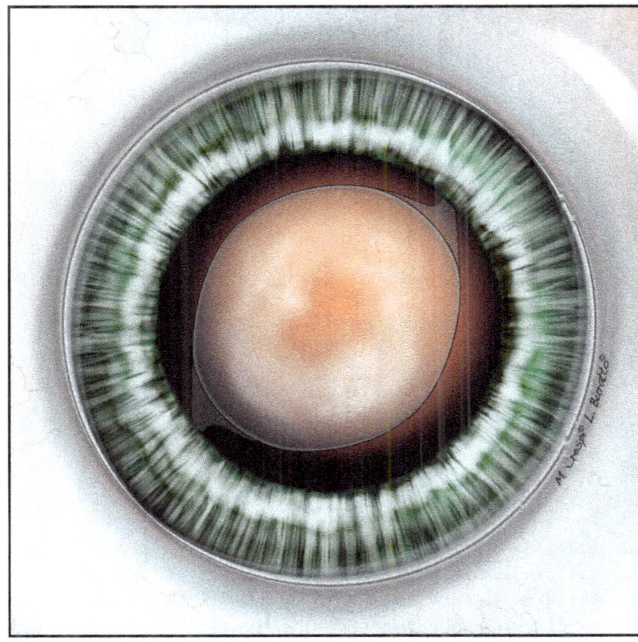

Figure 4-8. The Storz Hydroview Lens. This image illustrates the formation of hydroxyapatite crystals on the lens surface.

of the lens in xerogel (zero water hydrogel) during the manufacturing process (Figure 4-7).

The first clinical trials investigated model P422 UV, which has an optic diameter 6.0 mm, with a maximum length of the haptics of 13.0 mm, and an angle of 6 degrees. This model was then replaced with the model H60L, which had the same dimensions but more flexible PMMA haptics. The model H60M was a variant of this and had a maximum diameter of 12.5 mm. The Hydroview lens had the highest refractive index of all existing elastomers of hydrogel and silicone (1.474). To minimize water evaporation from the optic, this lens had to be used as quickly as possible following removal from the packaging or used when still immerged in water or BSS. Nevertheless, tests showed that, at room temperature, the lens could be used up to 3 minutes after it had been removed from water. The amount of time the lens had been folded determined the unfolding time of the lens inside the eye. Moreover, this lens had good hydrolytic stability, good photostability, and good resistance to the Nd:YAG laser.

Opacification was observed in numerous hydrogel IOLs (Hydroview H60M, Storz-Bausch + Lomb) with the formation of hydroxyapatite crystals on the lens surface. In 1995, implantation of the H60M lens began outside of the United States; early in 1999, this lens was approved by the FDA; and in May of that year, the first cases of opacification were reported (Figure 4-8).

Given that opacification of the lens was not seen in all patients, surgeons realized that the lens material was not the only factor responsible for the formation of hydroxyapatite crystals. These crystals caused the rough appearance of the opacity. This important complication was due to the high affinity of the polymer for calcium, irregularities of the lens surface, and possible interaction with some chemical substances during the surgical procedure.

Additional patient factors, such as diabetes mellitus, may also contribute to the appearance of this complication. The severity of these opacifications could actually reduce visual acuity significantly and justify explantation of the lens. Currently, these lenses are no longer commercially available.

Corneal Acrygel Lens

Acrygel is a copolymer of hydrophilic and hydrophobic methacrylates and is produced by the French company Corneal. It is thought that this material possesses biocompatibility equivalent to PMMA, combined with interesting hydrophilic properties. The water content of the ACR6D is 26%; the lens is one piece with an optic diameter of 6 0 mm and an overall length of 12.0 mm with a 0-degree angulation of the haptics. The refractive index is 1.47.

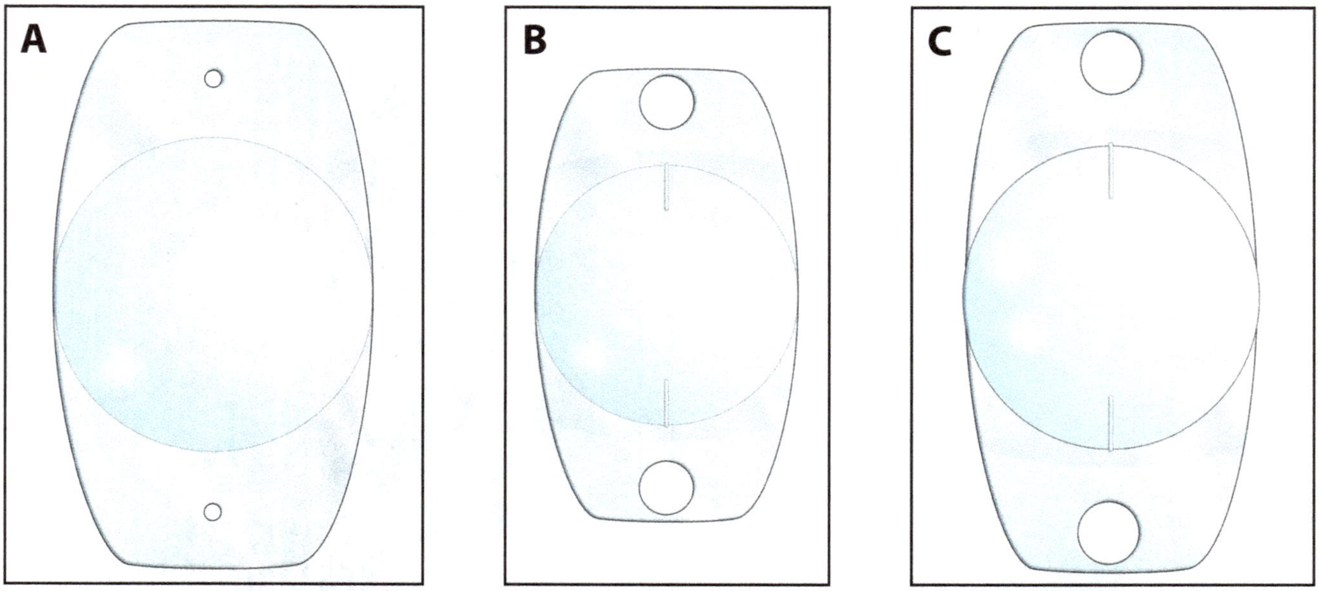

Figures 4-9. The IOL produced by STAAR. This image illustrates the IOL models produced by STAAR. The first (A) has been produced with smaller fenestrations, the second (B) has larger fenestrations, and finally, in the third model (C), the anteroposterior axis is longer.

STAAR IOL Foldable

STAAR was the first company to introduce lenses with flat haptics. It has a diameter of 10.5 mm. The foldable lens produced by STAAR is a biscuit- or cookie-shaped 1-piece silicone lens; the haptics or flanges are flush with the optic (of 6.0 mm for a maximum diameter of 10.5 mm). The plate haptics have a positioning hole of diameter 0.5 mm and small fenestrations. The refractive index is 1.41 (Model AA-4203).

In 1998, STAAR received FDA approval for its toric lens. The material was collamer, with an index of refraction of 1.44. The model of the lens was the AA4203-TF. One of the problems with this lens was that it decentered easily. A change in design significantly reduced the incidence of this early postoperative off-axis rotation; the manufacturer increased the overall length of the IOL from 10.8 mm (model AA4203-TF) to 11.2 mm (model AA4203-TL), and larger fenestrations allowed fusion between the anterior and posterior capsules. Cases of off-axis rotation became uncommon. These models of monofocal, toric, and implantable collamer contact lenses produced by STAAR Surgical are still commercially available (www.staar.com) (Figure 4-9).

References

1. Yang S, Lang A, Makker H, Zaleski E. Effect of silicone sound speed and intraocular lens thickness on pseudophakic axial length corrections. Allergan Medical Optics, Irvine, California 92718-2020, USA. *J Cataract Refract Surg.* 1995;21(4):442-446.
2. Elgohary M, Zaheer A, Werner L, Ionides A, Sheldrick J, Ahmed N. Opacification of Array SA40N silicone multifocal intraocular lens. *J Cataract Refract Surg.* 2007;33(2):342-347.
3. Wang JC, Tan A WT, Monatosh R, Chew PTK. Experience with ARRAY multifocal lenses in a Singapore population. *Singapore Med J.* 2005;46(11):616.

Suggested Readings

Dhaliwal RS, Mandira M. Update on intraocular lenses. In: Garg A, ed. *Advances in Ophthalmology* 2. New Delhi, India: Jaypee; 2005: Chapter 5.

Sachedev MS, Venkatesh P. Phaco intraocular lenses. In: *Phacoemulsification, Laser Cataract Surgery and Foldable IOLs.* New Delhi, India: Jaypee: Chapter 31.

5

Currently Used Lenses

Lucio Buratto, MD; Stephen F. Brint, MD, FACS; and Domenico Boccuzzi, MD, PhD

General Advantages of Foldable Intraocular Lenses

The use of foldable intraocular lenses (IOLs) is necessary for small-incision phacoemulsification, reducing the incidence of postoperative astigmatism, increasing the stability of the wound, and accelerating visual recovery and healing times.

There are 3 different types of incisions for phacoemulsification:

1. **Standard incisions:** Incisions with a wound diameter of approximately 2.75 to 3.2 mm
2. **Mini-incisions:** Incisions with the diameter for phacoemulsification reduced to 2.2 mm
3. **Microincisions:** Incisions with a diameter less than or equal to 1.8 mm

The value, therefore, is the minimum diameter of the incision that allows the passage of the ultrasound tip into the anterior chamber: 2.75 mm is the minimum gauge for the tip and the standard sleeve; 2.2 mm for the tip and the sleeve for the mini-incision; and 1.8 mm for the tip and the sleeve for the microincision cataract surgery (MICS). Incisions of 2.2 and 2.5 mm are considered to be mini-incisions because the minimum diameter for the ultrasound tip is 2.2 mm. In this case, a probe with a standard tip cannot be used, as this would require an incision of diameter 2.75 mm.

The same applies to MICS that can be performed with incisions of 1.8 and 2.0 mm.

Each of these methods requires appropriate instruments. Even IOLs must have the physical characteristics and be loaded into injectors that are suitable for introduction into incisions of increasingly small diameters (Figure 5-1).

Foldable IOLs can be produced with different materials, with the common denominator that they can be folded and rolled for loading into the narrow tunnels of the injectors. They will return to their original shape, with no abnormalities of the optic or the haptics over time. Moreover, the use of injectors and soft lenses increases protection for the corneal endothelium as compared to polymethylmethacrylate (PMMA) IOLs. With these rigid IOLs it was easier to have contact with endothelium or endothelial stripping during the insertion procedure.

As mentioned earlier, foldable IOLs can be produced of different materials: hydrophilic acrylic, hydrophobic acrylic, and silicone. Each of these materials has different characteristics and features that make it more or less suitable for implantation. An article published in the *Journal of Cataract & Refractive Surgery* analyzed the pros and cons of the various types of foldable lenses.[1] It examined uveal biocompatibility, inflammatory effect the material of the lens has on the eye, and capsular biocompatibility, or rather the capacity of determining the appearance of Elschnig's pearls and opacity of the posterior capsule.

Hydrophilic acrylic IOLs have good uveal biocompatibility but poor capsular compatibility. In other words, even though they cause little inflammation, they are responsible for early onset of posterior capsular opacification (PCO).

With silicone IOLs, more inflammation occurred in the anterior chamber (moderate degree), and there has been more severe anterior capsule opacification (ACO) as compared to acrylic lenses. In spite of this disadvantage,

Buratto L, Brint SF, Boccuzzi D.
Cataract Surgery and Intraocular Lenses (pp 23-26).

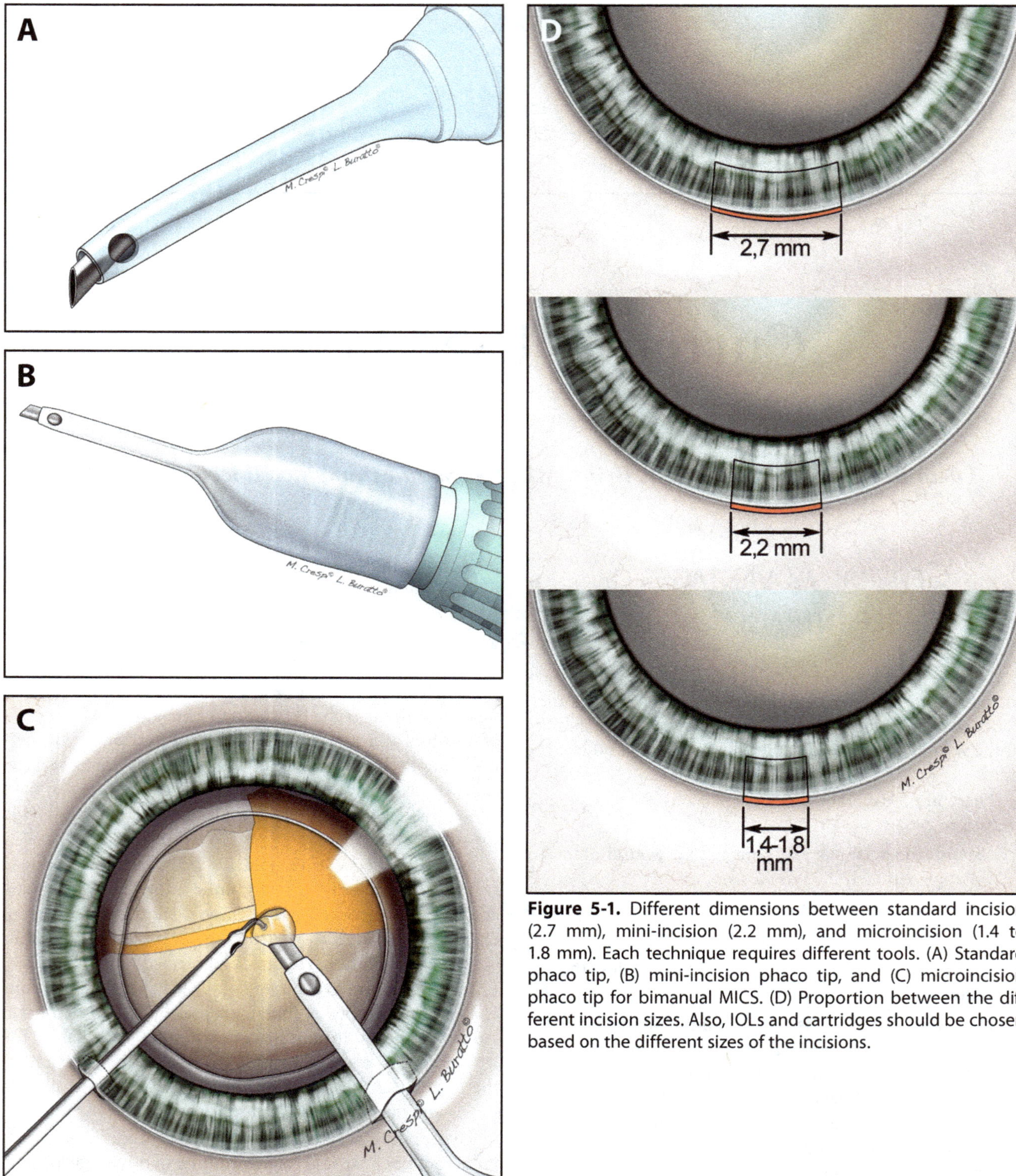

Figure 5-1. Different dimensions between standard incision (2.7 mm), mini-incision (2.2 mm), and microincision (1.4 to 1.8 mm). Each technique requires different tools. (A) Standard phaco tip, (B) mini-incision phaco tip, and (C) microincision phaco tip for bimanual MICS. (D) Proportion between the different incision sizes. Also, IOLs and cartridges should be chosen based on the different sizes of the incisions.

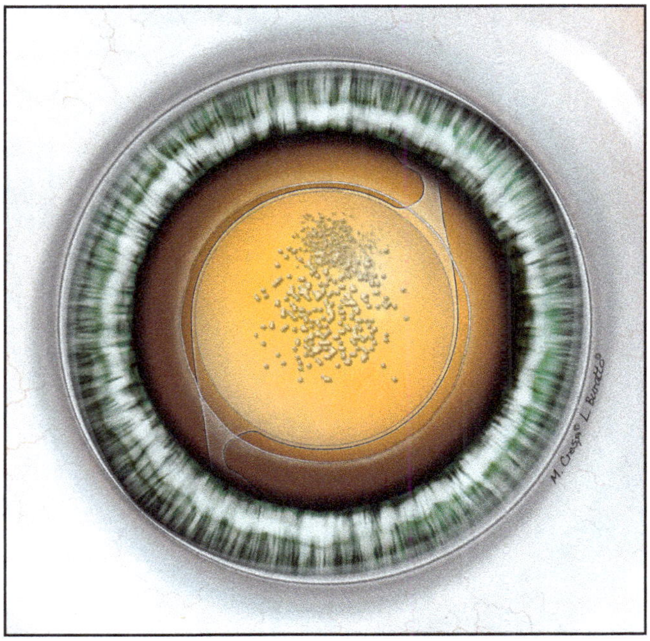

Figure 5-2. Damage to the IOL resulting from the YAG laser impact.

they have shown greater posterior capsular compatibility as opposed to hydrophobic acrylic IOLs.[2]

All of the foldable lenses are much easier to explant; this is not only because of their flexibility but also particularly because of less perilenticular fibrosis that leads to early mobilization in the capsular bag as opposed to PMMA IOLs.

The hydrophilic lens is the most straightforward foldable IOL used to explant. There is much less adhesion to the capsular bag and they are much easier to cut.

Foldable IOLs are generally associated with a lower incidence of PCO.

A paper published in 2009 in the *Canadian Journal of Ophthalmology* compared the incidence of PCO requiring neodymium:yttrium-aluminum-garnet (Nd:YAG) laser in relation to the 4 different types of lenses: square-edge PMMA (Aurolab), silicone (Tecnis Z9000), hydrophobic acrylic (AcrySof MA60AC and Sensar OptiEdge), and hydrophilic acrylic (Akreos Adapt) for a minimum follow-up of 2 years. It appeared that silicone IOLs have the lowest incidence of PCO requiring the Nd:YAG laser (1.4%), compared to 11.7% implanted with the PMMA IOL. In patients implanted with the square-edge acrylic IOLs, the incidence of PCO that required Nd:YAG laser treatment was 3.6% for AcrySof lenses, 4.8% for the group implanted with Sensar OptiEdge, and 6.8% for the group implanted with the IOL Akreos Adapt.[3]

However, YAG laser capsulotomy frequently damages the IOL. This damage is largely caused by the acoustic shock and the laser heat conduction, producing opacities in the IOL that can cause glare or a reduction in image quality. Each type of IOL showed a specific damage morphology following YAG laser impact (Figure 5-2).

PMMA IOLs have the lowest degree of compatibility with the YAG laser; cracks will radiate from the point of impact. IOLs in silicone, poly(2-hydroxyethyl methacrylate) (poly-HEMA), and acrylic IOLs containing HEMA (that have a high water content) have the highest resistance to the YAG laser with a lower incidence of damage. Generally speaking, foldable IOLs have better compatibility with the YAG laser compared to PMMA IOLs.[4,5]

Finally, advantages that apply to all foldable IOLs are their lower degree of biodegradability and reduced zonular stress; these are partly due to their reduced weight and the ease of insertion into the capsular bag.

Disadvantages of Silicone Intraocular Lenses

The properties of the material and the design and dimensions of silicone IOLs are extremely critical factors during their insertion in ocular areas other than the capsular bag. The implantation technique for this type of lens must be extremely delicate due to poor resistance of the lens material. Any damage to the surface of the optic caused by the injector or the holder-folder system can result in serious visual disturbances. Some postoperative problems have been reported with these lenses (silicone polymer by STAAR) such as clouding.

Foldable silicone lenses cannot be used with posterior capsule rupture. They are also contraindicated when there is a possibility that vitreoretinal surgery may be necessary, as silicone oil cannot be used as a tamponade under these conditions. The reason for this is that the tight interface that forms between the silicone oil and the IOL is extremely difficult to remove and would cause a significant drop in the patient's vision. For all of the previous reasons and because of the problems associated with difficult management and handling during folding and insertion, silicone IOLs are being abandoned by the majority of surgeons, and consequently, companies are shutting down their production (Figure 5-3).

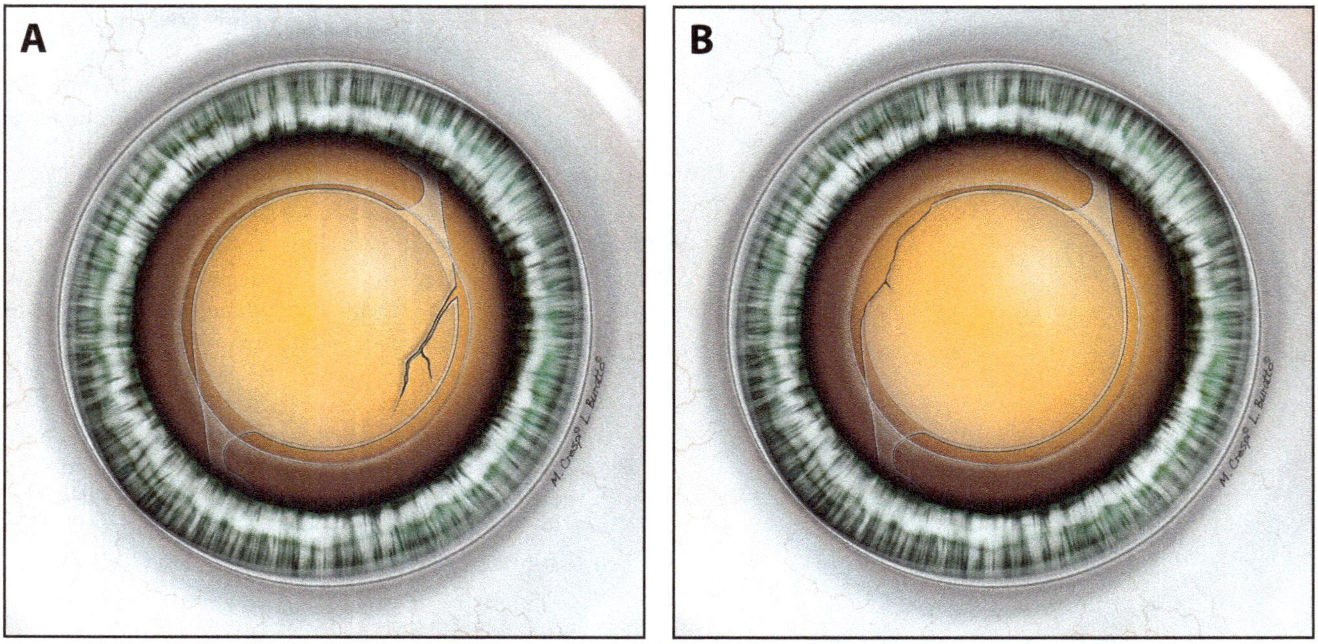

Figure 5-3. A silicone IOL with (A) a crack and (B) a structural defect occurred during insertion.

References

1. Abela-Formanek C, Amon M, Schild G, Schauersberger J, Heinze G, Kruger A. Uveal and capsular biocompatibility of hydrophilic acrylic, hydrophobic acrylic, and silicone intraocular lenses. *J Cataract Refract Surg.* 2002;28(1):50-61.
2. Abela-Formanek C, Amon M, Schauersberger J, Kruger A, Nepp J, Schild G. Results of hydrophilic acrylic, hydrophobic acrylic, and silicone intraocular lenses in uveitic eyes with cataract: comparison to a control group. *J Cataract Refract Surg.* 2002;28(7):1141-1152.
3. Ram J, Kumar S, Sukhija J, Severia S. Nd:YAG laser capsulotomy rates following implantation of square-edged intraocular lenses: polymethyl methacrylate versus silicone versus acrylic. *Can J Ophthalmol.* 2009;44(2):160-164.
4. Joo CK, Kim JH. Effect of neodymium: YAG laser photodisruption on intraocular lenses in vitro. *J Cataract Refract Surg.* 1992;18(6):562-566.
5. Dick B, Schween O, Pfeiffer N. Extent of damage to different intraocular lenses by neodymium: YAG laser treatment—an experimental study. *Klin Monbl Augenheilkd.* 1997;211(4):263-271.

6

Monofocal Intraocular Lenses

Lucio Buratto, MD; Stephen F. Brint, MD, FACS; and Domenico Boccuzzi, MD, PhD

This chapter will focus on spherical and aspheric monofocal intraocular lenses (IOLs). Toric IOLs will be examined later in the book.

The majority of lenses implanted today are monofocal. The reasons for this are easy power calculation and postoperative management, good visual quality, maintenance of good contrast sensitivity, absence of secondary effects, and low cost. When we speak of monofocal IOLs, the first distinction should be made on the basis of their design—3-piece vs single-piece IOLs. It is also possible to classify monofocal lenses on the basis of the material used in production, the shape of the optic, the presence or absence of asphericity, or the shape of the haptics. There are numerous criteria that can be used to classify this group of lenses; however, to keep things simple, we will refer to 3-piece IOLs and 1-piece IOLs, describing the characteristics of various lenses in detail later.

One-Piece and Three-Piece Intraocular Lenses

A desire for less invasive surgery has necessitated technological advancements in IOLs and insertion systems, so that increasingly smaller incisions may be used. Researchers have managed to produce IOLs that can be inserted through increasingly smaller incisions. They have stopped the production of 1-piece lenses with polymethylmethacrylate (PMMA) haptics or other materials that could be damaged during the folding process (Figure 6-1). One-piece IOLs for mini-incisional surgery have been developed that can be injected through incisions of up to 2.2 mm. The next step is the development of lenses for microincisional surgery (MICS) that can be injected through incisions of 1.5 mm.

Currently available 1-piece IOLs can be introduced through mini-incisions in cataract surgery. In terms of refractive characteristics, lens stability, incidence of tilt, percentage opacification of the posterior capsule, and the anterior capsule opening, 1-piece IOLs are identical to 3-piece IOLs.[1]

The only advantage 3-piece IOLs have over 1-piece IOLs is that, in the event of posterior capsule rupture, the 3-piece IOL can also be implanted in the sulcus, with good stability, if the overall length is 13 mm or at least 12.5 mm. Three-piece IOLs and 1-piece IOLs are currently available even though there is a growing tendency to implant the 1-piece versions.

The majority of the lenses are foldable; however, it is essential that surgeons are familiar with implantation techniques for PMMA IOLs as they may prove necessary in some specific cases, for example, anterior scleral fixation; however, they are gradually being abandoned (Figure 6-2).

Three-Piece Intraocular Lenses

If we compare 3-piece IOLs produced by the 5 main manufacturing companies that are currently available—Alcon, Abbott Medical Optics (AMO), Bausch + Lomb (B + L), Hoya, and Zeiss—it is apparent that the technical reasons for choosing this type of lens are more or less generally the same.

Buratto L, Brint SF, Boccuzzi D.
Cataract Surgery and Intraocular Lenses (pp 27-38).

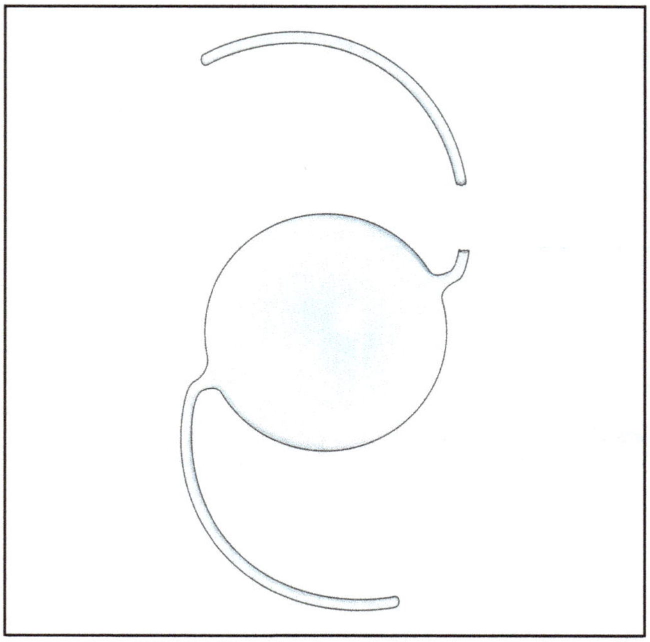

Figure 6-1. PMMA IOL with a haptic that was torn during the insertion procedure.

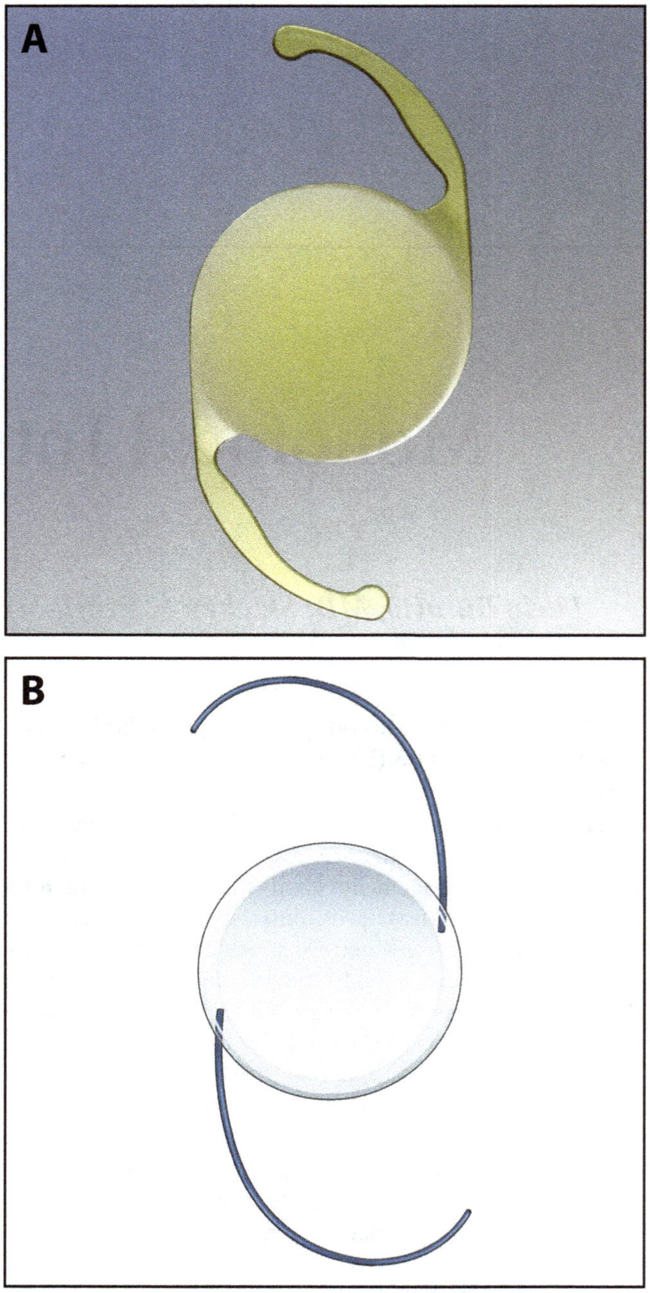

Figure 6-2. (A) One-piece hydrophobic acrylic IOL, Model AcrySof Natural by Alcon. (B) Three-piece hydrophobic acrylic IOL with PMMA haptics.

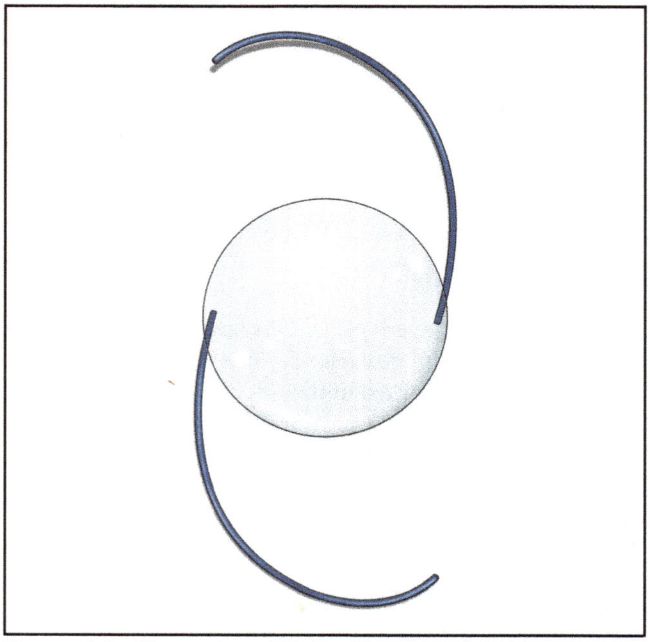

Figure 6-3. Three-piece IOL by Alcon, Model MA60MA. The first letter (M) of the code number indicates that the IOL is a 3-piece (M = Multipiece).

Alcon

Alcon produces several models of 3-piece lenses. They are made of hydrophobic acrylic with colored PMMA haptics (monoflex). This type of lens is identified by the letter M in the code (Multipiece) (Figure 6-3).

The 3-piece lenses produced by Alcon have different characteristics that are specific for each model: the color of the optic, the size and shape of the optic, the length of the haptics, and the vaulting of the haptics.

The lenses are available in 2 colors: the standard lens with a clear optic and the Natural lenses with a yellow-colored optic. The optic of the Natural is yellow so as to mimic the physiological color of the natural lens. With incorporation of the yellow chromophore, the Natural IOLs filter blue light at frequencies of between 400 and 550 nm that may damage the macula.

All of the Alcon IOLs (Natural and clear) have an ultraviolet (UV) filter (mandatory for Food and Drug Administration [FDA] approval).

The standard dimension of optics is 6.0 mm with a maximum diameter including the haptics of 13.0 mm. The inclination with respect to the optic plane is 10 degrees. The company produces models with 5.5-mm optics, a maximum diameter of the haptics of 12.5 mm, and a vaulting of the haptics of 5 degrees; it also produces models with 6.5-mm optics, haptics of 13.0 mm, and a vaulting of the haptics of 10 degrees.

The optic can be biconvex, anterior asymmetrical biconvex, or a meniscus. The meniscus is typical of the Expanded models that have a power of between –5.0 and + 5.0 D (low power levels). For lenses with the model Expanded of power between –10.0 and –4.0 D, the optic is plano concave. The diameter of the haptics varies between 11.5 and 13.5 mm with intervals of 0.5 mm. The haptics have a modified L-shape with an inclination of 5 degrees. None of the 3-piece lenses has an optic power greater than +30.0 D. For such high values, it is necessary to implant a 1-piece lens of dioptric power up to +40 D.

Abbott Medical Optics

AMO produces 3 models of 3-piece IOLs: the Sensar AR40 (with 3 versions available), the ZA9003, and the ZA9002.

The Sensar AR40 lenses are determined on the basis of the diopters: AR40M in powers between –10.0 and +1.5 D, AR40E in powers between +2.0 and +5.5 D, and AR40E in powers between +6.0 and +30.0 D.

The optic is hydrophobic acrylic with a UV filter and a diameter of 6.0 for all of the models; the shape of the optic changes—the AR40M (an IOL with a negative dioptric power) is a meniscus; the other 2 models are classical biconvex lenses.

The PMMA haptics are monofilament with blue core and a maximum diameter of 13.0 mm. The vaulting of the loops is 5 degrees, the same as for the other models of 3-piece IOLs discussed previously.

The ZA9003 IOL differs from the previous model because of the aspheric anterior surface of the optic. The optic (of diameter 6.0 mm) is always made of hydrophobic acrylic. The dioptric power ranges between +10.0 and +30.0 D.

The ZA9002 has a silicone optic; it also has an aspheric anterior surface, 3-piece with PMMA haptics. The dioptric power of this model varies between +5.0 and +30.0 D.

All of the AMO IOLs described have a square edge posterior to improve contact with the posterior capsule and to prevent cell migration and the formation of posterior capsule opacification (PCO). Moreover, they have a lateral margin that is sloped to reduce glare and a rounded edge for diffracting light.

The insertion involves the use of an Emerald C cartridge with a screw injector (Emerald Series) (model T or model XL).

Bausch + Lomb

The B + L 3-piece lens range is called SofPort. The characteristics of the silicone lenses (OG S2) are identical to those of other 3-piece IOLs—6.0-mm optic in silicone with a 360-degree anterior and posterior square edge, and PMMA haptics with a maximum diameter of 13.0 mm and 5-degree vault; the refractive index is 1.43.

The model SofPort SE is a classical spherical lens, while the model AO is the aspheric version with the profile of the optic hyperprolate and a spherical aberration value of zero. The objective of the aberration-free aspheric lenses is to respect the characteristics of the natural lens; in young patients, for example, they keep the positive spherical aberration of the cornea unchanged (generally +0.27 μm). In addition to improving the patient's visual quality, the advantage of an aberration-free (AO) aspheric lens is that it does not induce higher-order aberrations (HOA), for example, coma, with decentration.

Hoya (AF-1 Spheric Hydrophobic Intraocular Lens)

Hoya produces 6 IOLs: 4 models of 3-piece IOLs, one designed for mini-incisional surgery, and one for microincisional surgery (iSpheric IOL) (Figure 6-4).

Structurally, the 3-piece IOLs by Hoya are made of hydrophobic acrylic with PMMA haptics. The haptics are a modified C shape with a vault of 5 degrees. The diameter of the optic of these lenses is 6.0 mm with a maximum diameter of the loops 12.5 mm for the IOLs to be implanted in the bag, and 6.5 mm with a diameter of the loops 13.0 mm for IOLs to be implanted in the sulcus.

IOLs for implantation in the bag can be inserted through a 2.8-mm incision; the IOLs for implantation in the sulcus, with a larger optic diameter, require 3.0-mm incisions. All of these lenses have a step edge to prevent cell migration and PCO.

The IOLs for the bag and those for the sulcus both have a spherical optic available in 2 models: the YA models have a filter for UV rays and for light in the blue spectrum; the VA models have the filter for UV rays only. The IOL for implantation through a mini-incision has an optic of 6.0 mm, haptics of 12.5 mm, and is available only in the version with a filter for blue light; it can be inserted through incisions ≥2.5 mm.

The IOLs for introduction through a microincision have similar characteristics to the previous ones; the thickness of the optic is reduced, and there is greater flexibility that allows the insertion through incisions down to 2.0 mm.

Zeiss

The philosophy applied by Zeiss Meditec is slightly different from the other companies. Zeiss continues to produce just one type of 3-piece lens and has turned its attention now to a 1-piece lens, which we will examine later. The Hydromax lens is the only model to have an optic of

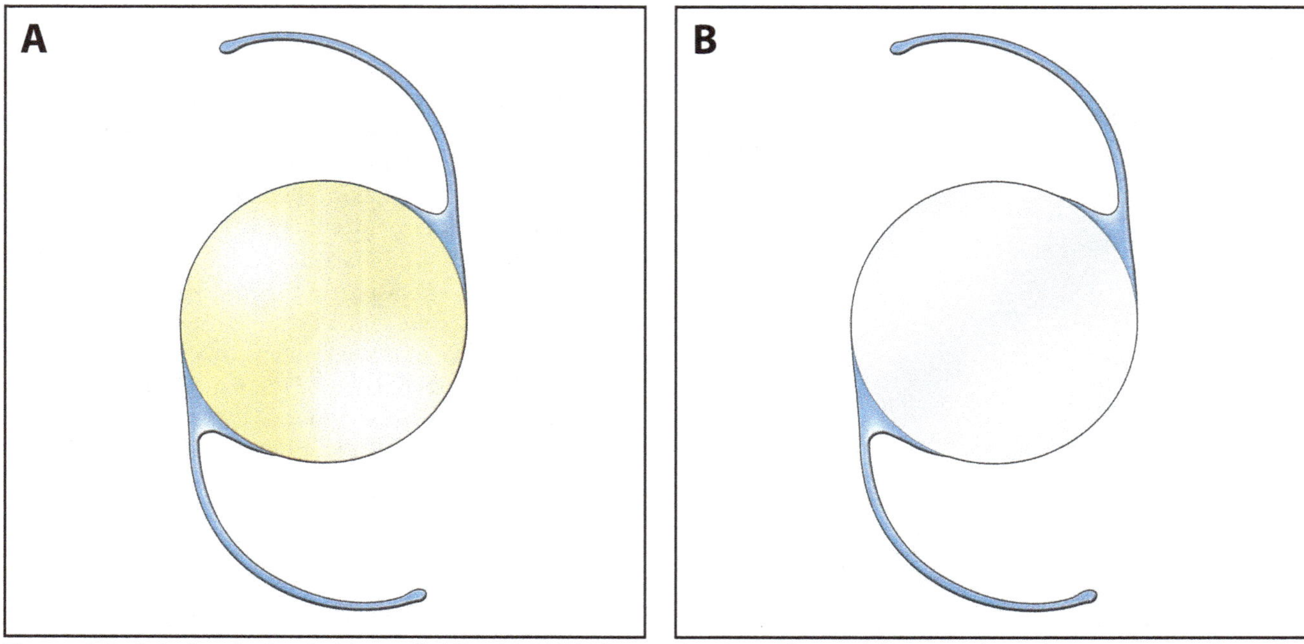

Figure 6-4. A 3-piece hydrophobic acrylic IOL with PMMA haptics by Hoya. The models are (A) the iSpheric YA60BB with a yellow optic to protect the eye against blue light and a UV filter and (B) the iSpheric VA60BB lens with a transparent optic and a UV filter.

hydrophobic acrylic, with a diameter of 6.0 mm and haptics of polyvinylidene fluoride (PVDF), a maximum diameter of 12.5 mm, and classical vault of 5 degrees. The refractive index of the lens is fairly high at 1.56, allowing a thinner optic.

The posterior square edge limits cell migration, reducing the incidence of PCO. The lens has a UV filter and can be injected through incisions of 2.8 mm.

One-Piece Intraocular Lenses

As mentioned earlier, foldable 1-piece IOLs can be described as the natural evolution of the IOL. This type of lens can be inserted using an injector with cartridges that have a very small bore diameter up to 1.8 mm, the dimension of the microincision. These developments are all part of the evolutionary pathway of cataract surgery that can be completed quickly by using increasingly smaller incisions.

One-piece IOLs must be implanted in the capsular bag because of the high risk of decentration and iris chafing if implanted in the sulcus.

Alcon

Alcon also produces a range of 1-piece lenses—monofocal, toric, multifocal, and toric multifocal (Figure 6-5). These lenses can be classified on the basis of their material, the color of the optic, the shape and size of the optic, the maximum diameter of the haptics, their shape, and the vault of the haptics.

The 1-piece lenses are foldable hydrophobic acrylic or rigid PMMA. The hydrophobic acrylic lenses are available in the version "N" (Natural) with yellow optics and a filter for blue light, and the version "A" (AcrySof) with a transparent optic. Both models also have a filter for UV rays (mandatory for FDA approval).

The standard dimension of the optic is 6.0 mm with a maximum diameter of the haptics of 13.0 mm. A 1-piece IOL with an optic of 5.5 mm and haptic diameter of 13.0 mm is also available. All of the 1-piece hydrophobic acrylic IOLs have modified L-shaped haptics with 0-degree vault. With the exception of the lens with an optic diameter of 5.5 mm and available in dioptric powers from +10.0 to +30.0 D, for all of the other models, the values available are +6.0 to +30.0 D with increasing intervals of 0.5 D, and +31.0 to +40.0 D with increasing intervals of 1.0 D. For the lenses of hydrophobic acrylic, the optic has an asymmetrical biconvex anterior surface; however, an aspheric version also exists (see following chapters) with a value of asphericity of −0.20 μm. All of the PMMA lenses have a clear optic of diameter varying between 5.0 and 7.0 mm with increasing intervals of 0.50 mm. The lenses with a 7.0-mm optic are for scleral fixation and have a fixation ring. The optic is biconvex.

Abbott Medical Optics

AMO produces a 1-piece monofocal lens: the Tecnis ZCB00. It is foldable and made of hydrophobic acrylic; it has a UV filter, an optic of 6.0 mm, and a maximum diameter of the haptics of 13.0 mm. The C-shaped haptics are planar with the optic (Figure 6-6).

The optic of the lens is biconvex with an aspheric anterior surface (hyperspherical with a value of −0.27 μm) and posterior square edge to prevent PCO. The lens is thinner at the center to facilitate implantation. AMO created

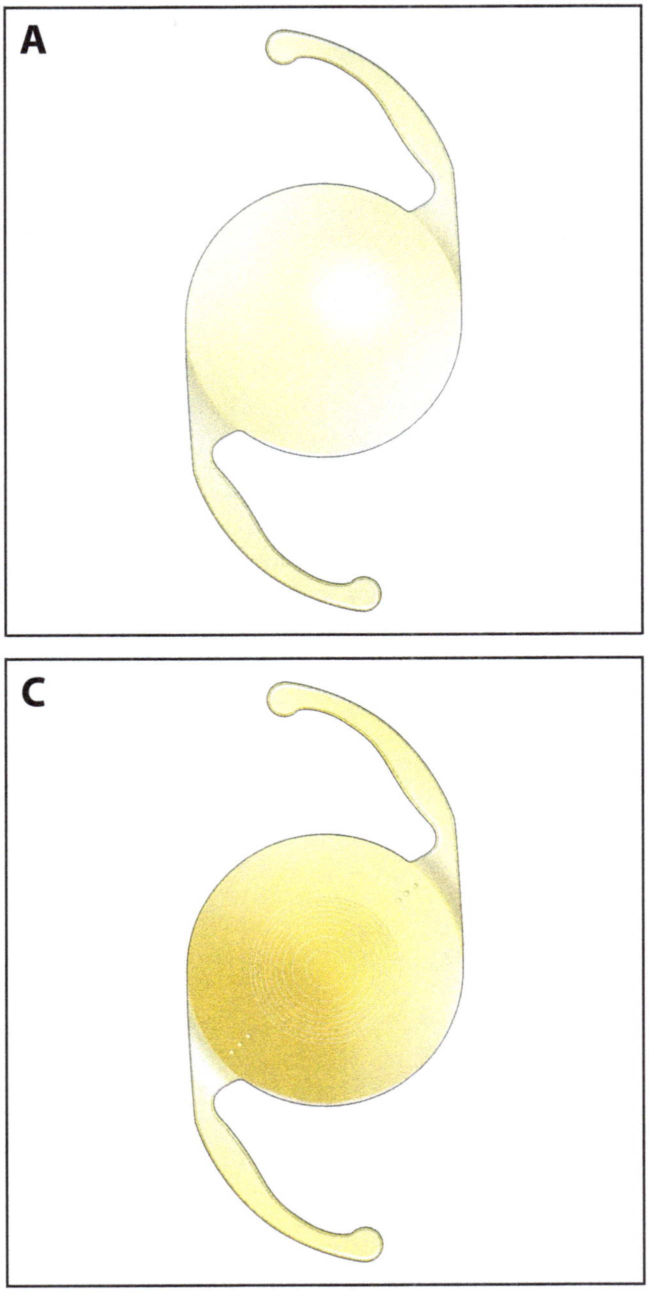

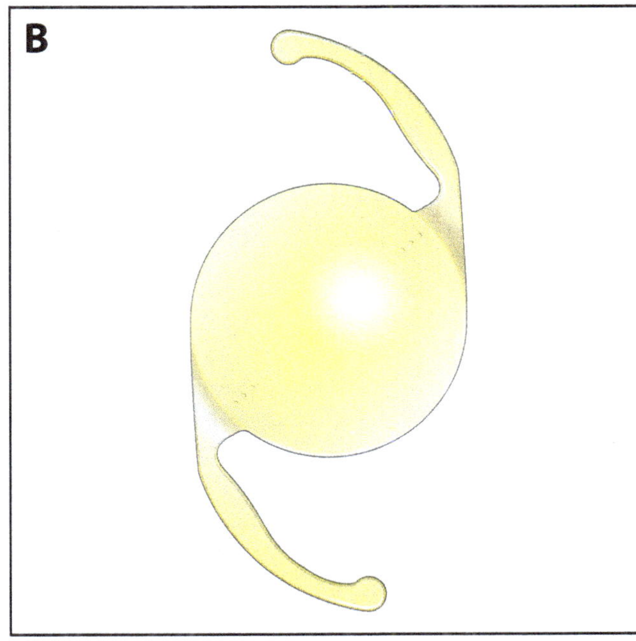

Figure 6-5. One-piece hydrophobic acrylic IOL produced by Alcon. All 3 lenses of the series have a yellow optic Model Natural, with a filter for blue light and a filter for UV rays. (A) Monofocal IOL Alcon. (B) Toric monofocal IOL. (C) Toric multifocal IOL Alcon ReStor with an apodized surface.

an aspheric lens with a negative spherical aberration of −0.27 μm with the objective of completely correcting the mean positive corneal spherical aberration (+0.27 is the mean value of the population) and achieving a value of zero.

Studies now demonstrate that elimination of corneal spherical aberration considerably improves contrast sensitivity, with reaction times approximately half-a-second faster than in a subject with a normal IOL. This is equivalent to being able to see an object on the road approximately 15 m sooner when driving at a speed of 90 km/h.

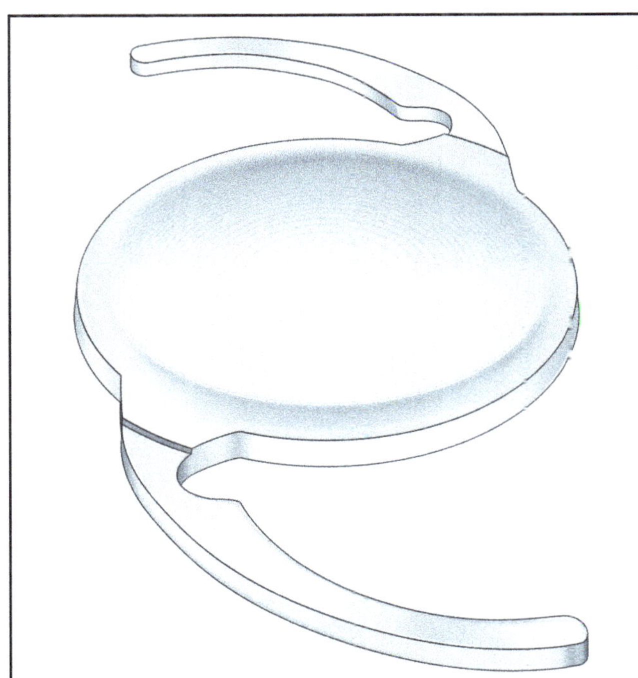

Figure 6-6. One-piece hydrophobic acrylic IOL. Tecnis Model ZCB00 with a UV filter. The Tecnis lens is produced with a characteristic square edge to prevent PCO; its anterior surface is hyperspherical with a value of −0.27 μm to compensate for the positive corneal spherical aberration.

Bausch + Lomb

The 1-piece IOL produced by B + L is called Akreos AO, as it is aberration-free, meaning that it has a spherical aberration equal to zero. There are 2 versions available: a standard lens and one suitable for MICS.

The Akreos AO (standard) is a 1-piece hydrophilic acrylic lens with a biconvex optic of diameter 6.0 mm and 4 fenestrated haptics coplanar with the optic plate. The maximum diameter of the haptics depends on the basis of the lens dioptric power.

For lens powers of between 0 and +15.0 D, the diameter of the haptics is 11.0 mm. For lens powers between 15.5 and 22.0 D, the diameter is 10.7 mm, while for lens powers greater than 22 D up to +30.0 D, the diameter is 10.5 mm. On the posterior surface, the optic has a square edge designed to prevent PCO (Figure 6-7).

The Akreos AO lens for MICS (MI60) has an unusual shape (Figure 6-8). Again, the material used was hydrophilic acrylic with an aberration-free optic of diameter 6.0 mm and designed with a posterior square edge.

The real innovative feature of the lens is the shape of the haptics. There are 4 haptics attached to this lens; they are positioned at a 10-degree angle to the optic with a more rigid proximal portion and a more flexible distal portion, called the "conforming tip." The end portion consists of 2 flexible offshoots that extend in a radial and longitudinal direction. These have the objective of allowing the contraction movements of the capsular bag without transmitting the movement to the central optic. This leads to excellent long-lasting stability and centration, even with asymmetric retraction (Figure 6-9).

For this type of lens, the maximum diameter of the haptics is also variable, and is based on the dioptric power of the lens. For lens powers of between +10.0 and +15.0 D, the diameter is 11.0 mm. For lens powers of between 15.5 and 22.0 D, the diameter is 10.7 mm, while for the values between +22.5 and +30.0 D, the diameter is 10.5 mm.

The B + L philosophy regarding asphericity is that the lens should be aberration free or rather with a spherical aberration that is equal to zero, leaving the corneal spherical aberration unchanged; which has a mean value

Evolution of the AcrySof From the Beginning to the Present Day

The AcrySof lens was the first hydrophobic acrylic lens introduced in the United States in 1994.

It was the first 3-piece lens with a 6.0-mm optic and haptics of diameter 13.0 mm; the C-shaped haptics were made of PMMA and formed an angle of 10 degrees with the optic. In 2000, Alcon introduced the 1-piece AcrySof, again of hydrophobic acrylic. The haptics of this lens were planar with the optic, of diameter 6.0 mm, and the maximum diameter of the haptics was 13.0 mm. In 2003, the company added a yellow chromophore (Natural model) to the AcrySof lens with the objective of reproducing the physiological color of the human lens, and more importantly, to introduce a filter for blue light that can damage the macula. In 2005, the 1-piece AcrySof was also produced as an aspheric lens, with a negative spherical aberration of −0.20 µm; this was to partially compensate the positive corneal spherical aberration (approximately +0.27 µm).

Since 2006, the AcrySof has also been available as a toric lens, with the possibility of correcting severe corneal astigmatism, up to 6 D of cylinder at the iris plane, a value that corresponds to approximately 4.11 D at the spectacle plane.

The AcrySof ReSTOR model D3 was introduced in 2007; this is a multifocal diffractive-refractive apodized lens with an additional component for near vision of +4.00 D at the iris plane (approximately +3.2 D at the spectacle plane). In 2008, the structure of the AcrySof ReSTOR was modified, with a reduction in the number of rings in the apodized portion and the addition of a component for near vision of +3.0 D at the iris plane, approximately +2.25 D at the spectacle plane (model D1). This lens can reduce the appearance of haloes and improve intermediate vision.

The latest addition to the Alcon family is the AcrySof ReSTOR Toric Multifocal lens; the design of the multifocal is that of the second generation of ReSTOR (model D1), with the additional correction of the cylinder. For the correction of the cylinder, currently, Alcon has restricted production to models that vary from +1.5 D at the iris plane (1.0 D at the corneal plane—model T3) to +3.0 D at the iris plane (+2.25 at the corneal plane—model T5). There is no doubt that this decision is fairly restrictive; however, Alcon is convinced that only a small percentage of patients are excluded.

The last newborn in the Alcon family is the multifocal IOL model SV. This IOL has the near addition of +2.5 D at the lens plane. This lens is suitable for far and intermediate vision and less suitable for near vision. This lens has new different features as compared to the D1 model. The apodized rings are 7 instead of 9 of the D1 model. Moreover, the central ring is for far vision while in the D1 model is for intermediate vision. The toricity of these IOLs is the same of the previous multifocal toric IOLs.

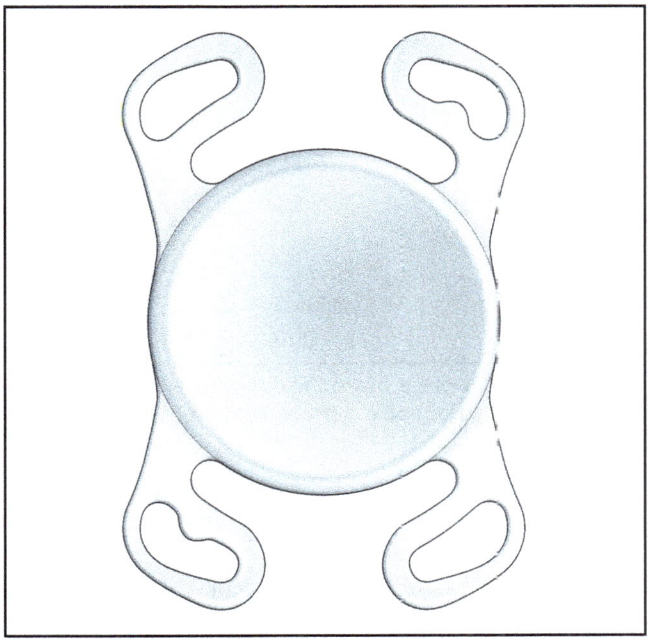

Figure 6-7. A 1-piece hydrophilic acrylic by Akreos AO, with a spherical aberration value of zero. The haptics are in the same plane as the optic.

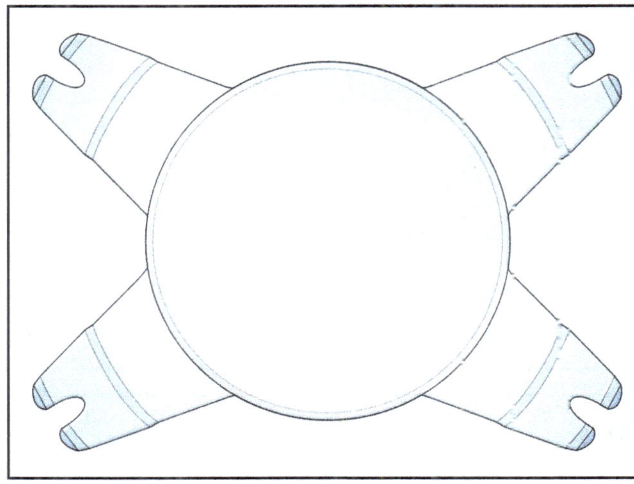

Figure 6-8. The Akreos AO IOL for MICS of hydrophilic acrylic.

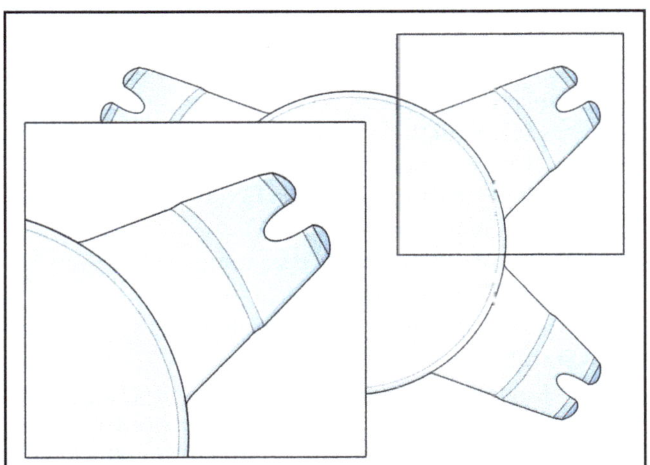

Figure 6-9. Close-up of the haptics of the Akreos AO lens for MICS.

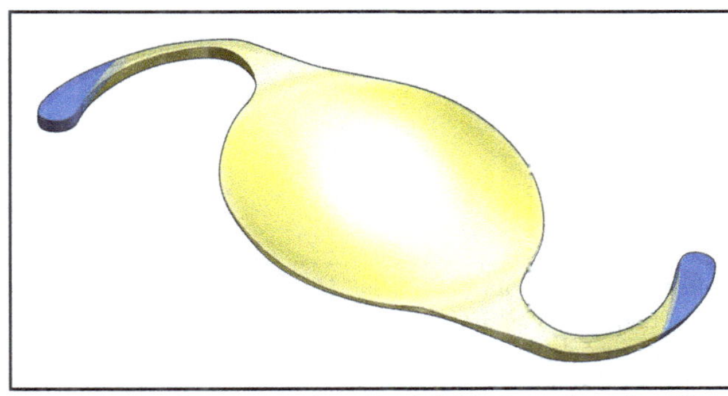

Figure 6-10. The 1-piece lens Model NY 60 produced by Hoya, with optic and haptics of hydrophobic acrylic; the end tips in colored PMMA facilitate the visibility of the lens as it is being inserted in the eye. The lens has a hyperspherical component of −0.18 μm.

of +0.27 μm in the population. The reason for this is that the B + L technicians believe that a small amount of positive spherical aberration (normally present in the cornea) provides an excellent depth of field, and as the IOL is aberration free, it will not generate any type of HOA in case of decentration of the lens.

As mentioned previously, the MI60 is a lens for use with a microincision; it can be inserted through 2.2-mm incisions with a standard insertion (with the cartridge entering the anterior chamber); it can also be inserted through 1.8-mm incisions with the linear method (meaning that the open tip of the cartridge and the corneal incision are brought close together with a second surgical instrument in the side-port incision to stabilize the eye and bring the cartridge into contact with the corneal tunnel).

Hoya

The 1-piece lens from Hoya is an innovative lens for insertion through a microincision (iMics NY 60); it can be inserted through sclero-corneal incisions of 1.8 mm and incisions in clear cornea measuring 2.0 mm. The lens is hydrophobic acrylic; the haptics are hydrophobic acrylic with a colored PMMA tip to improve visibility inside the bag and to avoid undesired adhesion of the haptic to the optic (Figure 6-10). The lens has a yellow 6.0-mm optic with filters for UV rays and blue light. The optic has a square-edge design to limit cell proliferation and prevent PCO. The optic is aspheric, with asphericity calculated as −0.18 μm; the idea is to partially reduce the positive corneal spherical aberration. The haptics are modified C shaped with a 5-degree vault. The maximum diameter is 12.5 mm. The lens power ranges from +6.0 to +30.0 D with intervals of 0.5 D.

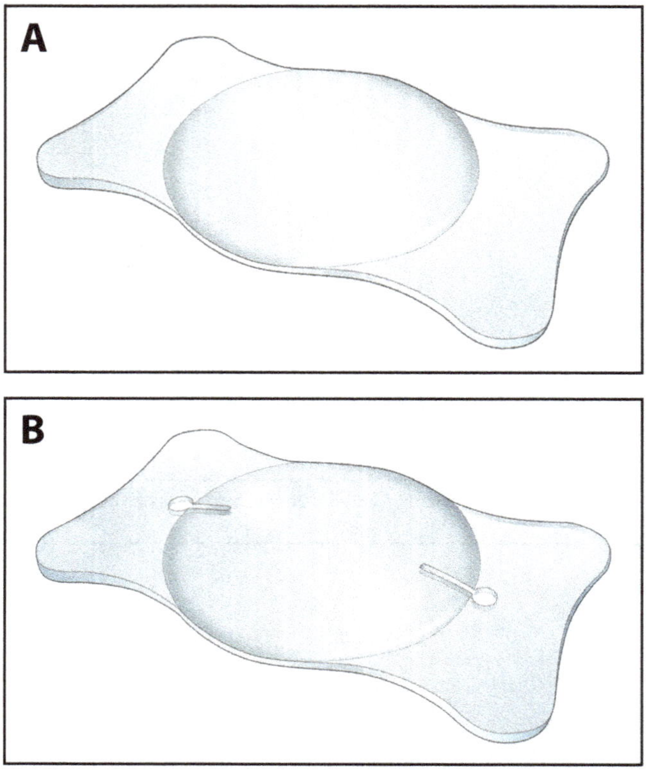

Figure 6-11. One-piece IOLs for MICS produced by Zeiss in hydrophilic acrylic with hydrophobic surface coating. (A) monofocal IOL available in 2 models: CT SPHERIS (monofocal spheric) or CT ASPHINA (monofocal aspheric) and (B) AT TORBI (monofocal bitoric aspheric). These lens can be inserted through 1.5-mm incisions.

Zeiss

Zeiss has taken an approach different from other companies; it has concentrated its efforts on the design and production of a range of monopiece lenses that account for the large majority of products in its portfolio.

Primarily, the material used to produce Zeiss IOLs is different: they are made of hydrophilic acrylic with a hydrophobic surface. The surface layer of the lens is not simply a dipped coating; the surface has been given a biochemical surface treatment. This is achieved by laser-cutting the lens; this procedure polymerizes the material into a hydrophobic substance.

The Zeiss IOLs are classified based on the lens type. The premium lenses belong to the AT (advance technology) group. There are aspheric multifocal optics and toric aspheric multifocal lenses (group—LISA; with these lenses, the light is distributed asymmetrically between distant [65%] and near focus [35%]), and the bitoric aspheric monofocal lenses (group—TORBI).

The monofocal lenses belong to the CT (cataract technology) group and include the monofocal spherical variant (-SPHERIS) and the monofocal aspheric variant (-ASPHINA). Two types of aspheric lenses are available:

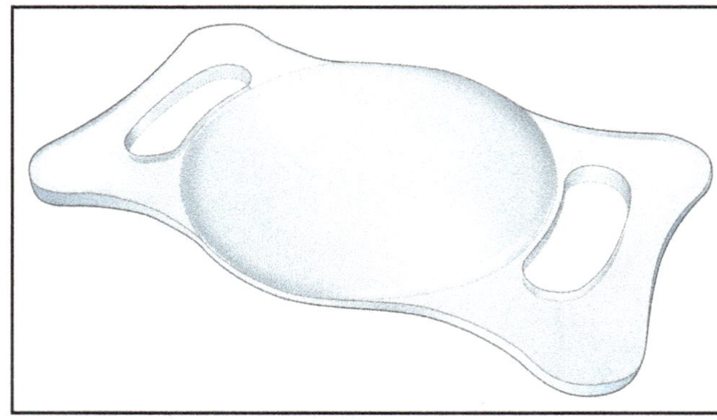

Figure 6-12. A 1-piece hydrophilic acrylic lens produced by Zeiss with a hydrophobic surface coating, 4-haptic design model.

those with neutral aberration and hyperaspheric with negative spherical aberration.

The Zeiss IOLs are classified into 3 main groups on the basis of design: MICS design, 4-haptic design, and 3-haptic design.

The MICS design group contains lenses suitable for microincisions measuring 1.5 mm (Figure 6-11). The lenses have an optic diameter of 6.0 mm; the haptics are planar with the optic, and the maximum diameter of the haptics is 11.0 mm. The models designed for MICS are available in the following models: AT (Advance Technology) as aspheric multifocal (LISA), toric multifocal aspheric (LISA-toric), and bitoric monofocal aspheric (-TORBI); and CT (Cataract Technology) as spherical monofocal (SPHERIS) and aspheric monofocal (ASPHINA).

A wide range of lens powers are available from –10.0 to +32.0 D with intervals of 0.5 D.

For the toric versions, the cylinder ranges from +1.0 to +12.0 D with intervals of 0.5 D.

The 4-haptic design group differs from the previous models as the haptics are planar to the optic but are fenestrated at the center. The maximum diameter of the haptics for all of these models is 11.0 mm (Figure 6-12).

Only the preloaded aspheric monofocal lens, the model Invent ZO, has 4 small and separate haptics, with a maximum haptic diameter of 10.5 mm. The 4-haptic design group is only available in the CT (Cataract Technology) version, either as spherical or as aspheric monofocal (Figure 6-13). A wide range of lens powers are also available for this type of lens, from 10.0 to +30.0 D with intervals of 0.5 D; on request, lens powers of +31.0 to +45.0 D with intervals of 1.0 D can also be produced. These lenses are ideal for mini-incisions and can be inserted through incisions of 2.2 mm, with the exception of the preloaded lens (Invent ZO), which requires an incision of 2.8 mm.

The final group is the 3-haptic design; it consists of 2 lens types and each has 3 fenestrated haptics positioned symmetrically around the optic. The haptics are not coplanar with the optic plate, but have a vault of 10 degrees and a

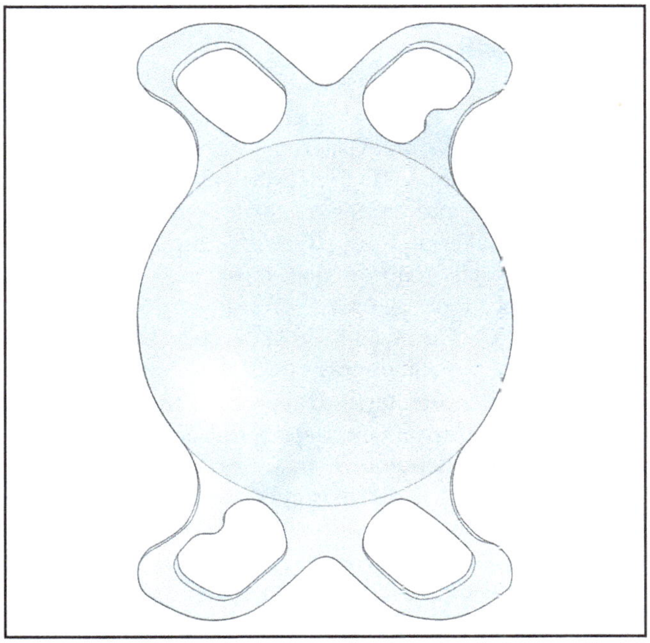

Figure 6-13. An aspheric monofocal preloaded lens, Model Invent ZO (Zeiss), with 4 small separate haptics. The 4-haptic design is only available in the CT (Cataract Technology) version, in other words as spherical or aspheric monofocal lenses.

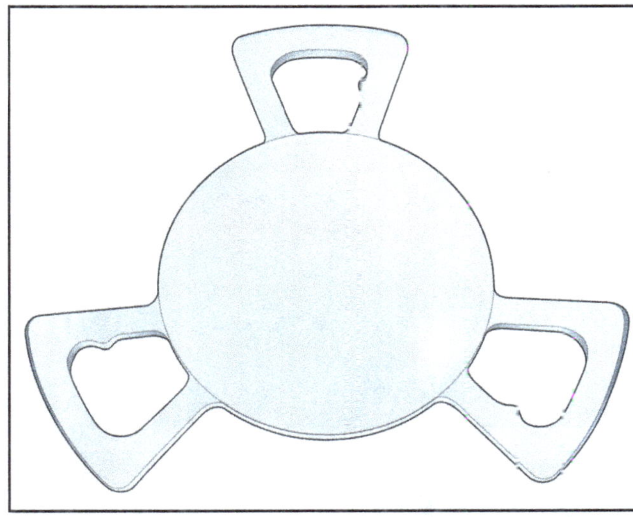

Figure 6-14. There are 2 models of the 3-haptic design, 1-piece IOL produced by Zeiss, with the fenestrated loops positioned symmetrically around the optic plate.

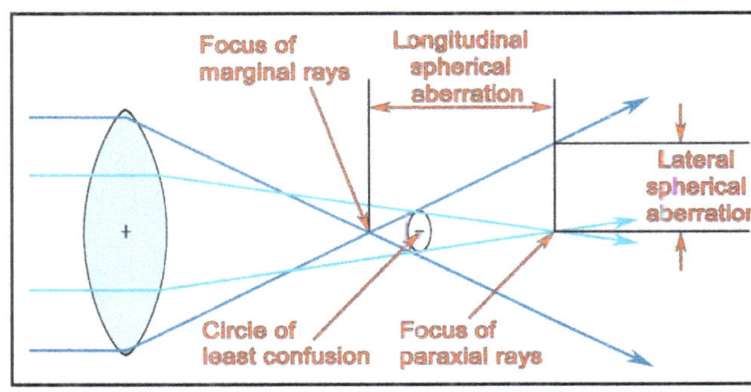

Figure 6-15. This drawing of the positive spherical aberration illustrates the longitudinal and lateral spherical aberration.

maximum diameter of 10.5 mm (Figure 6-14). The power of these lenses varies between +8.0 and +30.0 D. These 2 lens types are also preloaded and belong to the CT (Cataract Technology) group and are available in both the spherical and aspheric versions. These lenses can be inserted through incisions of 2.8 mm. Zeiss also produces 4 models of IOL that are available in yellow to filter blue light: AT LISA, AT LISA toric, CT ASPHINA for MICS, and CT ASPHINA 4-haptic design. The yellow filter for blue light is specific for light waves between 450 and 500 nm that are potentially damaging for the macula.

Aspheric Intraocular Lenses

Aspheric IOLs have a hyperprolate surface, which reduces positive spherical aberration, characteristic of all of the positive lenses (Figure 6-15). Negative spherical aberration of hyperaspheric IOLs can compensate for positive corneal spherical aberration. Wavefront analysis of the visual system has provided better information on optical aberrations that affect vision. Optical aberrations have been characterized using Zernike's polynomials (Figure 6-16).

An increase in ocular spherical aberration (SA) is highly correlated with a reduction in contrast sensitivity. The best contrast sensitivity was found in young patients between 20 and 30 years.

In 2004, a Japanese study[2] reported a progressive increase in positive spherical aberration Z(4,0) of the eye with aging. The high-order (up to the 6th order) corneal and ocular aberrations were calculated in the central 6.0 mm using a Hartmann-Shack aberrometer for a group of 75 eyes in 75 patients, mean age 43.5 ± 11.7 years (range, 18 to 69 years). Zernike's polynomials were used to calculate the root mean square (RMS) of the coma and the ocular and corneal spherical aberration. An age-related increase in RMS of coma and spherical aberration was seen. The results showed that an increase in ocular coma was correlated with a change in the cornea (an increase in the corneal coma correlated to an increase in ocular coma), with no variation in positive spherical aberration. An increase in spherical aberration is not correlated with modifications to the cornea but with changes in the internal structures of the eye. The anterior and posterior surfaces of the cornea, the lens, and the retina can generate HOAs in the phakic eye.

In the aphakic eye, 98.2% of the aberrations derive from the anterior surface of the cornea.[3]

In the pseudophakic eye, corneal aberrations are extremely important and are representative of the entire aphakic "ocular system." Zernike's polynomials for corneal HOAs derive from corneal topography. Scientific studies have demonstrated that the microincision required for cataract surgery does not change the corneal HOAs and this can be considered to be the same as the preoperative values.

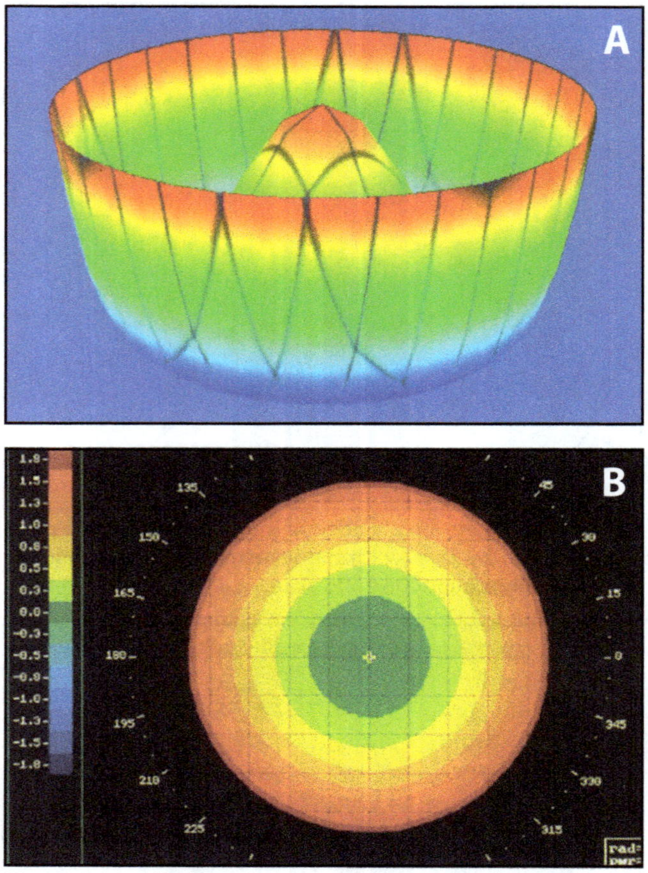

Figure 6-16. (A) The 3-dimensional illustration of the surface of the Z(4, 0) for primary spherical aberration (third order). (B) The refractive map of the anterior surface of the aspherical cornea with a radius of 7.695 mm (K-reading 43.86), the Q-value of −0.26, and a stromal refractive index of 1.376. The increase in the refractive power is indicated by the warmer colors. The additional refractive power is +1.00 D at a distance of 3.00 mm from the center.

Consequently, the choice of an aspheric IOL to compensate corneal aberrations and achieve the best visual acuity (BCVA) and the best contrast sensitivity is determined by careful study of the corneal HOA and its spherical aberration.

Presently, the FDA has approved 3 lenses for correction of positive spherical aberrations: Tecnis Z9000 (AMO), SofPort AO (B + L), and AcrySof IQ (Alcon). They each have a different strategy for the correction of spherical aberration.

The Tecnis Z9000 IOL has been designed with a negative spherical aberration of −0.27 µm, and this will compensate the total average positive spherical aberration of the cornea. The AcrySof IQ IOL has been designed with a negative spherical aberration of −0.20 µm, which partially compensates for the average positive spherical aberration of the cornea (approximately +0.27 µm measured at 6.0 mm). The SofPort AO IOL has been designed with a spherical aberration of zero, with the sole objective of eliminating the positive spherical aberration of the IOL, leaving the corneal component unchanged.

Different studies have shown that there is correlation between positive spherical aberration and "supervision" (considered to be natural visual acuity greater than or equal to 13/10).[4] Using an OPD Scan Nidek aberrometer (Nidek Co, LTD), Levy and colleagues quantified the total positive spherical aberration in patients with pupils dilated to a diameter greater than or equal to 6.0 mm, in 70 eyes of 35 patients of mean age 24.3 ± 7.7 years with supernatural vision (≥ 13/10). The mean RMS of the spherical aberration in this patient population was +0.110 ± 0.77 µm.

Other studies attempted to reproduce the same conditions of total positive spherical aberration in pseudophakic patients and determined that contrast sensitivity was greater in patients with a postoperative positive spherical aberration of +0.10 µm.

So how does the surgeon decide which aspheric IOL to implant? Why are there 3 different lenses to choose from? To understand the rationale of each individual company, it is essential to comprehend the population distribution of patients with spherical aberration. A study of 696 eyes[5] performed by Beiko et al found that the mean value of positive corneal spherical aberration was 0.274 ± 0.095 µm, and that its distribution followed a normal Gaussian curve.

Consequently, the IOL that allows a postoperative condition of positive spherical aberration of 0.10 µm is the Alcon AcrySof IQ (SA −0.20 µm) that leaves a slightly positive residual spherical aberration.

Actually, when the surgeon decides to implant an aspheric IOL, he or she should examine the eye using topography and measure the positive corneal spherical aberration (calculated at 6.0 mm). On the basis of the results achieved, he or she can choose the most suitable of the 3 aspheric lenses available; he or she should aim for a slightly positive result, with a value as close to +0.10 µm as possible (Table 6-1).

Aspheric Intraocular Lenses and Pupil Kinetics

The main function of aspheric IOLs is to eliminate or correct positive corneal spherical aberration to improve contrast sensitivity and to provide optimal vision. However, implantation of an aspheric as opposed to a traditional spherical IOL has specific requirements, particularly when the pupil diameter is much larger. Patients with scotopic pupil diameters larger than 5.0 mm are more likely to complain of haloes around light sources, caused by positive spherical aberration (Figure 6-17). In patients with small pupil diameters, visual and refractive results and visual comfort of an aspheric lens are identical to a traditional spherical lens. This phenomenon can be explained by a detailed analysis of the morphology of the aberration.

Spherical aberration is the physiological consequence when a positive lens is implanted. The incident rays on the central part of the lens will not converge at the same

Table 6-1

Spherical Aberration and Intraocular Lens

Hyperaspheric, neutral aspheric, and spherical intraocular lenses produce different aberration results according to the existing corneal asphericity

% OF PATIENTS	CORNEAL SA, µm	IOL SA, µm	OCULAR SA, µm	RESULTS
18	−0.06 to +0.18	−0.27	−0.33 to −0.9	Acceptable
		0	−0.06 to +0.18	Good
		+0.20	+0.14 to +0.38	Acceptable
69	+0.18 to +0.36	−0.27	-0.09 to +0.09	Good
		0	+0.18 to +0.36	Acceptable
		+0.20	+0.38 to +0.56	Poor
13	+0.36 to +0.48	−0.27	+0.09 to +0.21	Acceptable
		0	+0.36 to +0.48	Poor
		+0.20	+0.56 to +0.68	Poor

Results: ● Good ● Acceptable ● Poor

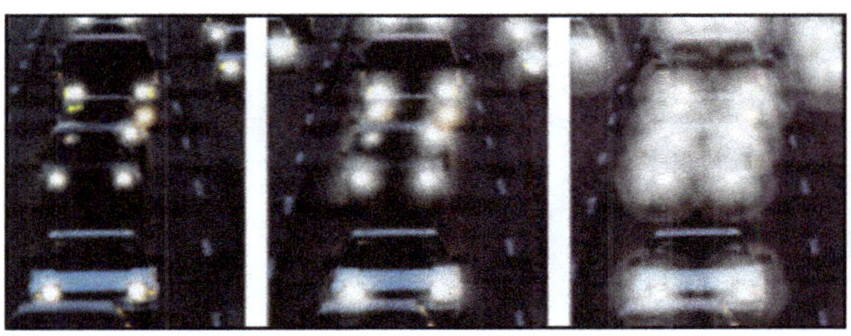

Figure 6-17. Spherical aberration is perceived as haloes around light sources that can create glare. An increase in the spherical aberration will lead to increasingly large haloes.

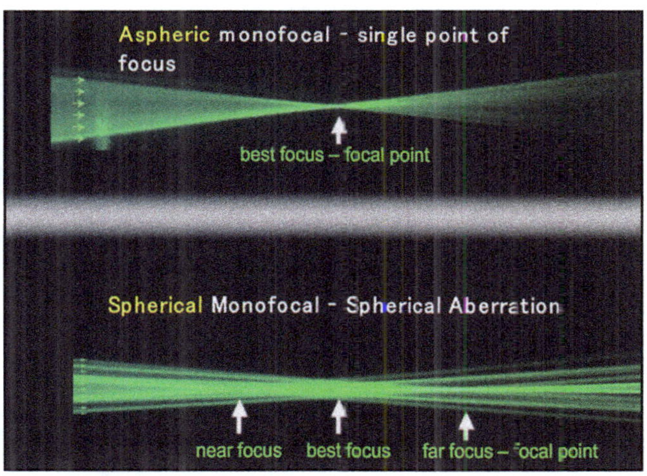

Figure 6-18. The luminous pattern when it passes through different IOLs, displayed by projecting a monofocal beam of green light (550 nm) through a lens positioned in water.

focal point as the peripheral rays, as these come into focus on points that are more anterior. This leads to a caustic, a 3-dimensional HOA symmetrical in its axis. It represents the Z(4,0) of Zernike's polynomial and is seen as a central focal point with an alternation of consecutive dark and clear haloes. This phenomenon can be decreased by an aspheric or hyperspheric lens that has a prolate or hyperprolate surface and can reduce or eliminate formation of positive spherical aberration (Figure 6-18). The greater the diameter of the opening that allows incident light, the greater the width of the caustic and the appearance of haloes. However, in small pupils with light passing exclusively through the central portion of the lens, the incident rays will focus at a single point, as the peripheral portion of the lens will not influence the situation in any way. The caustic will therefore be eliminated in the peripheral areas and haloes will not appear.

One important factor must be taken into consideration. The implantation of an aspheric IOL will unquestionably improve the patient's visual quality by correcting positive corneal spherical aberration. However, decentration of an aspheric IOL (aberration free) or a hyperspheric IOL (negative spherical aberration) decreases possible benefits of the aspheric lenses, creating HOA, such as coma, and reducing modulation transfer function.[6-9]

References

1. Nejima R, Miyata K, Honbou M, et al. A prospective, randomized comparison of single and three piece acrylic foldable intraocular lenses. *Br J Ophthalmol.* 2004;88(6):746-749.
2. Amano S, Amano Y, Yamagami S, et al. Age-related changes in corneal and ocular higher-order wavefront aberrations. *Am J Ophthalmol.* 2004;137(6):988-992.
3. Barbero S, Marcos S, Merayo-Lloves J, Moreno-Barriuso E. Validation of the estimation of corneal aberrations from video-keratography in keratoconus. *J Refract Surg.* 2002;18(3):263-270.
4. Levy Y, Segal O, Avni I, Zadok D. Ocular higher-order aberrations in eyes with supernormal vision. *Am J Ophthalmol.* 2005;139(2):225-228.
5. Beiko GH, Haigis W, Steinmuller A. Distribution of corneal spherical aberration in a comprehensive ophthalmology practice and whether keratometry can predict aberration values. *J Cataract Refract Surg.* 2007;35(5):848-858.
6. Sarver EJ, Wang L, Koch DD. The effect of decentration on high order aberrations. *Cataract Surgery Today.* 2006;Nov/Dec.
7. Altmann GE, Nichamin LD, Lane SS, Pepose JS. Optical performance of 3 intraocular lens designs in the presence of decentration. *J Cataract Refract Surg.* 2005;31(3):574-585.
8. Wang L, Koch DD. Effect of decentration of wavefront-corrected intraocular lenses on the higher-order aberrations of the eye. *Arch Ophthalmol.* 2005;123(9):1226-1230.
9. Krueger RR, MacRae SM, Applegate RA. In: Krueger RR, Applegate RA, MacRae SM, eds. *Wavefront Customized Visual Correction. The Quest for Super Vision II The Future of Customization.* Thorofare, NJ: SLACK Incorporated; 2004:363-373.

7

Toric Intraocular Lenses

Lucio Buratto, MD; Stephen F. Brint, MD, FACS; and Domenico Boccuzzi, MD, PhD

The development of toric intraocular lenses (IOLs) was an important evolutionary step in IOLs. This type of lens improves visual comfort for patients with astigmatism (even when the degree of astigmatism is high) and for patients who wish to eliminate spectacles and enjoy more natural vision. Astigmatism reduces visual acuity through meridian defocus; a corneal axis of a steeper curvature than the opposite axis will distort the images. Astigmatism, even when minimal, can lead to blurred vision, glare, ghost images, etc. A number of techniques are available for the correction of astigmatism.

Several techniques can be used to reduce postoperative astigmatism: astigmatic keratotomy (AK) and limbal relaxing incisions (LRI) are the easiest procedures to produce good refractive results and patient satisfaction. At the very beginning, the surgeon must evaluate the effect of the main incision and the side-port incision(s) on the corneal astigmatism. The corneal incision can have variable influence on the astigmatism, depending on the location of the incision, and the length of the corneal tunnel and its configuration. While planning the surgery, topography and corneal aberrometry are essential measurements for understanding the influence of the cornea on total astigmatism, and to determine the position of the main incision and the position and length of the relaxing incisions.

The sole keratometric measurement with the Javal keratometer is not always sufficient for the determination of the corneal astigmatism, as it is based on the measurement of 4 points positioned in the central 3 mm, and this fails to demonstrate any irregular astigmatism present.

It should also be pointed out that in young patients, a portion of the corneal astigmatism is compensated by opposite astigmatism of the anterior surface of the lens. The lens is removed during surgery, highlighting the corneal astigmatism.

Moreover, to ensure that the relaxing incisions do their job properly, a pachymetry map of the patient's eye is essential, as these incisions should be created at 90% of the corneal thickness.

The Role of the Corneal Incision

The corneal incision can influence postoperative astigmatism, depending on its location, on the location in relation to the limbus, tunnel length, width, shape, and depth.

This is a satisfactory method for the correction of small degrees of astigmatism and can aid the surgeon who prefers to leave pre-existing astigmatism unchanged.[1,2]

This is useful for patients who have no preoperative corneal astigmatism or in patients scheduled for implantation of a toric IOL.

In this last category of patients, it is essential to carefully plan the position of the incision and evaluate the effects on the corneal dynamics (surgically induced astigmatism [SIA]) to ensure the correct choice of IOL power and to precisely determine the axis for positioning the lens.[3]

A more posterior position of the corneal incision with longer corneal tunnels causes less astigmatism than more anterior incisions with short tunnels. Nomograms have been created that determine the influence of the main incision in relation to its location. However, each surgeon should learn from his or her own patients, on the basis of

Buratto L, Brint SF, Boccuzzi D.
Cataract Surgery and Intraocular Lenses (pp 39-52).

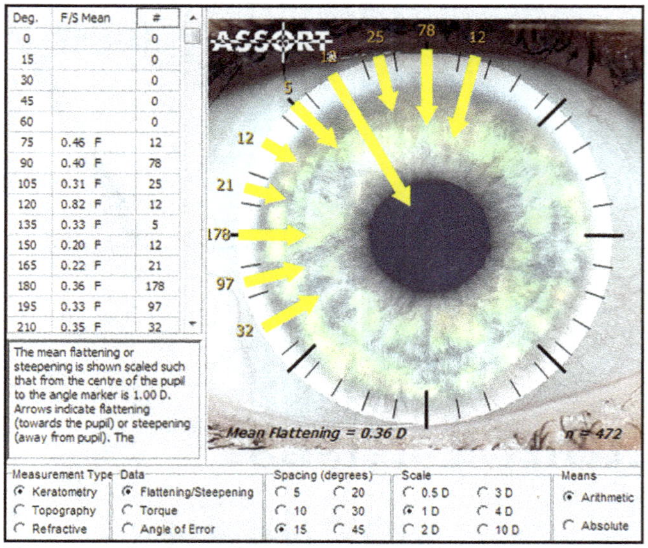

Figure 7-1. Moderate flattening measured by keratometry with incisions created on different meridians (on OD in the example). The numbers shown on every meridian indicate the number of eyes and the degree of flattening in diopters, as reported in the table on the left. (Reprinted with permission from Dr. Noel Alpins.)

his or her surgical techniques, and calculate the degree of SIA (Figure 7-1).

Larger corneal incisions lead to greater astigmatism as they cause greater relaxation of the meridian involved. A slight degree of induced corneal hyperopia is generated because the cornea is flattened. On the basis of the shape of the corneal incision, a cut that follows the curve of the limbus does not create changes in refraction if it is less than 3.0 mm. (A curved incision of <3.0 mm will not influence the astigmatism to any great degree.)

A straight incision created without considering the curved shape of the limbus will have greater influence on the astigmatism. Considering that the points are not all equidistant from the center of the cornea, the incision will exert an action that is not uniform. The points closer to the center flatten the cornea to a greater degree, leading to mild hyperopia. This method can be used to correct mild astigmatism; however, since the cornea will flatten itself, it will cause a hyperopic shift of 0.1 D. Therefore, the surgeon should target an extra 0.1 D of myopia.[4]

Regarding the depth of the incision, it should be pointed out that more superficial incisions will lead to greater induced astigmatism, as the superficial flap is elastic and will contract, thus flattening the cornea.[5,6]

With reference to the location of the cut, incisions at 12 o'clock are closer to the pupil that has shifted in a superonasal direction. Consequently, these incisions will have greater influence on astigmatism compared with temporal incisions that lie at a maximum distance from the pupil and consequently affect astigmatism to a lesser degree.

The use of a corneal suture also plays an important role in the management of astigmatism; a suture can increase the curvature of the meridian corresponding to the axis of placement, generating a myopic shift.

The cross-suture with normal tension is neutral in refractive terms as it creates retraction in both the longitudinal and the latitudinal directions.

Moreover, it should be pointed out that the choice of the location for the creation of the corneal incision plays a fundamental role in the postoperative development of higher-order aberrations (HOAs).[7]

When possible, creation of the corneal incision on the steeper meridian will reduce postoperative astigmatism and also reduce the appearance of HOAs, such as coma, trefoil, and secondary coma.

Relaxing Incisions

The techniques of AK and LRI are 2 important methods that can reduce postoperative astigmatism. Compared to AK, LRI allows the creation of more posterior incisions of greater length.

LRIs were introduced by surgeons who were hoping to create a technique that was easier to perform, was associated with a lower risk of overcorrection, and would not create irregular astigmatism if performed incorrectly.

The "coupling effect" allows the amount of relaxation at the incised meridian to be approximately the same as steepening at the opposite meridian.

When the LRIs are coupled (ie, when the incisions are created symmetrically on both sides of the meridian of greatest curvature), the coupling effect is 1:1; this means that the mean corneal power has not been changed, and consequently, it is not necessary to modify the power of the lens to be implanted. It should be pointed out that the correlation between the postoperative refractive error and an error in the calculation of the mean k is 1:1; this means that each diopter of error in the calculation of the corneal curvature will result in a refractive error of 1 D. The surgeon should refer to nomograms for the correct calculation of the size of the LRI.

One of the nomograms used is the Nichamin Age- and Pachymetry-Adjusted Intralimbal Arcuate Astigmatic Nomogram (NAPA) (Table 7-1). This method allows the correction of astigmatism between 0.75 and 3 D, and the use of this nomogram can correlate the size of the incision with the degree of astigmatism to be corrected and the patient's age.[8]

Donnenfeld introduced a second nomogram (Table 7-2). This method allows the treatment of astigmatism between 0.5 and 3.00 D. According to Donnenfeld, there is no correlation between the size of the incision and the patient's age, only with the amount of astigmatism.[9]

In both methods, the maximum size of the incision is 90 degrees.

Table 7-1

Nichamin Age- and Pachymetry-Adjusted Intralimbal Arcuate Astigmatic Nomogram[8]

PREOP CYLINDER (D)	PAIRED INCISIONS IN DEGREES OF ARC (WITH-THE-RULE ASTIGMATISM)					
	20 to 30 yr	31 to 40 yr	41 to 50 yr	51 to 60 yr	61 to 70 yr	71 to 80 yr
0.75	40	35	35	30	30	
1.00	45	40	40	35	35	30
1.25	55	50	45	40	35	35
1.50	60	55	50	45	40	40
1.75	65	60	55	50	45	45
2.00	70	65	60	55	50	45
2.25	75	70	65	60	55	50
2.50	80	75	70	65	60	55
2.75	85	80	75	70	65	60
3.00	90	90	85	80	70	65

PREOP CYLINDER (D)	PAIRED INCISIONS IN DEGREES OF ARC (AGAINST-THE-RULE ASTIGMATISM)					
	20 to 30 yr	31 to 40 yr	41 to 50 yr	51 to 60 yr	61 to 70 yr	71 to 80 yr
0.75	45	40	40	35	35	30
1.00	50	45	45	40	40	35
1.25	55	55	50	45	40	35
1.50	60	60	55	50	45	40
1.75	65	65	60	55	50	45
2.00	70	70	65	60	55	50
2.25	75	75	70	65	60	55
2.50	80	80	75	70	65	60
2.75	85	85	80	75	70	65
3.00	90	90	85	80	75	70

According to a method proposed by Nichamin, the incisions of phaco and the LRI can be combined. In order to correctly combine the LRI and the main corneal incision, it is sufficient to create a precut with a precalibrated blade to 90% of the corneal thickness, for a size corresponding to the length of the main incision. At this point, using the preincision, at half of the cut depth, the surgeon proceeds parallel to the corneal plane using the keratome to create the main entrance, and then enters the anterior chamber. Then, at the end of surgery, following implantation of the IOL and prior to removal of the viscoelastic substance (VES), the surgeon completes the relaxing incision for the length planned.

The Donnenfeld method, on the other hand, does not involve the combination of the incisions when the position corresponds to the entrance incision. It is also advisable to

Table 7-2

Nomogram for the Limbal Relaxing Incision[9]

Astigmatism in Diopters	Incision
0.50	1 incision, 1.5 hours (45 degrees)
0.75	2 incisions, 1 hour (30 degrees)
1.50	2 incisions, 2 hours (60 degrees)
3.00	2 incisions, 3 hours (90 degrees)
Add 5 degrees for against-the-rule astigmatism, add 5 degrees for younger patients, and subtract 5 degrees for older patients.	

leave a space of 10 degrees between the phaco incision and the relaxing incision.

For further information on the creation of the incisions, their position, and the extension, AMO has created a Web site (www.lricalculator.com) that provides access to a program called the LRI Calculator, containing all of the findings relative to the Nichamin and Donnenfeld nomograms. The surgeon specifies the type of nomogram he or she wishes to use, the biometry of the patient, the patient's age, the corneal thickness, the position of the main entrance for the cataract procedure, and the SIA; the program determines the position of the incisions and their length (in degrees).

Complications Associated With the Incisions

Complications rarely occur with this method; however, they are possible. The most frequent is the creation of incisions on an incorrect axis. This error increases pre-existing cylinder or creates irregular astigmatism.

Another complication, observed less frequently than the previous, is the possibility of corneal perforation. This may be caused by an incorrect setting of the blade depth or the incorrect calculation of the corneal thickness. With this complication, the perforations tend to heal rapidly and rarely requires sutures (when the perforations are small, they will not require sutures; when they are larger, it is advisable to place 1 or 2 loose sutures to close the wound but avoid inducing astigmatism).

Other possible complications are infections, reduction of corneal "sensitivity," irregular astigmatism, sensation of corneal discomfort, misalignment, and axial shift.

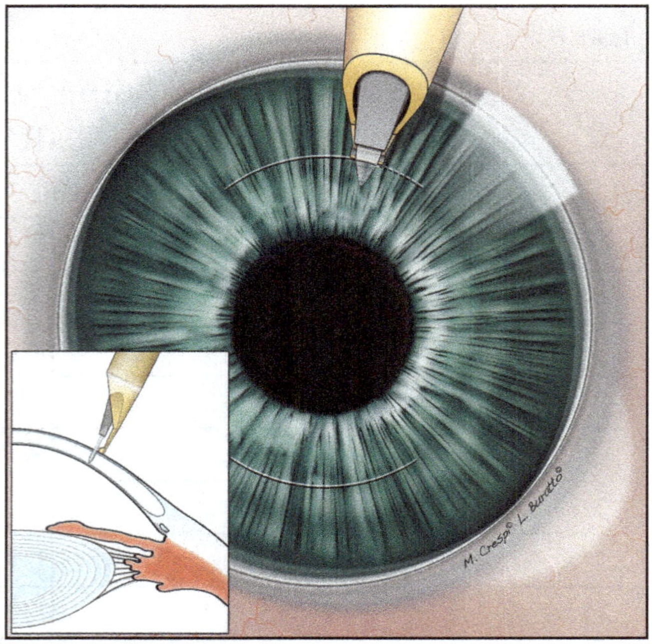

Figure 7-2. Free-hand AK using diamond blades.

Astigmatic Keratotomy

Corneal relaxing incisions (CRIs) were introduced in 1970 to reduce astigmatism in patients undergoing radial keratotomy. Good results depended largely on the surgeon's experience and the technique can correct even high amounts of astigmatism. These incisions must be created 3.5 to 4.0 mm from the optic center (a diameter approximately 7 to 8 mm) with precalibrated diamond blades. The problem with CRIs lies with the creation of perfect arches, of the correct length, and an even depth for the entire incision length.

Even expert surgeons have problems performing these incisions free-hand (Figure 7-2).

LRIs are also corneal incisions but positioned posterior near the limbus. These incisions should be created 5 mm from the optic center (of diameter approximately 10 mm) and require precalibrated blades that can cut incisions at 90% of the corneal thickness. LRIs are easier to create compared to the CRIs; however, because they are created in a more peripheral position, they correct smaller degrees of astigmatism (maximum 3 D). Moreover, LRIs are associated with fewer risks, including a lower risk of overcorrection and less irregular astigmatism (Figure 7-3).

Because of the risks associated with free-hand creation of CRIs, special mechanical knives were developed. These instruments function in the same way as the trephine used in the perforating keratoplasty technique; the difference is that the blade is precalibrated and the action of the trephine

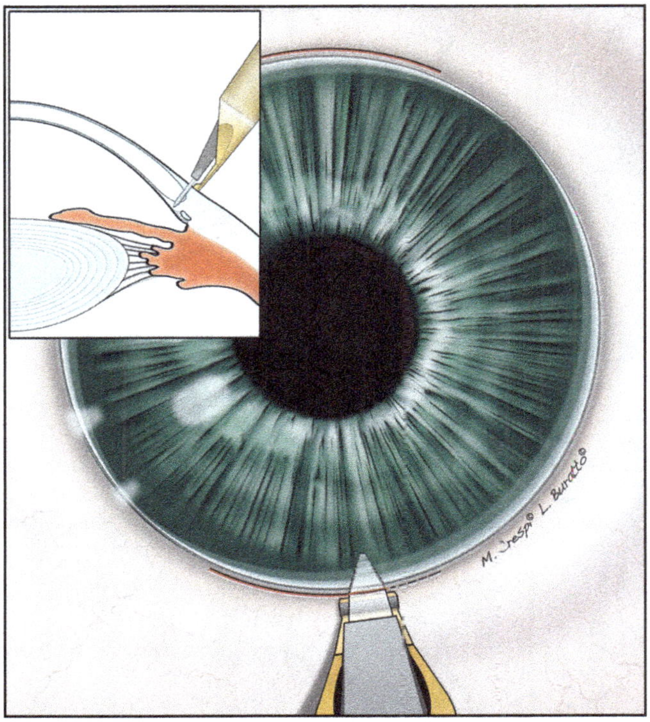

Figure 7-3. Creation of a LRI in the operating room with diamond blades. (The incisions must be performed at 90% of the corneal depth.)

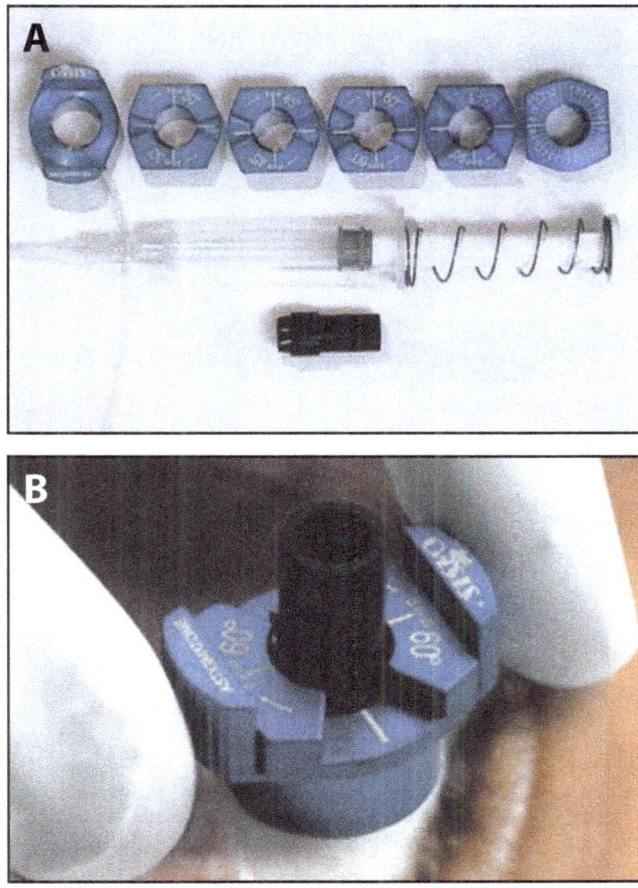

Figure 7-4. (A) Terry-Schanzlin Astigmatome Kit. (B) Aspiration alignment speculum positioned on the eye. (Reprinted with permission from Robbins AM. CRIs and the Terry-Schanzlin astigmatome. In: Chang DF, ed. *Mastering Refractive IOLs: The Art and Science*. Thorofare, NJ: SLACK Incorporated; 2008.)

does not lead to progressive penetration of the blade (that remains at the same depth). The instrument is also fitted with a calibrated ferrule that allows arcs of preset dimensions to be created.

One type of knife is the Terry-Schanzlin (Figure 7-4). It is fitted with a suction ring that is anchored on the eye through a suction syringe with air. The graduated stop marked with a range of arc widths can be inserted onto the suction ring. The stop will guide the extension of the cut and the blade, precalibrated at the desired corneal depth.

Nomograms have also been defined to determine the length of the incision required on the basis of the astigmatism to be corrected and the patient's age.[10]

Contraindications

Incisional surgery is a valid method for the correction of astigmatism during the cataract procedure. However, there are a number of conditions in which this type of technique is contraindicated. First is irregular astigmatism, as effects associated with this condition are not predictable. Moreover, all corneal pathologies must be excluded—keratoconus, peripheral corneal pathologies, marginal degeneration of Terrien, autoimmune pathologies (eg, rheumatoid arthritis), previous corneal surgery (particularly incisional surgery), and dry eye. With dry eye syndrome, the incisions can exacerbate this pathology and increase the corneal discomfort.

Astigmatism and Laser: Bioptics Technique

Residual postoperative astigmatism can also be corrected with well-known excimer techniques and all of its variations (LASIK, i-LASIK, photorefractive keratectomy [PRK]) (Figure 7-5). Excimer laser techniques have the enormous advantage of providing extremely precise and predictable results; they can also correct unexpected postoperative spherical refractive errors.

The operation can be performed in 2 ways. Prior to cataract surgery, the surgeon performs the lamellar cut. If this step is performed using a microkeratome, the flap does not need to be lifted; however, if it is performed with the femtosecond laser, the flap must be lifted (at the end of the cataract surgery) and then repositioned. Fifteen to 20 seconds after the lamellar cut, the surgeon completes the (preferably sutureless) cataract procedure, and when refraction has stabilized, the flap is lifted and the astigmatism and any residual spherical error are treated. The advantage of

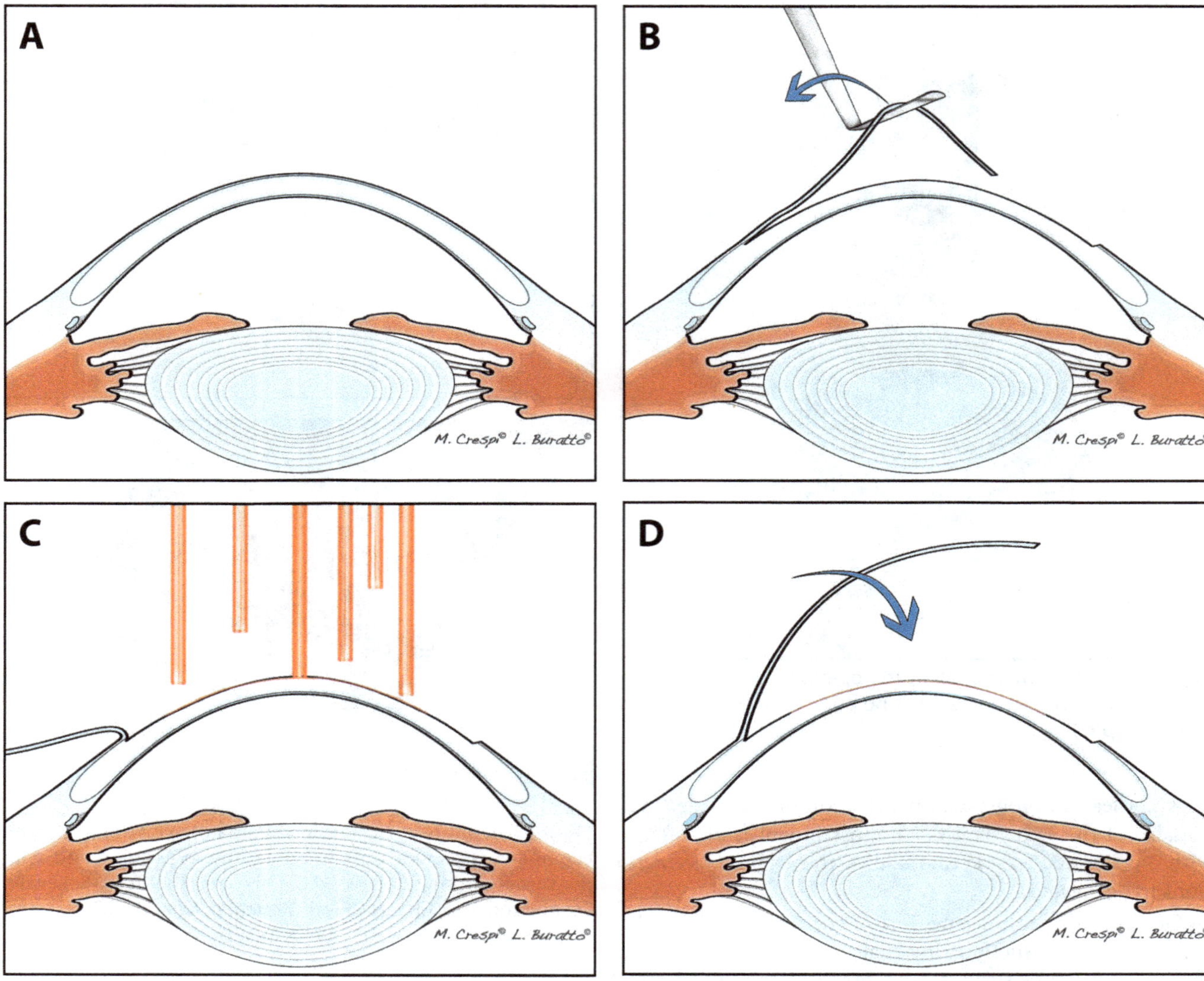

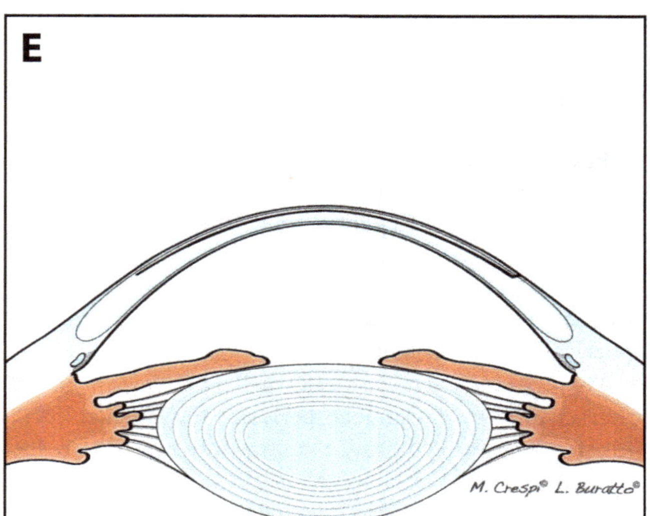

Figure 7-5. LASIK/i-LASIK method.

performing the refractive cut prior to the cataract surgery is that the astigmatism can be corrected early. Alternately, the surgeon should wait 3 months from the sutureless cataract procedure or until the suture has been removed and then proceed with a standard LASIK.

Toric IOLs are an important contribution to resolving the multiple problems associated with correction of astigmatism. They can be inserted in a single operation and provide an excellent refractive result that is highly predictable and stable over time.

Toric Intraocular Lens Preoperative Evaluations

The surgeon must make the decision to implant a toric IOL in his or her patient. He or she must inform the patient that a normal cataract procedure with the insertion of a monofocal IOL will not eliminate the need for spectacles. He or she must fully explain the advantages and drawbacks of this surgery.

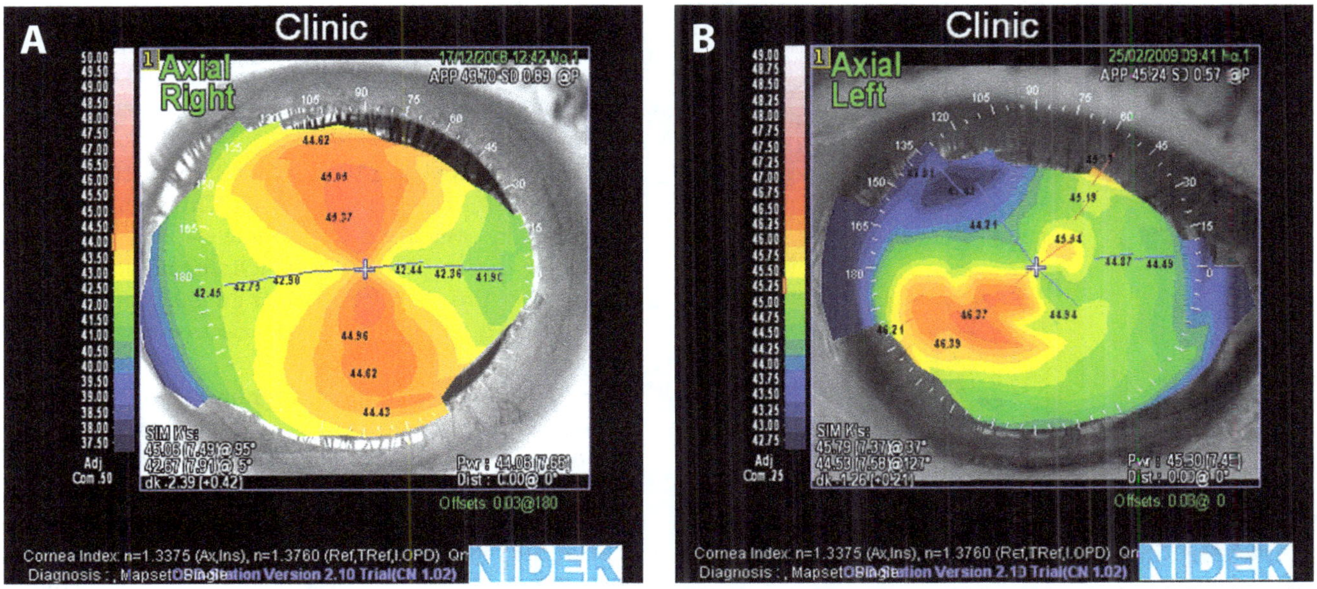

Figure 7-6. Corneal topography performed with the Nidek OPD Scan II topo-aberrometer. (A) The topography highlighted regular astigmatism. (B) In this case, the topography highlighted asymmetrical hourglass astigmatism. (Reprinted with permission from Dr. V. Orfeo.)

In order to do this properly, maximum attention must be paid to the evaluation of the ocular biometry parameters and the patient's refraction.

The aberrometers and tomographs may prove to be extremely useful; with a few simple steps this instrument can provide important parameters for surgeons who opt for surgery with premium IOLs.

In this type of surgery, indispensable data include topography, corneal and total aberrometry, pupillometry, and other parameters, such as corneal spherical aberration and asphericity.

When the surgeon performs cataract surgery, the eye will be liberated from all of the lens' influence on total refraction, including any compensation for corneal astigmatism, and the corneal cylinder will be fully revealed.

Topography is a great help as it can indicate whether the astigmatism is regular or irregular (Figure 7-6)

When choosing a toric IOL, it is important to exclude the presence of keratoconus, pellucid marginal degeneration, and the extremely irregular forms of astigmatism, with highly asymmetrical hourglass arrangements. The presence of keratoconus generates a HOA called *coma*. Coma is a deformation of the wavefront that assumes a sinusoidal appearance; it cannot be corrected with any type of lens. (Actually, toric lenses are increasingly popular for the correction of astigmatism caused by keratoconus as long as the keratoconus is stable and/or the patient has already had cross-linking and/or in patients who are over 50 and who have keratoconus in stages 1 to 2 with a fairly well-defined axis. This topic has not been covered in this chapter.)

One area in which toric IOLs play a fundamental role is correction of astigmatism in patients post perforating keratoplasty. There may be significant residual astigmatism in patients post corneal transplant and visual quality may be severely compromised.

In patients who are stable, after the suture has been removed (and having checked that the corneal flap is healthy, with no risk of rejection, and the topography is stable), the surgeon can implant a toric IOL that will partially or totally correct the residual corneal astigmatism.

Again, it is essential to examine the corneal flap with topography and ensure that the residual astigmatism has a certain degree of uniformity and is stable over time. The calculation methods are exactly the same; the only difference is that the corneal incision will correct higher amounts of astigmatism compared to traditional surgery. Consequently, it is advisable to close the incision with a suture; the surgeon should then adjust the refractive result and decide whether or not he or she needs to remove the suture sooner rather than later. Even if the correction is not total, the benefit for the patient will be significant with a major improvement in visual quality and in the patient's quality of life (Figure 7-7)!

Moreover, corneal aberrometry (not total aberrometry, a value that is not reliable as it is altered by the presence of the cataract) also allows the evaluation of the aberrometry axis of the cylinder and provides important information about the positioning axis of the IOL. The majority of aberrometers only measure the astigmatism present on the anterior face of the cornea; however, it should be remembered that there is also a posterior face and it can be determined by instruments that use the Scheimpflug camera.

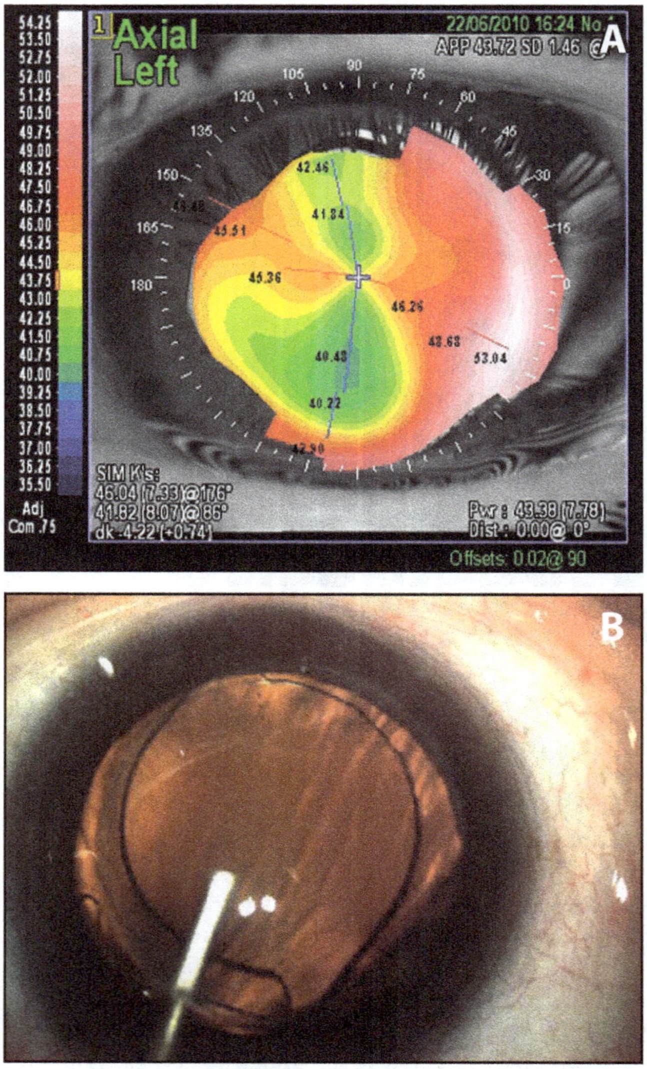

Figure 7-7. (A) Topographical image of a patient affected by cataract, with previous perforating keratoplasty. The astigmatism is not severe and has a regular profile. (B) An image of the same patient implanted with a toric IOL. The IOL has been aligned with the axis of greatest curvature, indicated by topography. (Reprinted with permission from Dr. V. Orfeo.)

Finally, when calculating astigmatism, it is essential that the surgeon is aware of the effects of the incision on the total cylinder. According to the technique used, each surgeon should calculate the astigmatism induced by the incision on at least 10 of his or her patients, to factor in the influence of his or her own incision into the calculation.

The choice of the IOL power, in terms of sphere and cylinder, can be calculated using specific software. For example, a Web site created by Alcon (www.acrysoftoric-calculator.com) allows surgeons to calculate the power of the lens to be implanted. All the surgeon has to do is input simple data such as the patient's eye, the power of the IOL, the power and the axis of the steepest and flattest meridians, the incision site, and the SIA. This Web site also produces an image of the eye to be operated, highlighting the steepest and flattest meridians, the incision site, and most importantly, the axis for positioning the IOL, a fundamental measurement for use in the operating room (Figure 7-8).

Also, AMO provides a Web site for the calculation of the Tecnis toric IOL at www.amoeasy.com. This Web site is easy to use, and by inserting a few parameters, it is possible to achieve the correct power of toric IOL (monofocal or multifocal). Also, this software provides an image of the eye to be operated, with all fundamental measurements needed in the operating room.

Zeiss also offers an online program for the calculation of the power of the toric IOL to be implanted, to evaluate the power of the cylinder, and to determine the positioning axis. Log on to https://zcalc.meditec.Zeiss.com/zcalc and register to gain access. In this case, it is not necessary to input the spherical power of the IOL (this can be calculated with the IOL Master or with an ultrasound method); a number of data are essential, including axial length, the instrument used to calculate the axial length (IOL Master, immersion ultrasound, contact ultrasound) and the relative constant, and the refractive index of the keratometer used to calculate K1 and K2.

For the calculation of the toric IOL, the values K1 and K2 must be inserted along with the relative axes of curvature and the incision site with SIA (Figure 7-9).

At the end of data input, a window appears showing an image of the eye to be operated, the incision site, the axes K1 and K2, and the positioning axis for the IOL.

This is an extremely precise instrument, but not as easy to use or as user-friendly as the AcrySof toric calculator.

AcrySof Toric Intraocular Lens

The design of the AcrySof Toric IOL is based on the platform of the 1-piece AcrySof Natural, a hydrophobic foldable acrylic lens with an optic measuring 6.0 mm. The acrylic material of the lens and the shape of the haptics contribute to preventing the rotation of the lens, ensuring excellent stability once it has been implanted in the capsular bag (Figure 7-10).

The posterior surface of the lens corrects the cylinder and carries the markers for correct positioning of the lens. The markers are 3 dots aligned at the 2 poles of the lens; they are positioned according to the corneal marking for the axis of cylinder.

Generally speaking, the markings should align with the steepest axis. The lens can correct corneal astigmatism that varies from 1.0 D (SN60T3: +1.50 D cyl at the lens plane, +1.03 D cyl at the corneal plane) up to 4 D (SN60T9: +6.0 D cyl at the lens plane, +4.11 D at the corneal plane) with steps of 0.75 D between one level and the next. The spherical powers of the lenses range between +6.0 and +30 D.

AcrySof TORIC SINGLE-PIECE NATURAL IOL — Alcon CE

Alcon does not receive or retain any patient data. Please print a copy of the final output for your records. Contact your Alcon representative for available AcrySof® Toric IOL models and diopter ranges.

Print

Lens Recommendation

Surgeon & Patient Information	
Surgeon Name	Surgeon
Patient Name	Patient
Additional Patient Information *(I.D., Case, etc.)*	
Lens Details	
AcrySof® Toric IOL	SN60T4
IOL Spherical Equivalent (SE)	20.5 D
Axis of Placement	17°
Cylinder Power (IOL Plane)	2.25 D
Cylinder Power (Corneal Plane)	1.55 D
Calculation Details	
Pre-Op Corneal Astigmatism:	2.00 D X 10°
Surgically Induced Astigmatism:	0.50 D X 60°
Crossed-Cylinder Result (corneal plane):	1.98 D X 17°
Anticipated Residual Astigmatism:	0.43 D X 17°

OD (Right)

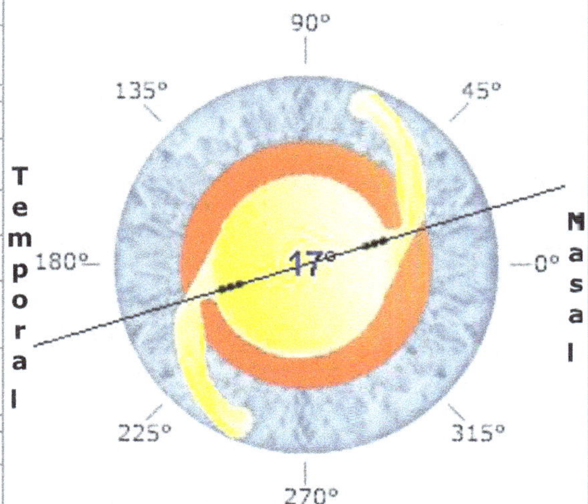

IOL: SN60T4 20.5D SE, Cyl:2.25D @ 17°

Flat K:43.50D @ 100° Steep K:45.50D @ 10°
P-IOL:20.5D SIA:0.50D IL:150° [V:3.4.3]
f251ba4914fa80eec983d52659868497 8/31/13 6:15:17

Pre-Op Information

Patient Data	
Flat K	43.50 D
@ Flat Axis	100°
Steep K	45.50 D
@ Steep Axis	10°
IOL Spherical Power (P-IOL)	20.5 D
Surgically Induced Astigmatism (SIA)	0.50 D
Incision Location (IL)	150°

Notes:

f251ba4914fa80eec983d52659868497 8/31/13 6:15:17

V: 3.4.3

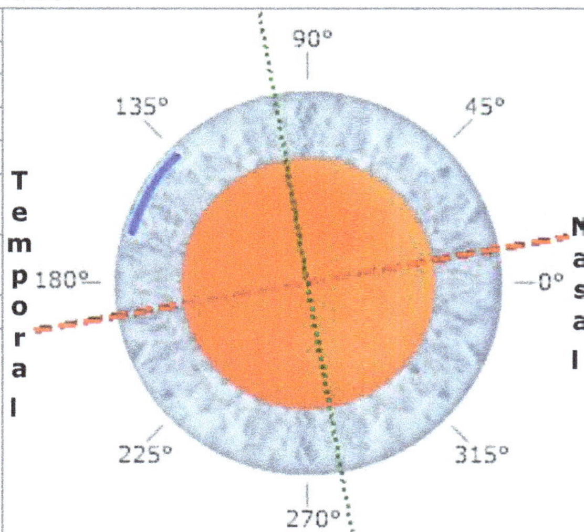

Flat K:43.50D @ 100° Steep K:45.50D @ 10°
P-IOL:20.5D SIA:0.50D IL:150° [V:3.4.3]
f251ba4914fa80eec983d52659868497 8/31/13 6:15:17

Steep Axis
Flat Axis
Incision

New Calculation | Tutorial | Help | Privacy Policy & Legal Terms

Figure 7-8. Image of the AcrySof Toric Calculator downloaded from www.acrysoftoriccalculator.com. It can be used to calculate the power of the IOL for implantation, the cylinder, and the axis of positioning on the basis of the incision site and the SIA. (Reprinted with permission from Alcon.)

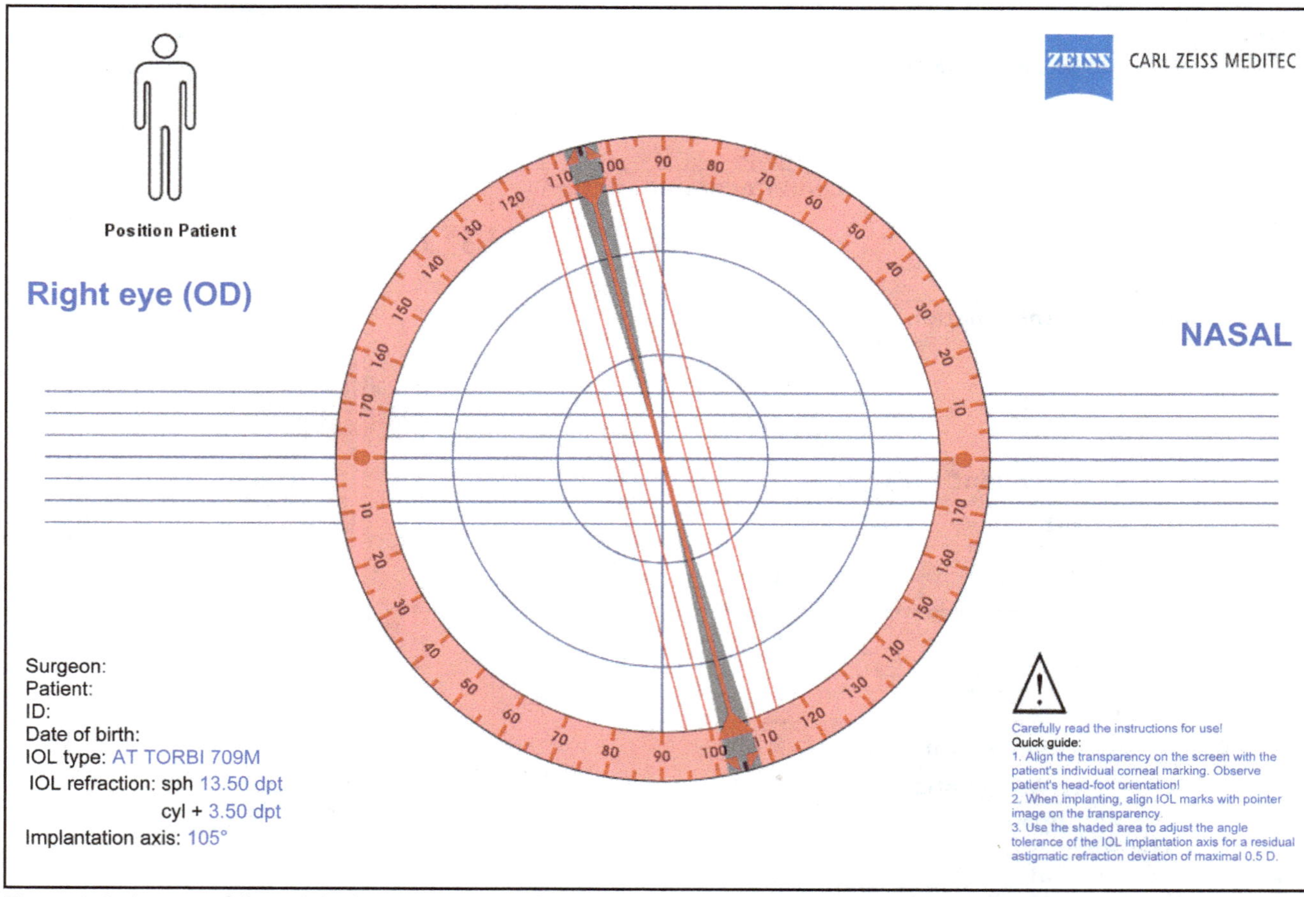

Figure 7-9. Images of the Z-Calc showing the axis of positioning of the IOL, taken from https://zcalc.meditec.zeiss.com. The printout shows the surgeon's name, the patient's name, the indication of the eye, and the type of lens to be implanted and its power.

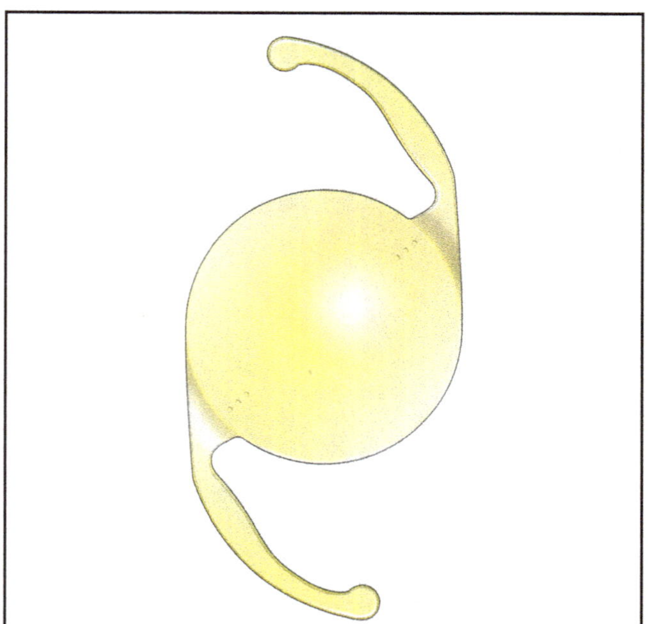

Figure 7-10. A toric IOL, AcrySof Model SN6ATx, a 1-piece aspherical hydrophobic acrylic IOL with a UV filter and a yellow optic (that acts as a filter for blue light). On the posterior surface of the lens, the 3 "landmarks" are visible on each side of the axis for positioning the lens.

The new model of the AcrySof Toric, called the IQ, is the aspheric version of the Natural lens, with a negative spherical aberration of –0.20 μm; it can partially compensate for positive spherical corneal aberration. The power of the IQ toric IOL varies from the model T2 with cyl +1 D at the lens surface corresponding to +0.68 D at the corneal plane, to the model T9 with cyl +6D, corresponding to +4.11 D at the corneal plane.

As mentioned before, the software for calculating the lens is available from Alcon (www.acrysoftoriccalculator.com). The package allows the simple and intuitive calculation of the power and cylinder of the IOL to be selected. By varying the incision site at the steepest or flattest meridians, it is possible to select the most suitable type of lens for a specific patient to correct the greatest amount of astigmatism.

Zeiss Meditec AT TORBI 709M

The AT TORBI is a 1-piece monofocal bitoric lens of hydrophilic acrylic with a hydrophobic coating, developed for insertion through a microincision. The diameter of the optic is 6.0 mm, and the maximum diameter between the haptics is 11.0 mm. The lens has a biscuit shape with the

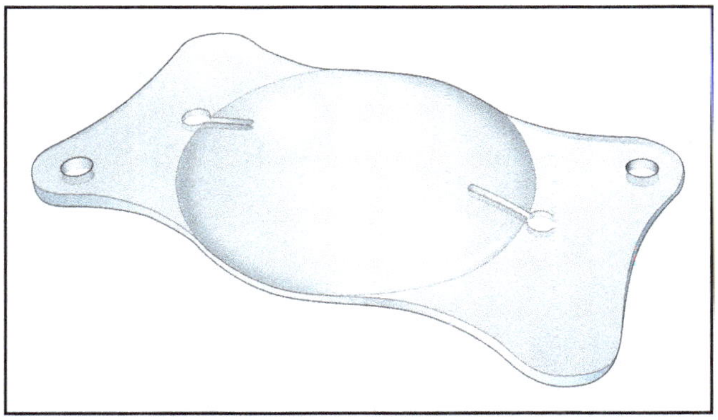

Figure 7-11. The IOL Model AT TORBI 709M is a hydrophilic acrylic lens with a hydrophobic surface coating. It is biscuit shaped with co-planar haptics and bitoric correction on both faces of the lens to reduce the thickness.

haptic plane and angulation of 0 degrees. The power of the lens varies between −10 and +32 D with cylinder varying between +1.0 D and +12.0 D with steps of 0.5 D. The lens was designed to be inserted through incision diameters of 1.5 to 1.8 mm. For high diopter values with high cylinder (approximately +30 D sph or greater), the surgeon should use injectors that can be inserted through incisions of diameter 2.75 mm because there may be problems injecting a lens of this thickness with injectors of such small bore.

The bitoric design allows a reduction in the thickness of the lens because it uniformly distributes the cylinder on the anterior and posterior surfaces; it creates a larger usable optic zone for equal central thickness and allows the manufacturer to create lenses with high values of cylinder.

For this reason, with this lens, the hydrophobic coating must be considered to be a different surface treatment; the hydrophobic coating has the markers for the correct positioning of the axis. The lens can be inserted using either a disposable or a reusable injector (Figure 7-11).

Abbott Medical Optics Tecnis Aspheric Toric Intraocular Lens

Using the Tecnis ZCB00 platform, AMO introduced its model of toric IOL. This 1-piece lens is manufactured of hydrophobic acrylic with aspheric surfaces; the diameter of the optic is 6 mm, and the maximum diameter of the haptics is 13 mm. The optic is biconvex with a toric aspheric anterior surface and has a negative spherical aberration of −0.27 µm to compensate for the positive spherical corneal aberration. The dioptric power of the lens varies between +5 and +34 D with steps of 0.5 D. There are 4 different options for the correction of cylinder (+1.00 D, +1.50 D, +2.25 D, +4.00 D). The positioning marks are found on the anterior surface of the lens; these are aligned on the steepest corneal axis. To prevent posterior capsule opacification (PCO), the lens has a square edge of 360 degrees called *ProTEC*. The lens has a 3-dimensional shape that increases the stability of the lens (even in terms of the rotation) called *Tri-Fix*, and has 3 anchor points for fixing the lens to the capsular bag. The lens has a UV-blocking filter, required for FDA approval.

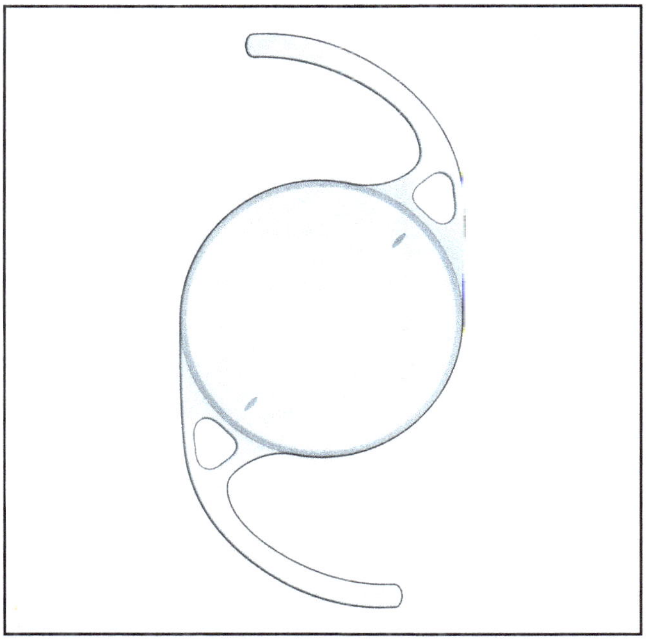

Figure 7-12. The enVista Toric IOL. This 1-piece lens is a glistening-free hydrophobic acrylic complete with a UV filter that has been designed with an aberration-free aspherical-toric biconvex surface.

Bausch + Lomb enVista Toric MX60T

Bausch + Lomb recently presented its toric IOL for the correction of astigmatism. This 1-piece lens in glistening-free hydrophobic acrylic complete with a UV filter has been designed with an aberration-free aspherical, toric biconvex surface (Figure 7-12). From a structural point of view, the diameter of the optic is 6 mm with a posterior square edge to prevent PCO and step-vaulted co-planar modified C haptics at a 0-degree angle; the maximum diameter of the lens is 12.5 mm. The haptics have been designed with calibrated fenestrated areas to allow a capsular contact of 120 degrees. There are 2 marks on the optic to ensure correct alignment of the lens. The spherical power of the lens varies between +6 and +30 D with steps of 0.5 D and a range of toric powers of 1.25, 2.00, 2.75, 3.00, 4.25, 5.00, and 5.75 D.

According to the Bausch + Lomb technicians, this lens has excellent rotational stability: rotation was ≤5 degrees in 100% of patients between 1 and 6 months and ≤5 degrees in 91% between 24 and 48 hours.

The power of the enVista Toric can be calculated using the enVista Toric Calculator available at the Web site https://envista.toriccalculator.com (Figure 7-13).

This calculator is intuitive and very easy to use; it requires the input of data relative to the surgeon and the patient.

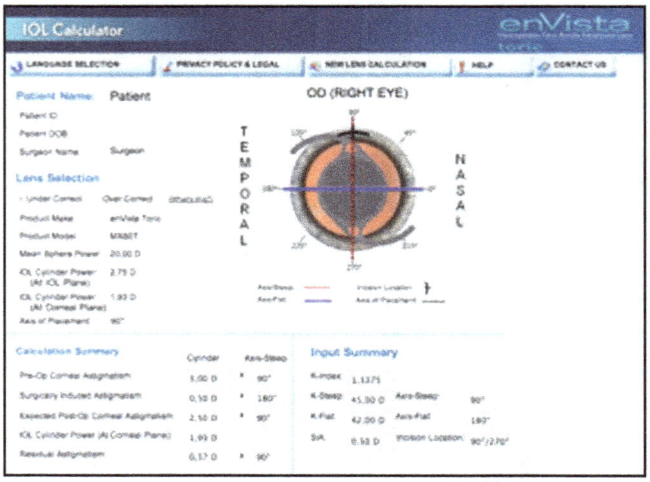

Figure 7-13. Image from the enVista Toric Calculator. This calculator is intuitive and very easy to use. It requires the input of data relative to the surgeon and the patient.

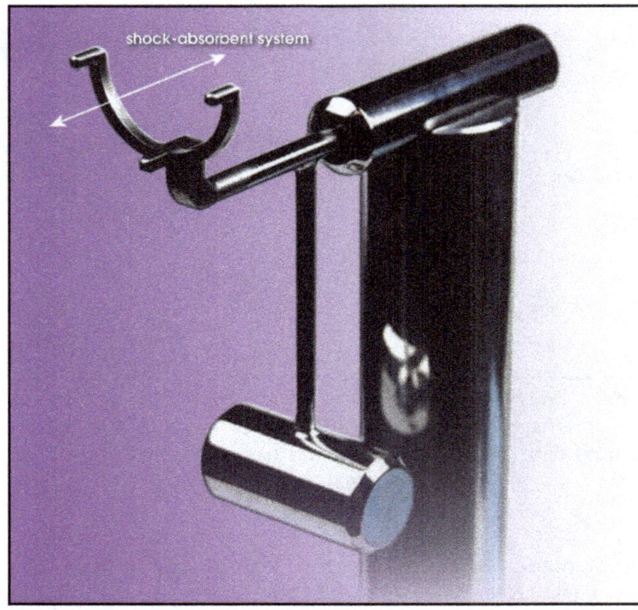

Figure 7-14. Buratto's marker. This marker has 3 corneal contact points that mark the 0-, 180-, and 270-degree axes. Moreover, this marker is fitted with a shock-absorbing system and a pendulum to ensure perfect positioning perpendicular to the floor. The marker can be hooked to the slit lamp by means of a special support device. (Reprinted with permission from Janach.)

The biometry data of the eye to be operated must be inputted to the calculator, selecting the right or left eye, the unit of measurement used to define the keratometric data (diopters or radius of curvature in millimeters), the power of the axis of greatest curvature with the specific axis, and the power of the axis of least curvature. Moreover, the calculator requires details about the incision site and the SIA to identify the precise axis for implanting the IOL. Finally, the spherical power of the lens must be selected on the basis of the biometry data. Once all of these data have been inserted, the calculator will produce a digital image of the eye, the planned incision site, the axes of greatest and least curvature, and finally the image of the IOL with the precise axis for the implant–indispensable information for the surgeon in the operating room.

Surgical Technique for the Toric Intraocular Lens

The first step involved in the process of implanting toric IOLs is marking the axis with the patient in an erect position (eg, at the slit lamp) to avoid cyclorotation of the eye when the patient is in a supine position. Ideally, the axes 0 to 180 degrees should be marked; then with a Mendez ring the precise axis for positioning the IOL is marked when the patient is supine on the operating bed.

There are a number of methods that can be used to mark the axis. For each method, the eye should be marked when the patient is erect. A number of markers are available: some use a mobile joint connected to a pendulum that positions itself perpendicular to the ground under the force of gravity (Elies 2- and 4-point pendulum marker); some markers can be attached to the Goldmann tonometer, like the Buratto Marker, to be used at the slit lamp.

In the first case, the pendulum markers are "free-hand" and this may lead to small degrees of decentration on the vertical axis. In the second case, the structure is connected to the slit lamp and the presence of a marker graduated for 360 degrees connected to the tonometer would appear to be more precise. In practice, the presence of the tubular structure attached to the tonometer makes it more difficult for the surgeon to visualize and center the eye, because of the physical volume of the marker. Buratto's pendulum marker is attached to the slit lamp. There are just 3 small elements for marking the axes at 0 to 180 degrees as well as to 270 degrees; the instrument has its own support and is not hooked to the Goldmann tonometer; the patient's eye is clearly visible with precise centering of the markings (Figure 7-14). Regardless of the method used, the surgeon must ensure that the patient's head is maintained in an erect position. For this reason, the patient should be placed against the headrest of the slit lamp to guarantee the correct position of the patient's eye.

The markers (pendulum and others) must be used to mark the main axes (0 to 180 degrees and/or 90 to 270 degrees) or definitively mark the axis for implantation of the IOL. If the surgeon decides to mark the primary axes alone, it will then be necessary to use a Mendez ring to determine the precise position for implanting the IOL (if this differs from the primary axes) (Figure 7-15). Some surgeons do not mark the eye but prefer to use the morphology of the iris vessels to identify the reference points. For example, in the process of calculating the axis of the astigmatism, followed by corneal topography and ocular aberrometry, many machines allow the production of an

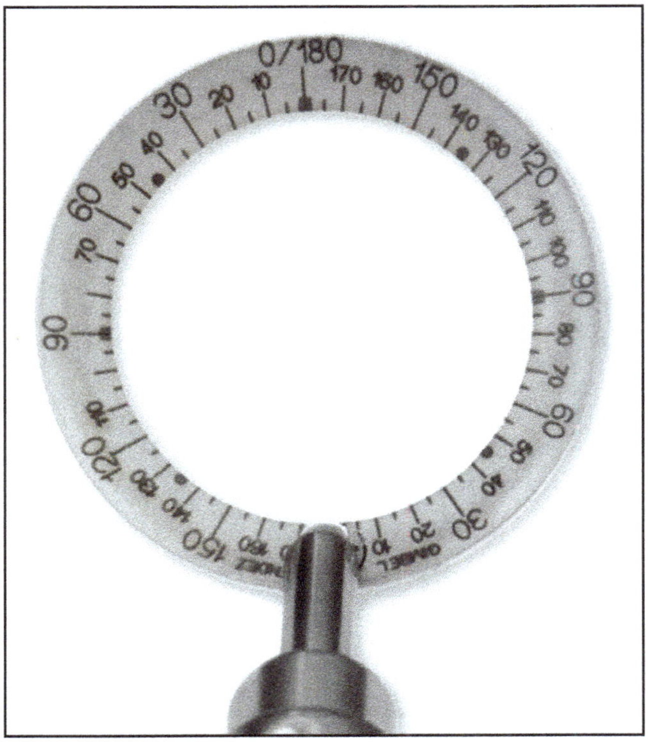

Figure 7-15. The Mendez ring. This is a graduated ring used to precisely mark the positioning axis for the IOL, using the reference points of 0 and 180 degrees obtained with the patient in an orthostatic position. (Reprinted with permission from Janach.)

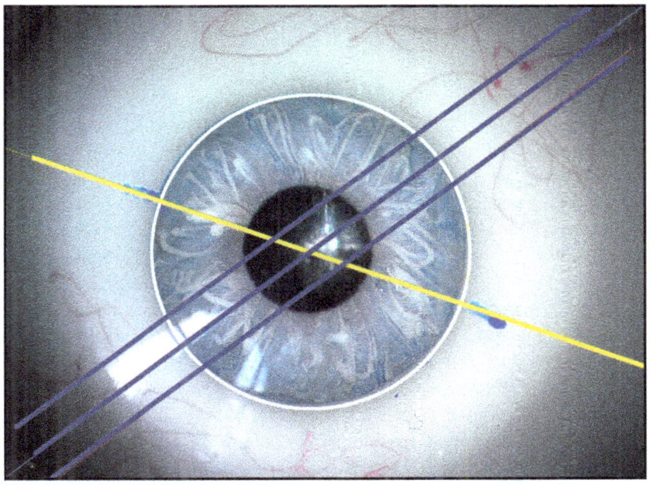

Figure 7-16. The computer system CALLISTO eye 3.0 produced by Carl Zeiss Meditec. This system allows the precise calculation of the axis for positioning the IOL on the basis of the patient's biometric values to recognize the marking sites (0 and 180 degrees) and to project this axis onto a screen. (Reprinted with permission from Carl Zeiss Meditec.)

image of the eye under photoptic and scotopic conditions for the measurement of pupillometry, in association with the crown calibrated in degrees. It is possible, therefore, to digitally overlap the 2 images and identify the reference iris markings even under scotopic conditions and use this as the reference for marking the axis. Finally, Zeiss has developed a system that avoids the need for intraoperative marking; it simply uses markings at 0 and 180 degrees and can project the correct axis for positioning the lens onto a screen. This system is called CALLISTO and it is an important technological innovation because, in the near future, it is probable that various electronic instrumentation (biometers, microscopes, positioning systems) will interact and simplify the life of the surgeon and his or her assistants (Figure 7-16).

Surgical Procedure for Correct Positioning of the Alcon Toric Intraocular Lens

When this IOL has been implanted under VES, it is advisable to position the lens counterclockwise by 10 to 15 degrees with respect to the definitive positioning axis. The VES is carefully aspirated, first from the posterior portion and then from the anterior portion of the eye. The IOL is then rotated into its definitive position, bringing the lens marks into correspondence with those of the cornea.

The Zeiss Toric lens requires a different implantation technique. The lens itself is biscuit shaped and the injector insertion method is slightly different.

The lens unfolds more rapidly due to the shape of the lens itself, and the surgeon must pay attention while directing the first haptic into the bag. Once the first haptic has been inserted inside the bag, the surgeon must continue to inject the lens into the anterior chamber, paying attention to slide the second haptic into the sulcus above the rhexis. Under these circumstances, half of the lens will be inside the bag and half will be sitting above the rhexis. At this point, the surgeon uses a hook to engage the hole located between the haptic and the base of the optic and rotate the lens into the planned position. At this point, the surgeon can place the second flange inside the bag and then aspirate the VES even from behind the lens; this will avoid any residue of VES that may rotate the lens. Once the lens has been positioned correctly, the surgeon can hydrate the main and side-port incisions.

If the lens is displaced during these procedures, VES must be reinjected, and the entire process of alignment repeated to the correct axis.

There are 2 steps that are essential for an excellent refractive result following the implantation of a toric IOL: the correct positioning of the lens on the axis and rotational stability over time.

References

1. Tejedor J, Murube J. Choosing the location of corneal incision based on preexisting astigmatism in phacoemulsification. *Am J Ophthalmol.* 2005;139(5):767-776.
2. Altan-Yaycioglu R, Akova YA, Akca S, Gur S, Oktem C. Effect on astigmatism of the location of clear corneal incision in phacoemulsification of cataract. *J Refract Surg.* 2007;23(5):515-518.
3. Bartels MC, Saxena R, van den Berg TJ, van Rij G, Mulder PG, Luyten GP. The influence of incision-induced astigmatism and axial lens position on the correction of myopic astigmatism with the Artisan toric phakic intraocular lens. *Ophthalmology.* 2006;113(7):1110-1117. Epub 2006 May 19.
4. Orfeo V, Boccuzzi D. ROL and SICCSO International Congress. Use of Perforating Incision for the Correction of Astigmatism in Cataract Surgery. Grosseto - 9 Luglio. 2011.
5. Ernest P, Hill W, Potvin R. Minimizing surgically induced astigmatism at the time of cataract surgery using a square posterior limbal incision. *J Ophthalmol.* 2011;2011:243170. Epub 2011 Nov 2.
6. Archana S, Khurana AK, Chawla U. A comparative study of sclera-corneal and clear corneal tunnel incision in manual small-incision cataract surgery. *Nepal J Ophthalmol.* 2011;3(5):19-22. doi:10.3126/nepjoph.v3i1.4273.
7. Jiang Y, Le Q, Yang J, Lu Y. Changes in corneal astigmatism and high order aberrations after clear corneal tunnel phacoemulsification guided by corneal topography. *J Refract Surg.* 2006;22(9 Suppl):S1083-S1088.
8. Nichamin LD. Nomogram for limbal relaxing incisions. *J Cataract Refract Surg.* 2006;32:1048.
9. Donnenfeld E, Solomon R. LRIs and refractive IOLs: my way. In: Chang DF, ed. *Mastering Refractive IOLs: The Art and Science.* Thorofare, NJ: SLACK Incorporated; 2008.
10. Robbins AM. CRIs and the Terry-Schanzlin astigmatome. In: Chang DF, ed. *Mastering Refractive IOLs: The Art and Science.* Thorofare, NJ: SLACK Incorporated; 2008.

8

Multifocal Intraocular Lenses

Lucio Buratto, MD; Stephen F. Brint, MD, FACS; and Domenico Boccuzzi, MD, PhD

Currently, multifocal intraocular lenses (IOLs) are the most interesting devices for correction of presbyopia in patients undergoing cataract surgery. They are available in 2 different types of designs based on the mechanism that leads to the multifocal properties: refractive and diffractive.

This type of lens is not always considered the gold standard for all patients. A precise and correct evaluation of the patient is essential, and the patient must be adequately informed about the benefits and side effects associated with these lenses.

Refractive—ReZoom

The Abbott Medical Optics (AMO) ReZoom lens is a 3-piece multifocal refractive lens with an optic of 6.0 mm with polymethylmethacrylate (PMMA) haptics and a maximum diameter of 13.0 mm. The 3-piece lenses can be implanted in the sulcus if there has been dialysis of the posterior capsule (and when a multifocal lens was previously implanted in the patient's other eye). This IOL is based on the principle of the Balanced View Optics Technology that exploits proportionate zones that are different for vision at a range of distances under different luminous conditions. The lens is divided into 5 optic zones that can provide good near, intermediate, and distance vision under different lighting conditions. The zones are concentric and have different diameters: zones 1, 3, and 5 are designed for distance vision; zones 2 and 4 are designed for near vision. An aspheric transition between the zones is responsible for intermediate vision.

The optic of the ReZoom lens consists of acrylic hydrophobic material. The addition for near vision is +3.50 D at the iris plane corresponding to +2.57 D at the spectacle plane. The ReZoom lens also uses the triple-edge design of OptiEdge.

The anterior part of the optic rim is rounded; the rim is squared in the posterior portion, creating a barrier (360 degrees) against posterior capsule opacification (PCO); it was also designed to reduce haloes to a minimum. This is extremely important because even early PCO can cause a sharp drop in vision; it can reduce contrast sensitivity and cause an increase in haloes (Figure 8-1).

Diffractive—Tecnis Multifocal ZMB00

The Tecnis ZMB00 lens by AMO is a 1-piece foldable diffractive multifocal IOL in a hydrophobic acrylic material with an optic of 6.0 mm and a maximum diameter between the 2 haptics of 13.0 mm. According to Food and Drug Administration (FDA) approval, this lens contains a filter for ultraviolet (UV) rays (Figure 8-2B).

The diffractive component is located on the posterior surface of the lens with a distribution of near/distance light of 50% and an addition for near vision of +4 D at the iris plane, which corresponds to +3.2 D at the corneal plane.

The powers vary between +5 and +34 D with intervals of 0.5 D. The anterior surface is prolate with a negative spherical aberration of −0.27 µm that compensates the average positive spherical aberration of the cornea.

Buratto L, Brint SF, Boccuzzi D.
Cataract Surgery and Intraocular Lenses (pp 53-72).

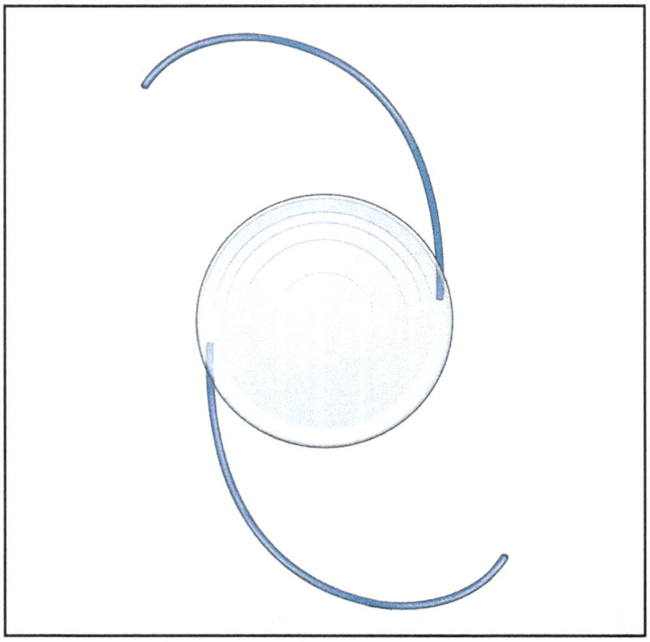

Figure 8-1. Refractive multifocal IOL AMO ReZoom, in which the multifocal properties are determined by different concentric optic zones. The multifocal properties are pupil dependent.

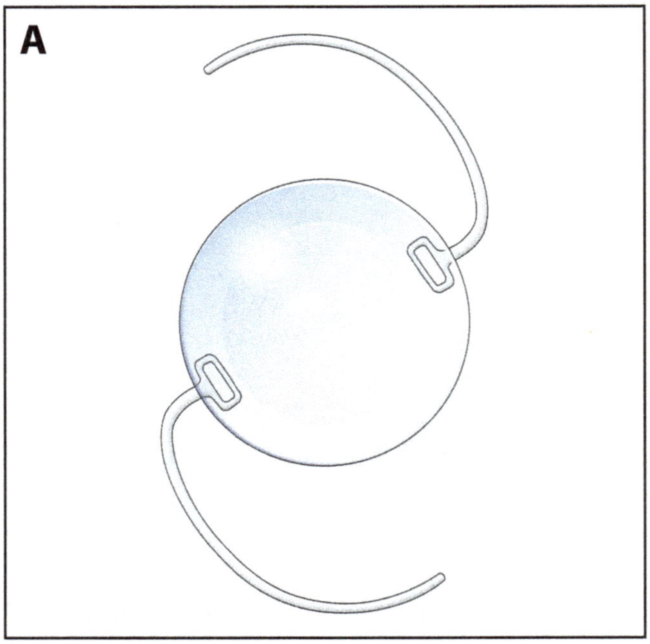

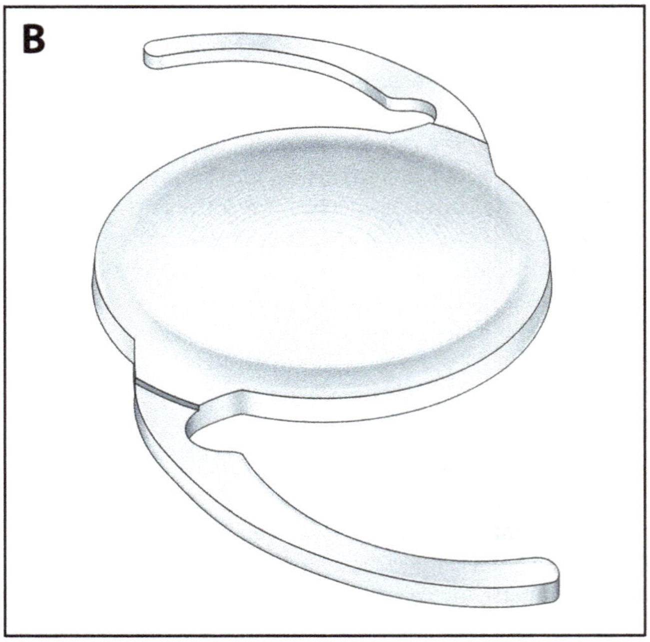

Figure 8-2. (A) Tecnis ZMA00—a 3-piece hydrophobic acrylic multifocal lens with a full diffractive optic. (B) Tecnis ZMB00, a 1-piece hydrophobic acrylic multifocal lens produced by AMO; it also has a full diffractive optic.

The technical innovation in the design of this new model of multifocal lens lies predominantly with the new shape ProTEC of the lens edge, which will reduce cell migration to a minimum with prevention of PCO and the Tri-Fix design system for precise centration of the lens in the capsular bag.

The IOL is diffractive and combines the anterior prolate surface of the well-known monofocal Tecnis lens with a diffractive posterior surface. The diffractive rings are all of the same width, meaning that the lens is independent of the pupil size; finally, the new acrylic material used in the manufacture of this lens has a larger number of Abbe, which results into a lower incidence of chromatic aberrations for distance vision.

One of the lenses produced by AMO is the 3-piece multifocal lens, known as the ZMA00 (Figure 8-2A). This lens has characteristics that closely resemble those of the 1-piece version. The difference is in the presence of modified C-shaped PMMA loops, with a tilt of 5 degrees at the optic plane. The structure of the optic is the same as that of the 1-piece lens; the only difference is that the posterior profile has a square edge (360 degrees) OptiEdge protected by a patent.

Diffractive—AT LISA

The AT LISA IOL by Zeiss is a monopiece aspheric diffractive multifocal hydrophilic acrylic lens with a hydrophobic surface. The external hydrophobic surface of the lens is not simply a coating but is a different biochemical treatment of the same material. This lens has a full-diffractive optic and is therefore independent of the pupil diameter, with smooth transition steps between the rings (SMP technology) for the reduction of haloes. This lens is complete with a UV filter (Figure 8-3) and has a negative spherical aberration of −0.26 μm that compensates for the positive spherical aberration of the human cornea. The distribution of the light is split into 65% for distance vision and 35% for near vision, with an addition of +3.75 D at the lens plane. This lens has an unusual biscuit shape with an

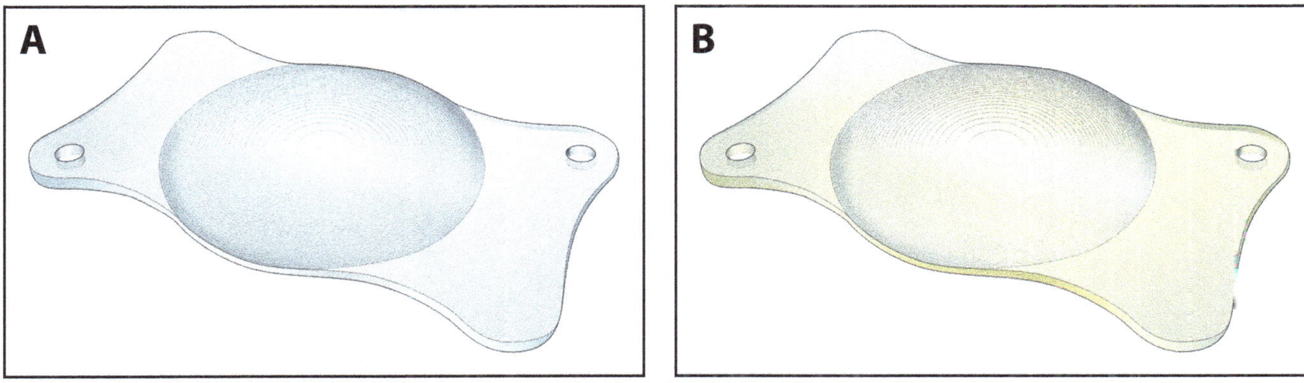

Figure 8-3. (A) AT LISA Model 809M (a transparent lens). (B) Model 809MV (a yellow lens). The lenses have an unusual biscuit shape (typical of the Zeiss IOLs) with coplanar haptics and full diffractive technology.

optic diameter of 6.0 mm and a total diameter of 11.0 mm. Its shape was designed to provide excellent centration in axial and radial terms.

From a technical point of view, the tilt of the haptics is 0 degrees, the lens has a square edge around the optic and in the haptics, and it was designed for insertion through a microincision; this lens can be inserted through incisions between 1.5 and 1.8 mm.

With the AT LISA lens, Zeiss has attempted to optimize the concept of the full diffractive multifocal lens, limiting the appearance of haloes around luminous sources, with the implementation of 3 small technological strategies: the presence of smooth steps, the optimal distribution of the distance-near luminous proportions, and the correction factor for reading. The smooth steps reduce light scattering, eliminating the presence of sharp corners on the lens surface.

The distribution of the light (65% for distance versus 35% for near) meant that this lens is ideal for distance vision under conditions of poor illumination, with less importance given to the conditions for "reading." It reduces the near vision image that overlaps the distance vision image and leads to the appearance of haloes when driving at night, when the pupil dilates and there are numerous point light sources.

Finally, the third element responsible for the appearance of haloes is the delta determined by the addition of near vision. An addition of +3.75 D is an intermediate value that partly compensates the reduced amount of the luminous portion dedicated to near vision (35%), without greatly increasing the width of the halo for reading.

AcrySof ReSTOR

The AcrySof ReSTOR (Model D3) is an apodized diffractive-refractive lens, a 1-piece lens of hydrophobic acrylic that can be inserted through incisions of 2.2 mm using an injector specifically designed for microincisions. The diameter of its optic is 6.0 mm, and the total haptic diameter is 13.0 mm. The additional near vision power is +4 D at the iris plane and this corresponds to +3.2 D at the spectacle plane. The design of the optic is anterior bi-convex in yellow hydrophobic acrylic that filters blue light (550 nm). The central diffractive diameter of the optic is 3.6 mm, and this is the apodized diffractive portion that creates zones of multifocal vision. The peripheral portion of 2.4 mm is the refractive portion dedicated exclusively to distance vision. The haptics are also produced of hydrophobic acrylic with a maximum diameter of 13.0 mm. It has a modified L-shape and a 0-degree angulation.

Iodization is defined as the gradual reduction in the height of the diffractive steps from the center toward the edges of the diffractive portion of the lens. This splits the light for near and distance vision. The gradual transition of the diffractive steps will reduce undesired photopic phenomena.

The ReSTOR lens has 12 diffractive steps of decreasing height; the thickness varies from 1.3 to 0.4 µm. This is the apodized diffractive portion in the central 3.6 mm of the lens and allows both near and distance vision (Figure 8-4).[1] The refractive region of AcrySof ReSTOR, on the other hand, is located on the peripheral portion of the optic surrounding the diffractive zone and this measures 2.4 mm; this area deviates light onto a specific focal point on the retina and was developed to reduce the appearance of haloes when the pupil dilates under conditions of poor illumination.

With near vision and a small pupil, the central region of the lens is used and the height of the steps will determine a delay in the light ray of one-half of a wavelength. Under these circumstances, the diffraction of light is 41% for distance vision and 41% for near vision (with 18% of the light lost through higher-order aberrations [HOA]).

When the pupil diameter increases, for example, during distance vision or under conditions of poor illumination, additional peripheral zones will be involved, the height of the diffractive steps gradually decreases, and the zones are less curved; this will extend to the monofocal refractive portion and results in a different distribution of the light

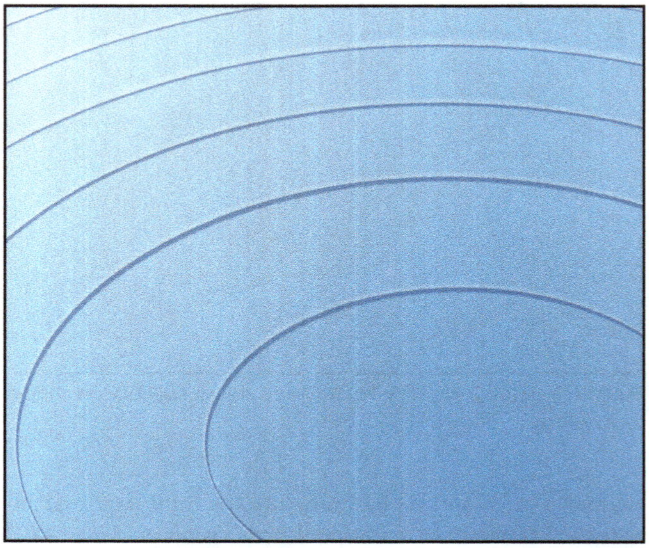

Figure 8-4. Magnification of the apodized region of AcrySof ReSTOR IOL. On the apodized diffractive surface of the lens, the steps are progressively shortened from 1.3 to 0.4 μm. (Reprinted with permission from Davison JA. Deciphering diffraction: how the Restor's apodized, refractive, diffractive optic works. *Cataract Refract Surg Today*. 2005;June:42-46.)

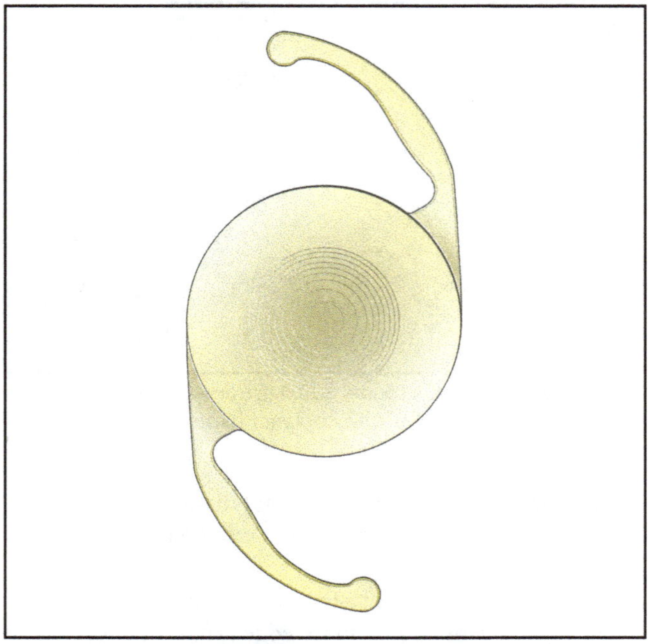

Figure 8-5. AcrySof ReSTOR Model D1 with a near addition of +3 D on the lens plane (+2.25 D on the spectacles plane). Note that the apodized concentric structure is found only in the central 3.6 mm; the peripheral areas of the optic become monofocal. With a variation of the pupil diameter, the ReSTOR modifies the percentage distribution of light for near and distance vision. With an increase in the pupil diameter, the lens increases the amount for distance vision and reduces the near vision amount.

intensity between near and distance vision with more light used for distance vision and less used for near vision.

The latest version of the ReSTOR (Model D1) has an additional power of +3 D at the iris plane, corresponding to approximately +2.25 D at the spectacle plane (Figure 8-5). This lens preserves the structure of the apodized diffractive central optic of 3.6 mm and the diffractive optic portion of 2.4 mm and has a different number of rings compared to the apodized portion. The number of rings changes from 12 in the D3 model to 9 in the D1; this is related to the previously mentioned +3 D for near vision instead of +4 D of the D3. This new version was developed to improve intermediate vision that was compromised with the previous +4 D version. It specifically enhances near vision. Moreover, it reduces the gap between the distance focus and near focus and reduces haloes and glare.

The toric ReSTOR lenses are exclusively D1 models; in other words, they have an additional near power of +3.0 D.

ReSTOR for Near Vision

The light from a near object reaches the cornea as diverging light. The diffractive lens uses the power of the lens and the additional 4 (or 3) D over the central 3.6 mm of the apodized zone to produce sharp images focused on the retina (eg, letters printed in a book). The portion of light focused for distance vision will create a second image, which will be severely blurred and disregarded by the patient's brain.

ReSTOR for Distance Vision

The light beams from a distant object reach the cornea as parallel light beams. In this case, the lens uses both the central diffractive portion of the lens and the peripheral refractive portion to produce sharp images focused on the retina (eg, a tree seen in the distance). The portion of the diffractive optic for near vision will create a second image, which will be severely blurred and disregarded by the brain.

General Vision With the ReSTOR

The ReSTOR lens has a very unusual structure that is difficult to explain. A number of factors are involved, for example, thickness of the optic, range of visible light wavelength, refractive indices of the optic media, and the anatomical structure of the foveola. Let us try and imagine that the 2 main focal points are created in an eye with this lens (following the diffraction of light): the first focal point will be located 19 mm from the lens (on the fovea) for distance vision; the second is closer and is located exactly 1 mm in front of the fovea (at a distance of 18 mm) for near vision. This is related to the +4-D power at the iris plane for near vision.

The distances can be measured in wavelengths. If we use green light (550 nm) in our reference eye, there will be approximately 46,000 wavelengths or cycles in the vitreous between the lens and the foveola (distance image) and approximately 44,000 between the lens and the near vision focal point located 1.0 mm closer (near vision).

Starting from the first diffractive step of the ReSTOR and moving outward with radial progression, the position

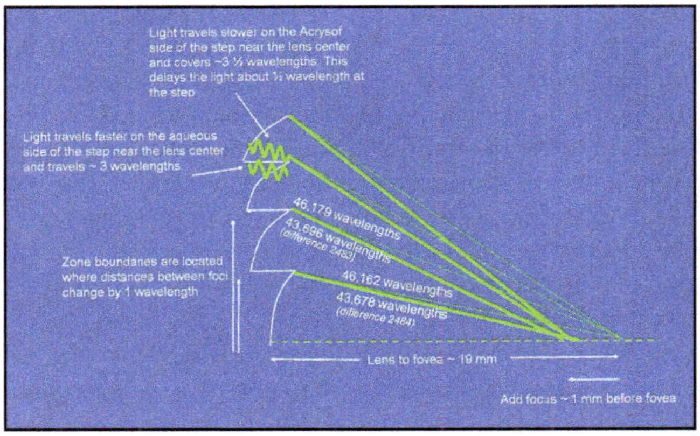

Figure 8-6. Light travels more slowly on the plastic portion of the step with respect to its speed through the aqueous. The consequent phase delay creates 2 focal points: one for distance vision and one for near vision. (Reprinted with permission from Davison JA. Deciphering diffraction: how the Restor's apodized, refractive, diffractive optic works. *Cataract Refract Surg Today.* 2005;June:42-46.)

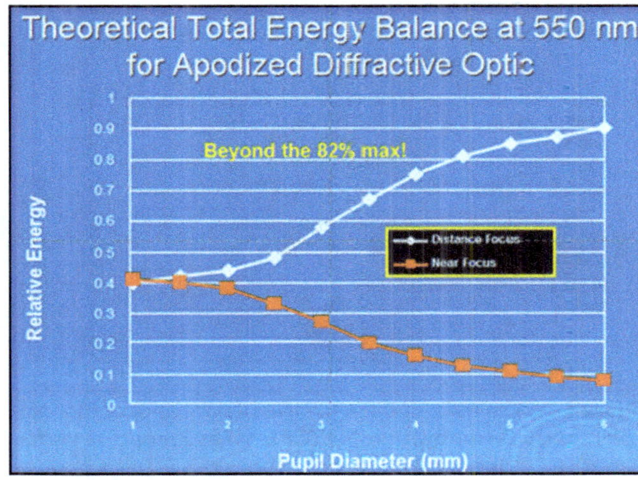

Figure 8-7. The apodization of the ReSTOR lens theoretically equalizes the portion of light for distance and near vision with small pupil diameters, while it increases the contribution for distance vision when the pupil increases in size and the peripheral portions of the lens come into play. (Reprinted with permission from Davison JA. Deciphering diffraction: how the Restor's apodized, refractive, diffractive optic works. *Cataract Refract Surg Today.* 2005;June:42-46.)

of the second step will be found precisely at the point in which the difference in the wavelengths between the 2 focal points for distance and near vision will differ by just one wavelength at the IOL plane. The same applies for the remaining 11 rings/steps; they will increasingly be closer but the difference between the wavelengths will always be 1 (in the version of the lens with a near addition of +3 D, there are 9 steps and not 12). The central steps of the diffractive zone are approximately 1.3 μm, and these will gradually decrease from the center of the optic toward the periphery by 0.2-μm steps to a minimum value of 0.4 μm.

The diffractive steps cause a delay in the light phase close to the rings. The height of the steps determines the amount of phase delay of the incident light, and the variation of the height modifies the surfaces of the optic itself. Even with the individual optic zones having an aspheric surface, the curvatures will be different and will differ from the optical curvature of the lens.

The shape of the surface of each zone determines the predominant direction of light that crosses each optic zone, while the small steps localized on the edges of each zone regulate the delay in the light phase. The surfaces of each zone and the delay in the phase determined by the height of the individual steps combine to create the overall optical properties of the lens. The height of the steps describes the optical properties of the ReSTOR IOL. When a light ray (green light) is incident on the edge of a step, the luminous portion that crosses the plastic side of the lens will travel more slowly than the portion of light that travels through the aqueous humor. There are approximately 3.5 wavelengths in the lens and approximately 3 wavelengths in the aqueous, meaning that there is a difference of approximately one-half of a wavelength, or the delay necessary to distribute approximately 41% of the light for each of the 2 focal points for distance and near vision (Figure 8-6).

In theoretical and practical terms, this is the best division of the light achievable with diffraction of these lenses with 2 powers and results from the complex interaction between the location of the edges of the optic zones and the structure of the zones themselves. The height of the steps basically determines how much light is directed for every image and determines the distribution of energy.

Higher steps at the center of the lens cause a delay of approximately one-half of a wavelength and split the light equally between 2 images (41% for each image or focal point with the remaining 18% of light lost through HOA). Lower steps, located progressively toward the edge of the lens, will decrease the optical delay to small fractions of wavelengths, directing less light toward the near image. This results in good near vision when the pupil is small (when the patient is reading, a convergence-miosis reflex is activated that is also induced by the light used for reading), and a greater proportion of light is directed to distance vision when the pupil diameter increases. This increase is enhanced further by the monofocal portion of the lens beyond the central apodized portion (Figure 8-7). This phenomenon translates into a variation in the percentage split for distance and near components, with variations in pupil diameter, increasing distance vision amount with a larger pupil diameter (Figure 8-8).

Understanding the Haloes

Multifocal lenses split the images into 2 focal points: a focal point for distance vision and a focal point for near vision. When we see an object at distance, the portion of the

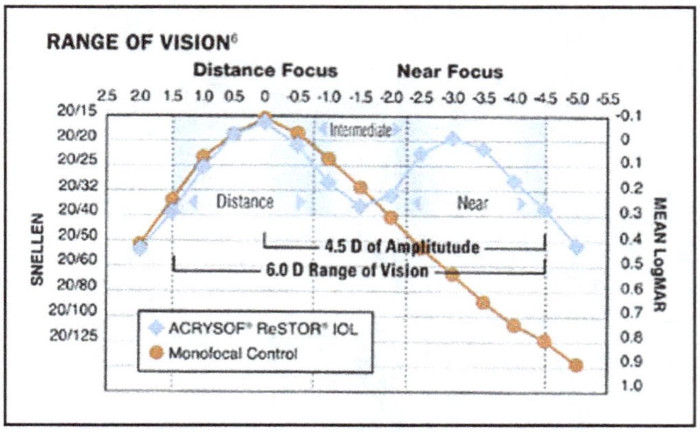

Figure 8-8. The spike of the refractive performance of monofocal lenses is 0 D. However, the ReSTOR lens has 2 refractive performance spikes: one at 0 D and a second one at –3 D. This is because the lens has one planar correction level and a second correction of +3 D. Consequently, this lens has a pseudo-accommodative range of 6.00 D compared to the 3.50 D of the monofocal lenses. (Reprinted with permission from Davison JA. Deciphering diffraction: how the Restor's apodized, refractive, diffractive optic works. *Cataract Refract Surg Today.* 2005;June:42-46.)

lens used for distance vision will bring the object into focus. Simultaneously, the portion of the lens for near vision will generate an analogous image that is out-of-focus or blurred. Overall, the person will be able to perceive the image he or she is observing, with small haloes that translate into a modest reduction in contrast sensitivity. The same thing happens when the person looks at a near object. Two images will be projected in this case, too: one will be in focus and the other will be blurred. In both of these situations, the undesired effect of the blurred image will reduce the contrast of the image that is in focus; the quality of the image is usually found acceptable for the patient with minimal reduction in contrast sensitivity. This situation is strongly influenced by pupil diameter (Figures 8-9 and 8-10).

The larger the diameter of the pupil, the greater the halo generated on the retina. On the other hand, when the pupil is small (between 2 and 3.5 mm) as seen in photopic conditions, or in near vision with the accommodation-miosis-convergence reflex, the haloes generated by the image overlapped with near over distance will be minimal.

Another factor that determines the severity and appearance of haloes is the amount of light dedicated to distance and near vision. When the light is split in a ratio of 50:50 for distance and near vision, the influence of the image that is out-of-focus on the object will be significant, and will lead to an image that is out-of-focus of the same intensity as the image in focus, generating evident haloes. On the other hand, when the ratio favors the distance vision, the intensity of the distance image predominates over the near image. It is extremely important to understand this concept because the various companies have adopted different strategies to manage this phenomenon. For example, AMO has developed the Tecnis with a constant 50:50 distance-near division of the light. In reality, the split is 41:41 with 18% lost through dispersion of the HOA. This characteristic, with an addition of +4 D at the lens plane, should be—or at least, that is how it seems on paper—the combination responsible for the greatest amount of haloes. This is because under every light condition and with any pupil diameter, the lens always offers the same balance between the 2 images, and the addition of +4 D for reading is responsible for formation of out-of-focus images of greater amounts (a high delta value in the addition for near vision).

Zeiss has developed a different strategy for the AT LISA. As mentioned earlier, the split of the light quota is 65% for distance vision and 35% for near vision. This tends to promote distance over near vision. To understand the basis of this decision, it is sufficient to consider that physiological pupillary mydriasis is in the evening or when driving at night. Under these circumstances, therefore, with a dilated pupil, in an environment with poor lighting where luminous spots appear in the dark, having just 35% of the luminous amount responsible for near vision will tend to significantly reduce the appearance of haloes and glare around light sources. With near vision, on the other hand, under good lighting conditions and with the smaller pupil reduced under the effects of the miosis-convergence stimulus, the 35% will be sufficient to achieve good reading ability, and the reduced pupil diameter will limit the appearance of haloes with the out-of-focus image in the lens dedicated to distance vision.

The third option is the system adopted by Alcon. With ReSTOR, Alcon has created a system with variable amounts. The lens is subdivided into a central apodized diffractive portion and into a peripheral refractive portion that can vary the amounts based on the pupil diameter. Decreasing width of the steps of the apodized portion can vary the luminous percentages based on the progressive involvement of the peripheral portions, until it exceeds the central 3.6 mm and uses only the peripheral monofocal refractive portion. With this type of lens, therefore, the vision amounts will be controlled by the degree of light stimulus and the convergence-miosis reflex. As mentioned, with distance vision, particularly in the evening with night driving, the pupil tends to dilate, progressively using the peripheral optic zones that increase the prevalence of the distance amount with respect to the near. When the pupil is dilated, the lens is split into 90% for distance vision and 10% for near vision; vice versa, when the pupil is small, the amounts are 50:50 (41% distance vision, 41% near vision, and 18% lost in HOAs), and this achieves maximum balance for reading and daytime vision. This amount uses reduced pupil diameter to reduce formation of haloes that are otherwise more evident because of "influence" of the out-of-focus image with respect to the image in focus.

Finally, an important element is the addition for near vision; the greater the addition for near vision, the greater

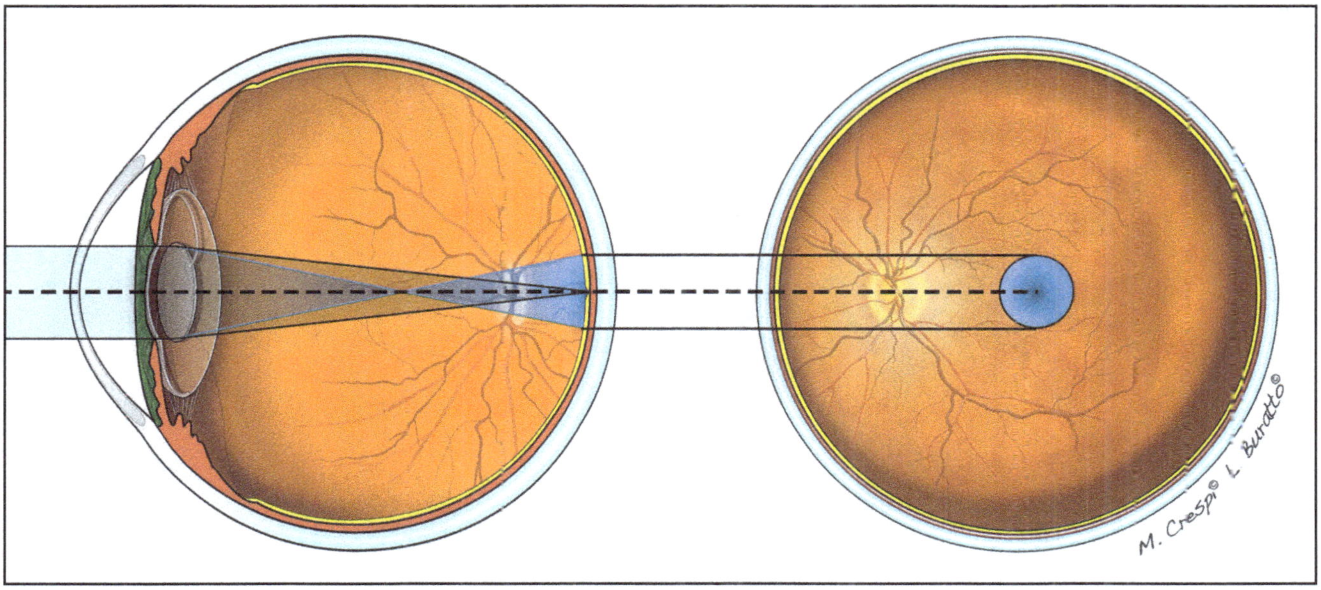

Figure 8-9. With the multifocal lenses, when the patient sees an item positioned at a distance, a sharp image is formed on the retina, created by the portion of the lens responsible for distance vision (F1), and another blurred image generated by the other areas of the lens (F2). These 2 images will overlap on the retina, generating diffusion haloes that reduce the visual quality and the contrast sensitivity.

the distance between the 2 focal points (near and distance) and the greater the diffusion of the halo created on the retina.

This explains why diffractive IOLs with a high addition for near vision (+3 D, +3.5 D) produce greater glare and more haloes compared to refractive lenses that have a smaller addition and allocate a smaller percentage (approximately 20%) to near vision.

Zonal Multifocal Lenses—The Oculentis Mplus

Oculentis has recently launched a new type of multifocal lens that is completely different from diffractive, refractive, and accommodative multifocal lenses.

The Mplus (Lentis Mplus LS-312/LS-313) is a "zonal" lens that consists of an asymmetric aspheric lens for distance vision, combined with a sector of +3.00 D located in an inferior position, for near vision, structured in such a way as to allow smooth and continuous transition between the 2 zones. The Mplus lens combines the presence of 2 spherical surfaces with different radii of curvature: a principle surface and a second surface incorporated with the first to provide the 2 focal points. The 3-dimensional structure of this type of lens (the presence of the segment for near vision incorporated in the segment for distance vision) means that these lenses are independent of the pupil diameter. Another characteristic of this type of lens is that the light incident on the transition zone between the 2 lenses is reflected away from the optic axis, to prevent the appearance of diffraction and superimposition of interferences.

Structure of the Lens

The Oculentis Mplus LS-312 MF or LS-313 MF (Figures 8-11 and 8-12) is manufactured with Hydrosmart, a material with a high water content (25%) and a hydrophobic surface. It has a refractive index of 1.46 and an incorporated filter for blue light.

The lens is available in 2 different shapes: the traditional lens with an optic of diameter 6 mm, C-shaped haptics with a 0-degree tilt, and a maximum overall diameter of 12 mm (LS-312 MF); and the biscuit-shaped lens with an optic diameter of 6 mm, a plane fenestrated optics with a 0-degree tilt, and a maximum overall diameter of 11 mm (LS-313 MF).

The lens powers available are between 0 and +36 D with intervals of 0.5 D.

The lens has an asymmetrical 3-dimensional structure, and consequently the implantation must respect the position of the anterior face and the rotational orientation. The surface is marked to ensure correct positioning of the lens.

In the traditional version of the lens, the orientation of the anterior and posterior surface is dictated by the haptics that are positioned in a classical manner (with the possibility of rotating the lens in a clockwise direction).

In the biscuit version of the lens, an asymmetrical appendix on the superior fenestration provides the

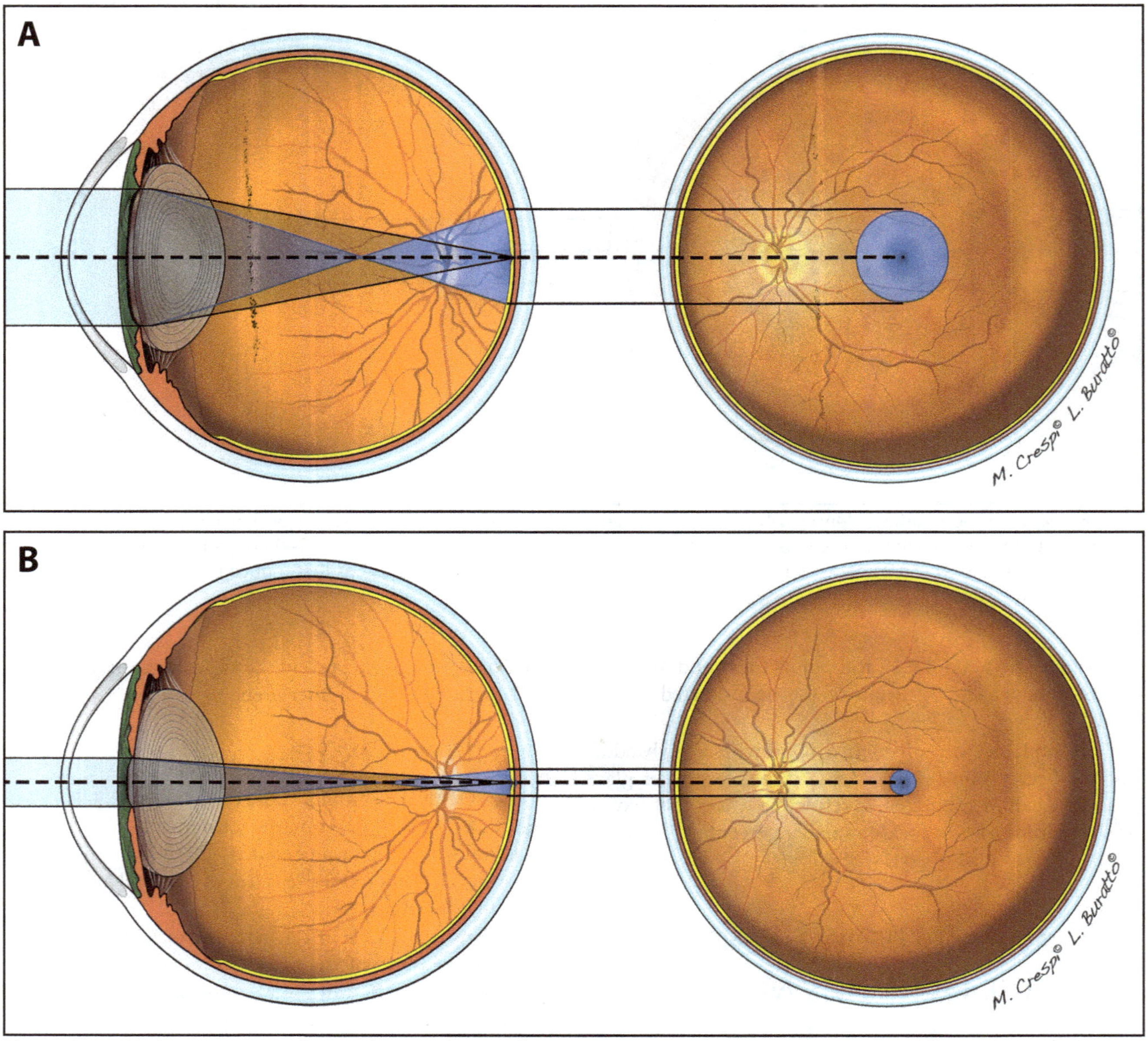

Figure 8-10. Under scotopic conditions, the near focus will generate an overlapping image, creating a diffusion halo on the main focus point of the distance vision (B). The dimensions of this halo are greater than those of the halo created when the pupil is small under photopic conditions (A). This will explain the increase in the depth of field in an eye with a miotic pupil.

reference points for the correct front-rear orientation of the lens.

The markings on the optic of the lens (similar to those present on the toric IOLs) allow correct positioning of the lens at the 0- to 180-degree axis, necessary for orienting the portion for near vision in the lower part of the visual field.

Finally, the lens has a square edge (360 degrees) that prevents PCO.

Oculentis Multifocal Toric Intraocular Lens

In addition to the standard multifocal lenses, the Oculentis Mplus is also available for the correction of astigmatism (Figure 8-13). The toric version of the Oculentis Multifocal is produced only with the haptics in the biscuit form (LS-313 MFT). It has a biconvex optic with a toric aspheric posterior surface. As with the standard multifocal version, the toric version also has a portion of add for near vision (+3.00 D) located in the inferior portion. Because of the 3-dimensional structure of the lens, and its

One-Piece Multifocal Posterior Chamber Lens
With Aspherical Surface
For Capsular Bag Fixation

oculentis®

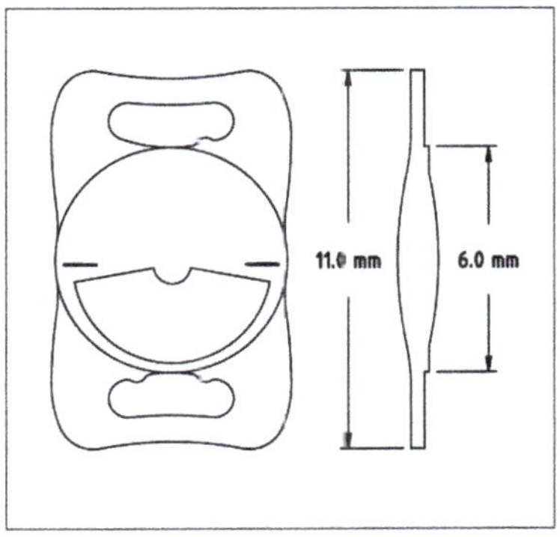

LENTIS® Mplus
LS-313 MF

Type	One-piece multifocal acrylic IOL
Optic size	6.0 mm
Overall length	11.0 mm
Haptic angulation	0°
Optic	Biconvex Aspherical surface - posterior Sector-shaped addition of +3.0 Diopters
Central thickness	0.98 mm (+22.00D)
Design	Optic and haptics with 360 degrees square edge
Material	HydroSmart copolymer consisting of acrylates with hydrophobic surface, UV absorbing
Sterilization	Steam autoclaved
Available diopters	± 0.0D to +36.0D (0.5D)
Refractive index	1.46
Estimated A-factor (acoustic)	118.0
Estimated A-factor (optic)	118.1 (SRK/T)
Estimated anterior chamber depth	4.97 mm
Recommended incision size	2.6 mm
Recommended injector (reusable)	Injector: Viscoject-1-hand: LI604205 Viscoject-2-hand: LI604215 Cartridge: Viscoject 1.8 Cartridge-Set: LP604250M (*) Viscoject 2.2 Cartridge-Set: LP604240M
Recommended injector-sets (disposable)	Viscoject-Injector + Viscoglide 1.8 Cartridge LP604350 (*) Viscoject-Injector + Viscoglide 2.2 Cartridge LP604340

* max. +27.0D

CE 1275

03/2011

Oculentis GmbH
Am Borsigturm 58
13507 Berlin
www.oculentis.com

Figure 8-11. Information for Lentis LS-313 MF. (Reprinted with permission from Topcon.)

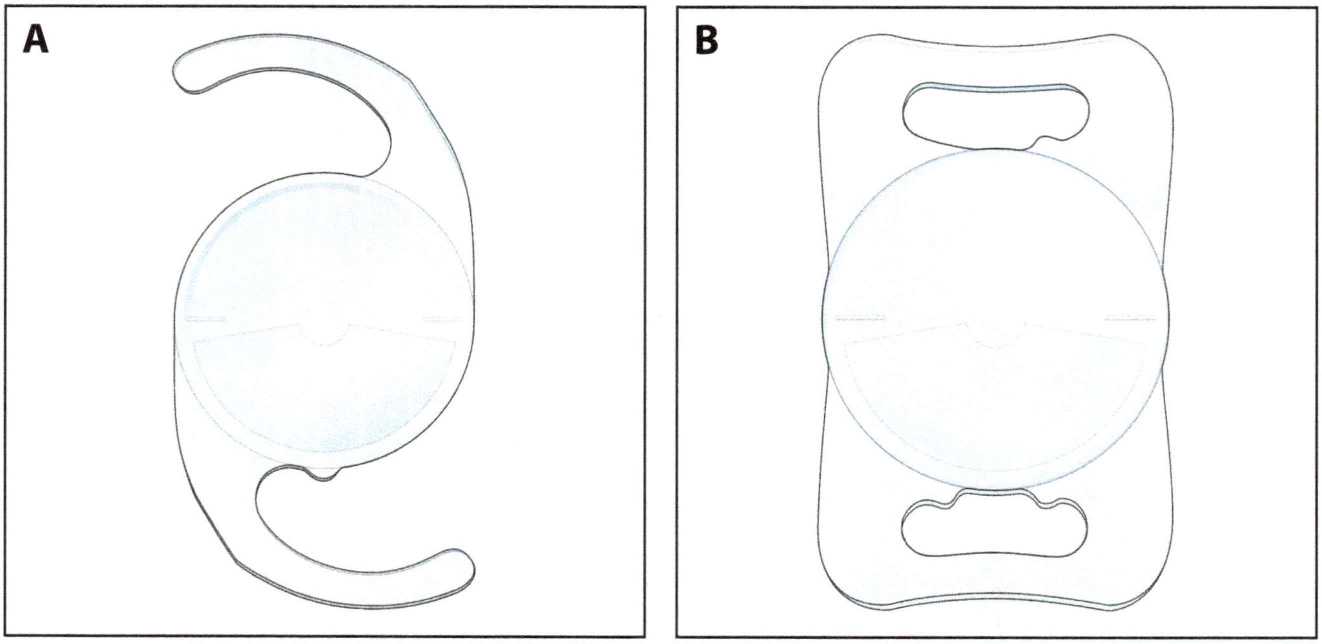

Figure 8-12. The 2 photographs present the 2 models of the Oculentis Mplus lens. (A) The model with the traditional haptics (LS-312 MF) and (B) the model with the biscuit-shaped haptics (LS-313 MF). The reverse D-shape section localized on the lower portion of the optic can be seen with the 2 markings used for positioning the lens.

obligatory orientation because of the additional portion for near vision, the orientation of the toric is personalized for every patient and is programmed when the lens power is calculated. The toric lenses produced by Oculentis (Mplus toric) are always positioned at 180 degrees to ensure that the portion of the lens for near vision is positioned at the bottom. The difference with this lens is that the toric power of the posterior surface will be oriented based on the patient's astigmatism. In reference to the range of cylinder powers, Oculentis produces a wide range of corrections that vary between 0.25 and 12.0 D.

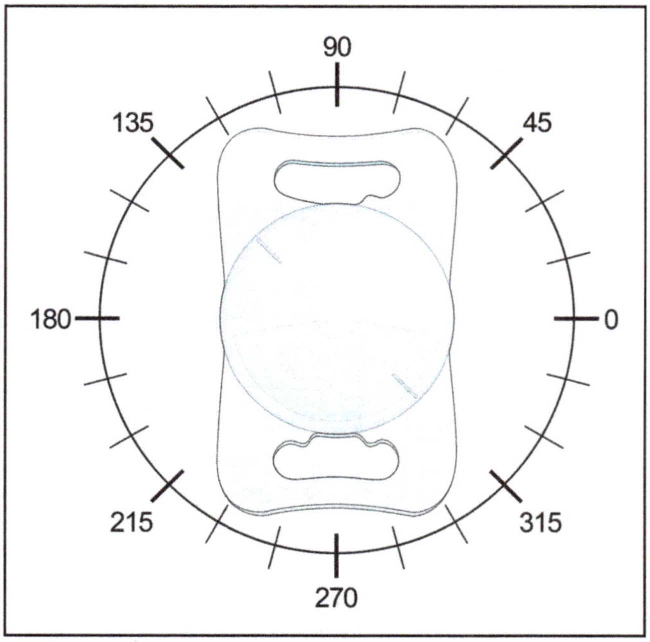

Figure 8-13. Design of the Oculentis LS-313 MFT (the T indicates a toric lens). The lens has the same shape of the multifocal lenses of the opulent family; however, the posterior surface contains the toric portion. The lens has 2 pairs of markings: one for the correct orientation of the lens at 180 degrees and the second pair to indicate the posterior torque, programmed in the phase of lens calculation.

Comparison With Other Multifocal Intraocular Lenses

Presently, there are no significant findings on the efficacy of this new type of lens. Clinical trials suggest that this category of innovative and highly functional lenses can provide the patient with good distance and near vision, without the occurrence of serious disturbances such as glare and haloes.

Currently, there are very few papers that compare this type of lens with the other multifocal lenses available. In an article published in *Journal of Cataract & Refractive Surgery* in January 2012, the Oculentis lenses were compared with lenses that are considered to be the market reference, the AcrySof ReSTOR.[2]

From a study performed on 90 eyes implanted with the Oculentis Mplus LS-312 and 143 control eyes implanted with the ReSTOR, the Oculentis is comparable to ReSTOR for uncorrected distance visual acuity and for appearance of dysphotopsias. However, the ReSTOR lenses have better visual performance at 30 and 40 cm.[2]

Patient Selection

A fundamental part of the implantation of multifocal IOLs is careful patient selection. A patient who seems suitable for implantation of a multifocal IOL must be carefully informed of the advantages, expectations, and disadvantages involved following implantation of this type of lens (see Chapter 10).

Presently, in order to eliminate or reduce the need for spectacles and improve near and distance vision, the surgeon can choose from 5 different implantation options: bilateral implantation of refractive, diffractive, or accommodative IOLs; a mixture of different types of lenses; or monofocal aspheric IOLs for monovision. When the surgeon and patient have agreed on the decision to implant a multifocal lens, there are several steps that need to be followed.

Pathologies to Avoid

The decision to implant a multifocal IOL must exclude pathologies that can compromise a good surgical outcome—corneal pathologies, severe astigmatism, retinal degeneration, etc.

It should always be remembered that implantation of a multifocal IOL reduces contrast sensitivity by about 50%, as the light will be diffracted in the 2 portions relative to distance and near vision. Any factor that leads to a further reduction in contrast sensitivity will affect the surgical outcome and the optimal performance of this type of lens.

Keratoconus and pellucid marginal degeneration are 2 examples of corneal pathologies that contraindicate implantation of a multifocal IOL. In some cases, these 2 pathologies may be misinterpreted by the patient who will often seek the surgeon for cataract surgery. The 2 pathologies may be in a nonprogressive phase; both will create HOAs such as coma and trefoil, which can compromise the "purity" of the visual signal transmitted to the retina. Modulation transfer function (MTF) expresses the variation in contrast sensitivity during the passage of the light information through the media. If there are HOAs that affect MTF, there will be a greater dispersion of light information in HOAs and the visual quality will be reduced to such a degree that the function of the multifocal IOL will be compromised.

The following equation shows how the contrast sensitivity function (CSF) depends on the MTF and on the neuroretinal transfer function (NTF), according to Dr. Martin A. Mainster and Dr. Patricia L. Turner.[3]

$$CSF = MTF \times NTF$$

The clinical applications are direct: if the NTF is unchanged after cataract surgery, the postoperative visual function (CSF) depends directly on the improvement of the MTF (ocular dioptric media). However, there are other factors that can modify the MTF (eg, keratoconus or pellucid marginal degeneration). As a result, the CSF (the postoperative visual function) will be reduced.

Following detailed analysis, the same applies to the presence of macular degeneration. In this case, however, the NTF will be compromised. Under these circumstances, the reduction in NTF will result in an overall reduction of CSF, compromising good outcomes with implantation of a multifocal IOL.

Our objective is to customize the procedure to suit the individual patient, adapt our experience to the patient's needs, and, with multifocal lenses, provide the patient with more that he or she expected, namely good-quality near and distance vision.

Patient Requirements

Customization of cataract surgery, or personalization of the surgery, must begin with an understanding of the patient's needs, routine activities, and visual expectations.

The decision to implant a multifocal IOL is based on the patient's desire to live without spectacles for most routine activities. It is essential, therefore, that the surgeon is fully aware whether the patient is an avid reader and whether he or she drives a lot; this information is important while deciding which lens to implant. In addition to studying the anatomical-functional characteristics of the patient's eye (eg, astigmatism, pupil dynamics, the dominant eye), the surgeon should also understand whether the patient would prefer to have better distance vision with good intermediate vision or whether optimal near vision is preferable. All this information will be useful in the choice of lens to implant as specific characteristics can satisfy the type of vision required.

Selection of the Lens Based on Pupil Dynamics

In the patient selection process, the surgeon should carefully examine pupil size under photopic and scotopic conditions, ocular dominance, amount of astigmatism, refraction, vision, and type of cataract.

TABLE 8-1

TABLE FOR SELECTING THE INTRAOCULAR LENS BASED ON THE PUPIL

	GOOD PUPIL KINETICS	POOR PUPIL KINETICS	LARGE PUPILS
Distance vision and driving	ReSTOR D1 (Alcon), Acri.LISA (Zeiss), Crystalens (B + L)	ZMB00 (AMO) = ReSTOR D1 (Alcon), Acri.LISA (Zeiss)	Acri.LISA (Zeiss) = ZMB00 (AMO)
Near vision and reading	ReSTOR D3 (Alcon), ZMB00 (AMO)	ReSTOR D3 (Alcon), ZMB00 (AMO)	ZMB00 (AMO)
Intermediate	ReZoom (Alcon), ReSTOR D1	ReSTOR D1, Crystalens (B + L)	Crystalens (B + L)

Patients with poor pupil kinetics cannot be implanted with a refractive IOL such as the ReZoom, as this would compromise the effect of the lens itself.

A diffractive lens should be implanted in patients with small pupils.

For patients with large pupils, even under normal light conditions, the ReSTOR lens should not be considered as a diffractive IOL, as this can compromise the quality of near vision. The ReSTOR distributes light on the basis of pupil diameter. In photopic conditions with a small pupil, the IOL distributes the light 42% for far vision and 42% for near vision with 18% lost in HOAs. In mesopic conditions with larger pupils, light focuses more on the far focus.

For patients who frequently use a computer, intermediate distance vision should predominate; consequently, a refractive lens should be implanted (eg, ReZoom) in both the eyes, although this may affect the quality of night vision.

Recently, Alcon introduced a new version of the ReSTOR lens with a near vision addition of +2.5 D. Because of the innovative features of this lens, the way it distributes light and the addition for near vision, it is an excellent IOL for intermediate distance, and ideal for people who work on a computer. However, reading smaller characters may prove to be more difficult as this requires a specific lens for very near vision.

For the avid reader, a diffractive lens is preferred as this improves near vision (and decreases intermediate distance). Here, the surgeon can implant either the Tecnis ZMB00 multifocal full diffractive or the AcrySof ReSTOR D3. Both of these lenses have an addition for near vision of +4 D at the lens plane, corresponding to +3.2 D at the spectacle plane.

If the patient wishes to be completely independent of spectacles, the surgeon may opt for the "mix and match" option to combine the properties of the various types of lenses. Mix and match means deciding to implant 2 multifocal lenses with different characteristics to take advantage of the different characteristics and reduce associated problems (Table 8-1).

MULTIFOCAL INTRAOCULAR LENS AND ASTIGMATISM

The correction of astigmatism during cataract surgery using toric IOLs can achieve excellent results. The use of these lenses significantly improves the patient's quality of life through a significant increase in visual performance. The decision to correct astigmatism with toric IOLs is valuable when the surgeon opts for the implantation of multifocal lenses. To allow perfect functioning of multifocal lenses, it is necessary to correct even small amounts of astigmatism. If astigmatism greater than 0.5 D exists postoperatively, it may compromise the patient's independence from spectacles and the success of surgery. Therefore, patients with residual postoperative astigmatism greater than 0.5 D must be corrected with relaxing limbal or corneal incisions by implanting a toric multifocal lens or through a second refractive laser surgery. For astigmatism in excess of 0.68 D at the corneal plane, currently available toric multifocal lenses can correct corneal cylinder and also have multifocal performance.

The belief that mild astigmatism can be corrected with relaxing incisions or clear corneal incisions is challenged by 2 important factors. The first is the unpredictability of the refractive result. For limbal relaxing incisions, it is essential to create a curved limbal incision of even depth 90% of the corneal depth, with a precalibrated blade or an adjustable diamond blade, of variable length depending on the amount of the astigmatism. For CRIs, on the other hand, the maximum power that can be achieved with an incision of 2.75 mm is approximately 0.75 D, with a slight hyperopic shift because of the mild alteration in the coupling ratio. In both cases, the result is not totally predictable.

The second is that this procedure creates HOAs; this increases light dispersion, further reducing contrast sensitivity that has already been reduced through the use of diffractive multifocal lenses.

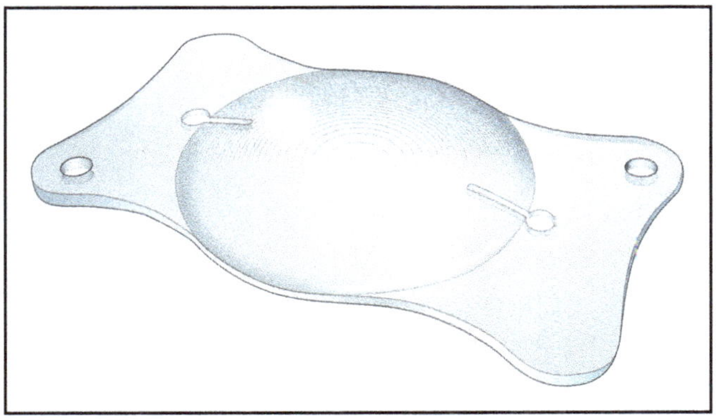

Figure 8-14. IOL AT LISA Toric 909M. The Zeiss lens has coplanar haptics with 0-degree tilting. This lens can be implanted through a microincision.

Despite the fact that there are no data reported in the literature regarding the increase of HOAs with limbal relaxing incisions, some findings demonstrate that creation of perforating incisions is responsible for increase in HOAs, coma in particular (not statistically significant) and trefoil (statistically significant).[4] The use of multifocal toric lenses is, therefore, the natural evolution of the concept of multifocal lenses, as they correct cylinder defects with a method that is safe, predictable, and physiological appropriate. Astigmatism is no longer a limitation to the use of multifocal lenses. Now the surgeon can decide to correct presbyopia with reduced risk of patient dissatisfaction.

Currently, there are 3 types of toric multifocal lenses available: the Zeiss Meditec AT LISA toric, the Alcon ReSTOR Toric IOL, and the new Tecnis Multifocal Toric lens recently launched by AMO. This increases the number of patients whose vision can be corrected with multifocal lenses.

There are 2 main problems associated with implantation of a toric multifocal IOL: rotational stability and centration in the bag.

It is essential that the lens is stable in the bag and is perfectly centered on the visual axis to achieve a good result for distance and near vision and maximize the multifocal properties.

Zeiss Meditec AT LISA Toric

The AT LISA toric is a 1-piece lens of hydrophilic acrylic; it is aspheric, diffractive, multifocal, and coated with a hydrophobic layer. The lens has a toric anterior surface and a multifocal diffractive aspheric posterior surface with negative spherical aberration. The platform is the AT LISA, and thus this lens has a full diffractive optic, independent of pupil diameter, with smooth transition steps between the rings (SMP technology) for reduction of haloes.

The power of the lens varies between −10.0 and +32.0 D with steps of 0.5 D, and cylinder variable between +1.0 and +12.0 D with steps of 0.5 D. The lens has a biscuit shape with a 6.0-mm optic and a total diameter of 11.0 mm. Markers are present on the surface of the lens for correct positioning along the axis of cylinder (Figure 8-14).

Its shape was designed to ensure optimal axial and radial centration. Tilt of the haptics is 0 degrees, it has a square edge on the optic and haptics and was designed for implantation through a microincision; it can be implanted through incisions between 1.5 and 1.8 mm. For lens powers not between +16.0 and +24.0 D with cylinder in excess of 3 D, the lens cartridge is different from the standard lens and is supplied along with the lens from Zeiss.

The wide range of powers available to correct spherical and astigmatic errors means that the surgeon can also correct a wide range of cylinder errors. Sometimes, in patients post penetrating keratoplasty, the surgery itself may have been perfect; however, an extremely high amount of residual astigmatism persists. This may be with-the-rule in terms of shape with a low incidence of HOAs. In this situation, Zeiss IOLs are indicated for correction of the error. As with monofocal toric IOLs, the type of multifocal IOL can be calculated using the online Zeiss software package, ZCALC (https://zcalc.meditec.Zeiss.com/zcalc).

As mentioned previously, it is possible to calculate the power of the IOL and its axis by using the software and adding the patient's biometry, the incision site, and the surgically induced astigmatism.

Alcon AcrySof ReSTOR Toric Intraocular Lens

The technology of the ReSTOR multifocal lens (apodized refractive-diffractive aspheric) has been combined with Alcon's experience in toric lenses, resulting in a toric multifocal lens. The basic platform is the ReSTOR. This is a 1-piece hydrophobic acrylic lens (acrylate/methacrylate copolymer); the optic is 6.0 mm and the maximum diameter between the haptics of 13.0 mm with powers that vary between +6.0 and +30.0 D with steps of 0.5 D. The modified L-shaped haptics are flexible acrylic with zero tilt; it is produced in Stableforce that produces rotational stability and excellent centration in the bag. The lens has a high refractive index, is extremely thin, and has filters for UV and blue light. Presently, the lenses available have 4 different powers for correction of the cylinder (+1.0 D, +1.50 D, +2.25 D, and +3.00 D at the lens plane). The range of powers is fairly limited as compared to Zeiss; according to Alcon philosophy, this range satisfies the clinical requirements of the majority of astigmatic patients. There are very few patients with corneal astigmatism > 2.5 D.

This lens is a biconvex aspheric apodized diffractive-refractive multifocal lens with the toric component on the posterior surface of the lens (Figure 8-15). This type of lens has the features of the ReSTOR D1; the code is SND1T, where the suffix D1 indicates that the near vision addition is +3.0 D at the lens plane, corresponding to approximately 2.25 D at the spectacle plane. The letter T attached to the number expresses the power of the cylinder. T2 corresponds to a value of +1.0 D; T5 corresponds to a value of +3.0 D. There are 3 marks on the posterior surface of the lens (3 on each side of the lens) and these allow precise alignment of the axis of the cylinder.

As with the latest generation of ReSTOR multifocals, these lenses have a central diffractive portion of 3.6 mm with 9 concentric steps (instead of 12) and the monofocal refractive peripheral 2.4 mm to improve distance vision in poor illumination.

With this type of lens, the lower addition for near vision (+3.0 D as opposed +4.0 D) produces better intermediate vision and also reduces perception of haloes around light sources with poor illumination.

Like the toric IOLs, there is also an online program available for calculation of the power of the multifocal toric IOLs. Log on to www.acrysoftoriccalculator.com. The software package is very simple and intuitive and gives the surgeon the ability to program the surgery, selecting the incision site, visualizing the steepest and flattest refractive axes, and evaluating the possibility of implanting a multifocal toric IOL.

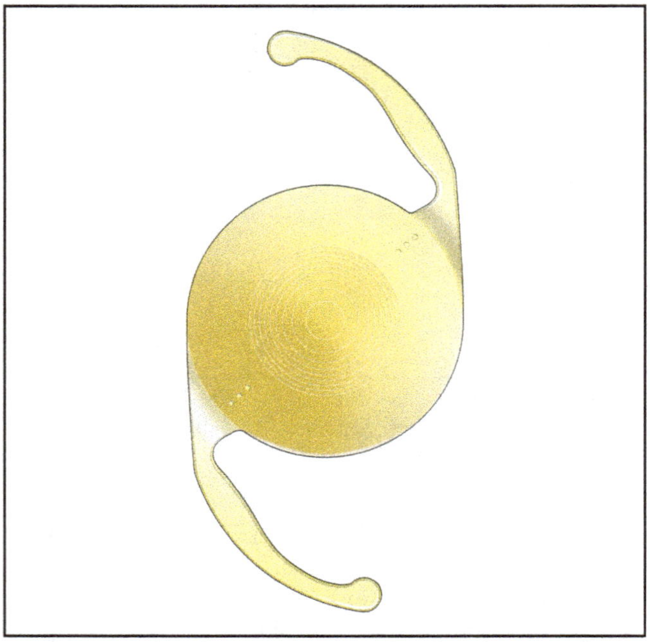

Figure 8-15. The Alcon ReSTOR Toric lens has the same characteristics as the ReSTOR D1 (7 rings in the apodized portion and an additional +3 D for near vision) with the additional correction of astigmatism.

AMO Tecnis Multifocal Toric Intraocular Lens

AMO recently launched a new multifocal toric IOL, increasing the number of patients who can be implanted with a Tecnis multifocal lens. The basic platform is the multifocal Tecnis ZMB00. This 1-piece lens is manufactured from hydrophobic acrylic with an aspheric surface; the diameter of the optic is 6 mm, and the maximum diameter of the haptics is 13 mm. The optic is biconvex with a toric aspheric anterior surface, with negative spherical aberration of −0.27 μm to compensate positive spherical corneal aberration. The full diffractive surface is on the posterior side of the lens, with a 50% distribution of light for distance/near vision and an addition of +4 D for near, and this corresponds to +3.2 D at the corneal plane. The power of the lens varies between +5 and +34 D with steps of 0.5 D. There are 4 different options for the correction of cylinder (+1.00 D, +1.50 D, +2.25 D, and +4.00 D). The positioning marks are found on the anterior surface of the lens; these are aligned on the steep corneal axis. The lens has a square edge of angulation 360 degrees to prevent PCO called *ProTEC*. The lens has a 3-dimensional shape that increases the stability of the lens (even in terms of rotation) called Tri-Fix, with 3 anchor points for fixing the lens to the capsular bag. The lens has a UV-blocking filter, required for FDA approval.

Patient Selection for Multifocal Intraocular Lenses

Careful patient selection is important for the successful outcome of the implantation procedure for multifocal IOLs.

Only careful examination of the patient's clinical and psychological characteristics and the patient's lifestyle can avoid a poor result—a good surgical procedure but considerable patient dissatisfaction!

Now we will look at some of the more important patient inclusion criteria.

- **Preoperative refraction:** The preoperative refraction is one of the factors that have greater influence with the patient's postoperative satisfaction when a multifocal IOL is implanted. Patients with large refractive errors will be really happy with the elimination of spectacles and will gladly accept some minor compromises; these patients have severe myopia or hyperopia and have to wear spectacles for all distances (distance vision and reading). Patients who have good uncorrected distance vision and use spectacles for reading only and mildly myopic patients who use spectacles only for distance vision will not have the same enthusiasm for the advantages of multifocal lenses because of the reduction in contrast sensitivity.

- **Good preoperative vision:** Preoperative visual performance will affect patient satisfaction. Patients with poor vision and reduced contrast sensitivity induced by the cataract will be more satisfied than the patient who still has good vision with spectacles or contact lenses. In practical terms, the greater the postoperative improvement, the greater the patient satisfaction.
- **Bilateral surgery with respect to unilateral surgery:** It is essential to inform the patient that the result with multifocal IOLs will improve when bilateral implants are performed. If just one of the patient's eyes has a cataract, the implantation of just one multifocal IOL will not produce the same satisfaction as bilateral implants.
- **Pupil size:** There is no doubt that pupil size has an important influence on the choice of the multifocal IOL. For appropriate selection of the type of IOL, it is essential to pay special attention to the variation of the pupil diameter with changes in light conditions.
- **Alterations of the eye surface:** Good quality of the lacrimal film and excellent uniformity of the corneal surface are essential for a good outcome with implantation of multifocal lenses. Pathologies that result in irregularities of the basement membrane, corneal scars, or leukomas will reduce MTF, generating HOAs responsible for reduction in contrast sensitivity.
- **Other ocular pathologies:** In addition to the anomalies of corneal surface (dry eye syndrome), corneal pathologies such as keratoconus, pellucid marginal degeneration, severe irregular astigmatism, or pathologies that can alter the NTF (age-related macular degeneration, macular pucker, diabetic macular edema, chronic glaucoma) are contraindications for implantation of a multifocal IOL (see the successive paragraphs).
- **Patient's age:** Compared to young patients who have greater demands, elderly patients will be more satisfied with the results of surgery. Young patients, with early cataracts, have not had experience with presbyopia and therefore will not fully appreciate the advantages of a presbyopic-correcting IOL. It should always be remembered that an artificial IOL, and particularly a multifocal IOL, will never be able to mimic the performance of the natural crystalline lens. In these patients, the surgical outcome will be excellent but the patient will be dissatisfied.
- **Tolerance to haloes:** The perception of haloes is one of the side effects associated with implantation of refractive or diffractive IOLs. Haloes following implantation of the latest generation of IOLs are limited to certain specific circumstances; however, the doctor should always warn the patient of this possibility. The patient should be questioned about sensitivity to light and intolerance to haloes that may appear when driving at night or under conditions of poor illumination. With these patients, it is better to avoid implanting multifocal IOLs as the visual results may leave them even more dissatisfied.
- **Work, hobbies and lifestyle:** This information is important for patient selection and the correct choice of a multifocal IOL. The surgeon must understand whether the patient's professional activities involve significant driving at night or prolonged use of a computer; whether his or her work predominantly involves middle or near vision; or if the patient is an avid reader or a passionate golfer. All of these findings are important for the choice of IOL to be implanted.
- **Personality:** If the individual is easygoing and can adapt to changing conditions, he or she will be more likely to accept the minor problems associated with a multifocal IOL and to be able to see without spectacles. People who are set in their ways, stubborn, perfectionists, or people who are used to maximum precision because of their profession (engineers, architects) will not tolerate any deficit in their vision and will be extremely unhappy with this type of lens.
- **Realistic expectations:** The implantation of a multifocal lens can be described as a compromise for vision. The slight drop in contrast sensitivity and the perception of haloes around light sources is the price the patient will have to pay to enjoy independence from spectacles in the majority of everyday situations. If the patient has expectations of perfect vision under any lighting conditions and at any distance, this is unrealistic. Consequently, the surgeon should carefully select these patients, as they are not ideal candidates for the implantation of presbyopic-correcting IOLs.

The criteria above are guidelines that will assist the surgeon in his or her selection of the patient considering multifocal IOLs.

Conclusion

Multifocal lenses offer patients good independence from spectacles for near and distance vision. Careful patient selection is an essential component of surgical success determining the patient's degree of satisfaction.

The compromise associated with multifocal lenses and the increase in side effects when the pupil diameter increases suggest exclusion from implantation of this type of lens in patients whose professional activities are performed under poor illumination (eg, long-distance truck or bus drivers). It is equally important to exclude all patients who expect to achieve perfect vision or who still have good spectacle-free vision with early signs of presbyopia and who cannot come to terms with the idea of having to wear corrective lenses for near vision.

It should always be remembered that an artificial IOL, and particularly a multifocal IOL, can never reproduce the effect of the natural crystalline lens. The outcome of the surgery is likely to be perfect but the patient will not be satisfied with the results.

Ideal Patients

Hyperopic patients with age-related cataracts and with-the-rule astigmatism are ideal subjects for the implantation of multifocal lenses. These patients have to wear corrective lenses at all times for both near and distance vision, and the cataract will cause significant reduction in visual acuity and contrast sensitivity. For these patients, the possibility of eliminating spectacles for near and distance vision is an enormous advantage and a great improvement for their quality of life; consequently, they are more inclined to accept a certain degree of compromise.

It should also be remembered that for maximum benefit from implantation of these lenses, bilateral implantation should be planned with a short interval between the first and second procedures. The process of neuroadaptation will be optimized with bilateral multifocals.

The moderately myopic patient is the most difficult to satisfy; these patients have always had excellent near vision and no blurring, so they will be much more intolerant to the appearance of haloes.

Generally, hyperopic patients prefer overcorrection of their refraction. This means that a part of the incident light will focus behind the retina, creating a small circle of light around the central image. The moderately myopic patient, however, prefers to be slightly undercorrected so that his or her existing near and distance vision has less chance of haloes and aberrations.

The Preoperative Interview

The surgeon should talk to the patient at length prior to surgery and describe the advantages and compromises associated with the implantation of multifocal IOLs; this will save a lot of time postoperatively. The surgeon should explain that haloes are an integral part of multifocal lens implantation, and that, in time, the process of neuroadaptation will reduce their impact and attenuate the degree of discomfort. The surgeon should also explain that it sometimes might be necessary to use spectacles, for example, when using the computer (particularly for patients with bilateral ReSTOR or Tecnis ZM900) implants.

In healthy subjects, the visual apparatus produces sharp images, despite the presence of optical aberrations that might blur them. Every eye has aberrations that produce a specific luminous pattern of an object: this is known as the point spread function (or PSF). When the brain adapts to specific aberrations and produces sharp images, each person's vision should improve and be sharper even with intrinsic aberrations under unfamiliar conditions. If this theory is true, it has important implications in all those procedures that modify the optical properties of each and every eye (eg, refractive surgery and cataract procedures).

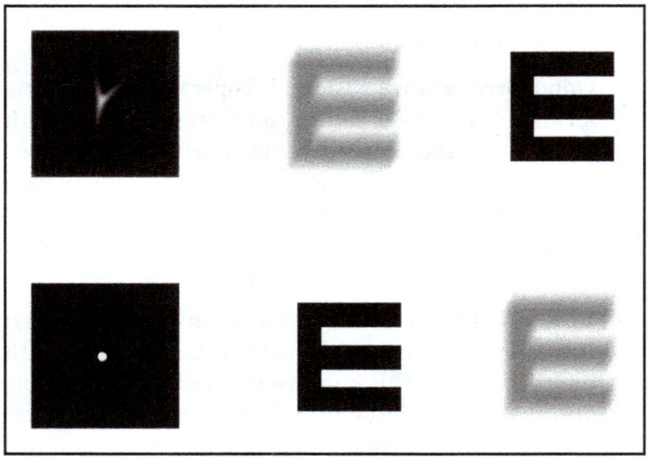

Figure 8-16. This image illustrates the possible effects of the neuroadaptation process in the retinal images before and after their ideal correction. (Reprinted with permission from Artal P. Neuroadaptation and multifocal IOLs. In: Chang DF, ed. *Mastering Refractive IOLs: The Art and Science.* Thorofare, NJ: SLACK Incorporated; 2008.)

Many patients report progressive improvement over time in some of the optical phenomena for no particular reason. Common situations of neuroadaptation include the frequently observed adaptation to blurred vision, to distorted vision, and to alteration of colors. One very simple example is the correction of presbyopia using spectacles. Initially, when the patient wears reading spectacles for the first time, he or she is aware of the lenses and the distortion of the retinal image; however, just a few days later, these sensations disappear and the patient will be more than happy with this correction. Time plays an important role in the process of neuroadaptation. In customized refractive surgery, wavefront guided, the correction of the aberrations will immediately lead to a phase of visual discomfort. This phenomenon comes from the fact that the brain is already used to a specific type of aberration. Immediately after surgery, the neurosensory adaptation process is still "programmed" to compensate for the previous aberration pattern. If the brain is programmed to produce a modified image, initially there will be a deterioration of the corrected image (Figure 8-16). Neuroadaptation is important because it allows our visual-brain system to adapt to new visual conditions. It is essential to fully understand these processes, particularly when attempting to improve binocular vision.

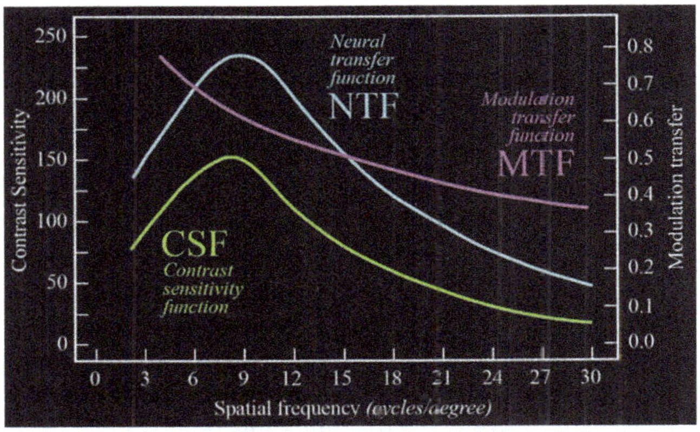

Figure 8-17. The process of contrast sensitivity of the human eye is described by the CSF that illustrates how sensitive the eye is to different spatial frequencies. The NTF describes the visual sensitivity of the retina and the brain independently of the eye's optical factors. The MTF describes how the information transfer process relative to contrast from the eye's optics decreases as the spatial frequencies increase. The CSF reduces with an increase in the spatial frequencies (smaller targets) because the retina and the brain have a lower sensitivity to high spatial frequencies (NTF) and the cornea, the crystalline, and the other dioptric media transfer less contrast sensitivity information to the retina at higher frequencies with respect to the low frequencies (MTF). (Reprinted with permission from Mainster MA, Turner PL. Multifocal IOLs and maculopathy—how much is too much? In: Chang DF, ed. *Mastering Refractive IOLs: The Art and Science.* Thorofare, NJ: SLACK Incorporated; 2008.)

Multifocal Intraocular Lens and Maculopathy

Age-related maculopathy (AMD) and diabetic maculopathy are the 2 most common forms of the condition. AMD is the main cause of severe and irreversible sight loss in the industrialized world. Patients with an intermediate degree of AMD (numerous drusen of intermediate dimensions and one or more large drusen lines) have an 18% probability of progressing to the advanced stage of AMD within 5 years. This probability increases to 26% if the large drusen are found in both eyes.

Treatment of diabetic retinopathy can reduce the risk of severe vision loss by 90%; however, this condition (diabetic retinopathy) is still the main cause of blindness in developing countries.

The duration of the diabetes and severity of the hyperglycemia are important risk factors in diabetic retinopathy. In less than 5 years, retinopathy affects 40% of Type 2 diabetes patients controlled with insulin, and 24% of patients controlled with oral hypoglycemic drugs. Moreover, the condition is found in 25% of the population affected by Type 1 diabetes for more than 5 years. The percentage of progression or development of diabetic retinopathy over a period of 1 year varies between 5% and 10%.

In these (and other) forms of retinopathies, loss of visual acuity and contrast sensitivity can compromise the patient's everyday life.[5,6]

A reduction in contrast sensitivity can greatly influence the patient's quality of life and he or she will have difficulty moving around, recognizing faces, reading, and driving.[5,7-9] A 25% reduction in contrast sensitivity can seriously affect night driving and reaction times.[10]

A 50% reduction in contrast sensitivity and visual acuity in patients over 65 years of age is associated with a 3- to 5-fold probability that the patient's everyday routine will be affected, irrespective of the loss of visual acuity.[5] A 90% reduction in contrast sensitivity is a criterion of visual debilitation.[11]

On the contrary, with normal vision, a 10-fold reduction in contrast sensitivity is responsible for a 2-fold reduction in reading capacity; moreover, walking generally requires low spatial frequencies not compromised by multifocal lenses.[12,13]

Tests to determine contrast sensitivity can highlight a reduction in visual performance that is not normally observed when just the visual acuity is measured.[9,14,15] Numerous studies have shown that AMD produces a reduction in contrast sensitivity, even in the initial stages.[9,14] As AMD progresses, contrast sensitivity decreases. The situation is similar for diabetic retinopathy. Contrast sensitivity is reduced in diabetic patients compared to patients without diabetes; the same applies to diabetic patients with retinopathy compared to diabetics without retinopathy.[16,17]

As suggested by Dr. Martin A. Mainster and Dr. Patricia L. Turner, CSF provides a general description of the visual function.[7,18,19] It analyzes the degree of contrast a subject requires to distinguish the sine wave grating of a specific dimension (spatial frequency). Wide and fine gratings have a low and a high frequency, respectively. The spatial frequency is measured in cycles per degree (cpd) of visual angles. Six, 15, and 30 cpd correspond to 1/50, 5/10, and 10/10 of visual acuity.

The spatial frequency for recognition of simple outlines or for reading a newspaper is 3 and 12 cpd, respectively, corresponding to a visual acuity of 1/10 and approximately 4/10, respectively.[20] Greater contrast is required for visualization of finer details compared to larger, more obvious ones; consequently, contrast sensitivity will be reduced with an increase in the spatial frequency from the spike between 3 and 6 cpd (Figure 8-17). Moreover, contrast sensitivity drops as the distance from the fovea increases (retinal eccentricity).[21]

Independent of the eye's optic, neuroretinal visual sensitivity can be described as NTF.[8] NTF and CSF have the same graphic pattern (on a Cartesian grid with the spatial frequency on the x axis and the contrast sensitivity on the ordinate). The methods for the measurement of the NTF include projection of the sinusoidal grids directly onto the patient's retina using methods that exclude the eye's optical aberrations.

CSF decreases with an increase in the spatial frequency (finer targets) for 2 basic reasons:

1. The retina and the brain are less sensitive to high spatial frequencies.
2. The cornea, the lens of the eye, and all of the media transfer less contrast information at higher compared to lower frequencies.

MTF describes how the contrast information transferred is reduced as it passes through the eye's media, when the spatial frequency increases.[18] In practice, the media filter the information on contrast and provide more efficient transmission or transfer of the low spatial frequencies as opposed to the higher frequencies. This situation is comparable to the process of color transmission that is affected by age and the yellowing of the lens; in this case, the transmission of lower optic frequencies (longer wavelengths in the red spectrum) is more efficient than the transmission of the higher wavelengths (shorter wavelengths in the blue spectrum).

Dr. Mainster and Dr. Turner used the following equation to show how the CSF depends on the eye's optic (MTF) and on the neuroretinal function (NTF).[18]

$$CSF = MTF \times NTF$$

They demonstrated how clinical applications are direct: if the NTF has not been modified following cataract surgery, the postoperative visual function (CSF) depends on the improvement of the eye's media (MTF).

If the MTF is unchanged following implantation of multifocal IOLs, the improvements seen in visual function (CSF) in the months following surgery are proportional to the increase in NTF, due to neuroadaptation. This will allow us to quantify the process of postoperative neuroadaptation.

If the eye's ocular media (MTF) are unchanged with appearance of macular changes, the loss of visual function (CSF) will be proportional to the degeneration of the neuroretinal complex (NTF).

Activities that require a low spatial frequency (large details) are more tolerant to defocus as opposed to fine-detailed activities, which require sharp vision of fine details, involving high spatial frequencies. For this reason, patients with reduced visual acuity have greater tolerance to defocus as opposed to patients with normal vision. However, loss of contrast sensitivity is a serious issue and correlated to the problems with everyday activities faced by patients with maculopathy (reading, moving about, etc). Patients with poor vision with maculopathy frequently benefit from devices that magnify the images (eg, lenses or screens). As described, the transfer equation discussed previously provides a practical method for understanding the simultaneous loss of contrast sensitivity caused by maculopathy in patients implanted with multifocal IOLs. The decreases in contrast sensitivity can be expressed as percentage losses or logarithmic decreases. For example, a loss of 2 points (log) (50%), 4 points (log) (75%), and 10 points (log) (90%) correspond to a reduction of 6, 12, and 20 dBm, respectively.[9,14]

The transfer equation illustrates that reduction in CSF is additive when expressed in logarithmic units. For example, a uniform reduction in optic sensitivity of 6 dB (50%) produced by a multifocal IOL should be fairly acceptable to normal subjects without macular alterations; a reduction in neuroretinal sensitivity of 6 dB caused by maculopathy should be well tolerated by patients with AMD. In theory, these should be combined to produce a decrease in contrast sensitivity of 12 dB (4 logarithmic units or 75% reduction). Patients with maculopathy can benefit from cataract surgery even if their visual acuity does not improve.[22,23]

The loss of contrast sensitivity caused by opacity of the lens is cumulative with the macular abnormalities. Consequently, the implantation of an IOL can improve visual performance under intermediate luminous frequencies, even when alterations of the macula have compromised vision with high frequencies (fine details). The implantation of aspheric IOLs with a higher MTF (or higher ability to transfer the images to the retina) should produce a greater visual improvement.[24,25] The wavelength at the center of the visible spectrum allows the vision of intermediate and high spatial frequencies in pseudophakic subjects; this would explain why the blue-blocking filters fail to clinically improve contrast sensitivity.

The sensitivity of the rhodopsin photoreceptors is reduced in subjects with AMD and diabetic retinopathy, which creates significant difficulty in the patient's ability to perform normal activities, such as walking and night driving.[26-30] Circadian dysfunctions increase with age; they are associated with insomnia, depression, and a number of systemic disorders. Cataract surgery can improve the stimulation of the rhodopsin receptors, improve circadian cycles, and reduce insomnia.[31-34] Non-blue-filtering multifocal lenses can preserve this improvement. Dr. Mainster believes that blue-blocking filters decrease rod and circadian photoreception by 14% to 21% and 27% to 38%, respectively, reducing the important benefits obtained from cataract surgery.[31,35,36]

Numerous recent studies performed by Swiss and Chinese researchers showed that cataract surgery is not an important risk factor for the advanced forms of AMD.[37-39]

Neuroadaptation can compensate for some changes appearing on the visual input structures to the brain centers of sight. The brain creates visual images by capturing small portions of the retinal images and processing this information in small channels of reduced spatial frequency. The monocular information is initially transferred from the eye to the visual cortex and successively to the higher-order neurons, which process binocular vision and other complex information. Knowledge on how the brain defines the images in patients implanted with multifocal IOLs with or without maculopathy is still fairly basic. The clinical information highlights the process of neuroadaptation, which can be accelerated by perceptive learning.[40,41]

Dr. Mainster and Dr. Turner concluded that the majority of pseudophakic subjects following implantation of multifocal IOLs and free from retinal problems are generally extremely satisfied with their vision. The small reduction in contrast sensitivity is well accepted considering their independence from spectacles. Patients with vision loss (AMD, diabetic retinopathy) will tolerate image defocus; however, their contrast sensitivity is an important indicator for their ability to read and perform their normal everyday activities. A loss in contrast sensitivity induced by multifocal IOLs is cumulative with the loss caused by the maculopathy, and it is possible that the combination of these 2 phenomena alters normal vision, leading to further reduction in the visual capacity of the patient with maculopathy, particularly under poor lighting conditions. Everyday activities may prove to be a major problem for these patients.

References

1. Davison JA. Deciphering diffraction: How the ReSTOR's apodized, refractive, diffractive optic works. *Cataract Refract Surg Today.* 2005;June:42-46.
2. Van der Linden JW, Van Velthoven M, Van der Meulen I, Nieuwendaal C, Mourits M, Lapid-Gortzak R. Comparison of a new-generation sectorial addition multifocal intraocular lens and a diffractive apodized multifocal intraocular lens. *J Cataract Refract Surg.* 2012;38(1):68-73. Epub 2011 Nov 10.
3. Mainster MA, Turner PL. Multifocal IOL and maculopathy—how much is too much. In: Chang DF, ed. *Mastering Refractive IOLs. The Art and Science.* Thorofare, NJ: SLACK Incorporated; 2008.
4. Orfeo V, Boccuzzi D. Use of Perforating Incision for the Correction of Astigmatism in Cataract Surgery. ROL and SICCSO International Congress - Grosseto 7-9- Luglio 2011.
5. West SK, Rubin GS, Broman AT, Muñoz B, Bandeen-Roche K, Turano K. How does visual impairment affect performance on tasks of everyday life? The SEE Project. Salisbury Eye Evaluation. *Arch Ophthalmol.* 2002;120(6):774-780.
6. Rubin GS, Bandeen-Roche K, Huang GH, et al. The association of multiple visual impairments with self-reported visual disability: SEE project. *Invest Ophthalmol Vis Sci.* 2001;42(1):64-72.
7. Owsley C. Contrast sensitivity. *Ophthalmol Clin North Am.* 2003;16(2):171-177.
8. Wolffsohn JS, Cochrane AL. Design of the low vision quality-of-life questionnaire (LVQOL) and measuring the outcome of low-vision rehabilitation. *Am J Ophthalmol.* 2000;130(6):793-802.
9. Eperjesi F, Wolffsohn J, Bowden J, Napper G, Rubinstein M. Normative contrast sensitivity values for the back-lit Melbourne Edge Test and the effect of visual impairment. *Ophthalmic Physiol Opt.* 2004;24(6):600-606.
10. Ginsburg AP. Contrast sensitivity and functional vision. *Int Ophthalmol Clin.* 2003;43(2):5-15.
11. Leat SJ, Legge GE, Bullimore MA. What is low vision? A re-evaluation of definitions. *Optom Vis Sci.* 1999;76(4):198-211.
12. Legge GE, Rubin GS, Luebker A. Psychophysics of reading—V. The role of contrast in normal vision. *Vision Res.* 1987;27(7):1165-1177.
13. Akutsu H, Legge GE, Showalter M, Lindstrom RL, Zabel RW, Kirby VM. Contrast sensitivity and reading through multifocal intraocular lenses. *Arch Ophthalmol.* 1992;110(8):1076-1080.
14. Wolkstein M, Atkin A, Bodis-Wollner I. Contrast sensitivity in retinal disease. *Ophthalmology.* 1980;87(11):1140-1149.
15. Marmor MF. Contrast sensitivity versus visual acuity in retinal disease. *Br J Ophthalmol.* 1986;70(7):553-559.
16. Arend O, Remky A, Evans D, Stüber R, Harris A. Contrast sensitivity loss is coupled with capillary dropout in patients with diabetes. *Invest Ophthalmol Vis Sci.* 1997;38(9):1819-1824.
17. Ismail GM, Whitaker D. Early detection of changes in visual function in diabetes mellitus. *Ophthalmic Physiol Opt.* 1998;18(1):3-12.
18. Mainster MA. Contemporary optics and ocular pathology. *Surv Ophthalmol.* 1978;23(2):135-142.
19. Amesbury EC, Schallhorn SC. Contrast sensitivity and limits of vision. *Int Ophthalmol Clin.* 2003;43(2):31-42.
20. Nio YK, Jansonius NM, Wijdh RH, et al. Effect of methods of myopia correction on visual acuity, contrast sensitivity, and depth of focus. *J Cataract Refract Surg.* 2003;29(11):2082-2095.
21. Frisén L, Glansholm A. Optical and neural resolution in peripheral vision. *Invest Ophthalmol.* 1975;14(7):528-536.
22. Adamsons I, Rubin GS, Vitale S, Taylor HR, Stark WJ. The effect of early cataracts on glare and contrast sensitivity. A pilot study. *Arch Ophthalmol.* 1992;110(8):1081-1086.
23. Elliott DB, Situ P. Visual acuity versus letter contrast sensitivity in early cataract. *Vision Res.* 1998;38(13):2047-2052.
24. Holladay JT, Piers PA, Koranyi G, van der Mooren M, Norrby NE. A new intraocular lens design to reduce spherical aberration of pseudophakic eyes. *J Refract Surg.* 2002;18(6):683-691.
25. Piers PA, Fernandez EJ, Manzanera S, Norrby S, Artal P. Adaptive optics simulation of intraocular lenses with modified spherical aberration. *Invest Ophthalmol Vis Sci.* 2004;45(12):4601-4610.
26. Brown B, Brabyn L, Welch L, Haegerstrom-Portnoy G, Colenbrander A. Contribution of vision variables to mobility in age-related maculopathy patients. *Am J Optom Physiol Opt.* 1986;63(9):733-739.
27. Sunness JS, Rubin GS, Applegate CA, et al. Visual function abnormalities and prognosis in eyes with age-related geographic atrophy of the macula and good visual acuity. *Ophthalmology.* 1997;104(10):1677-1691.
28. Owsley C, Jackson GR, Cideciyan AV, et al. Psychophysical evidence for rod vulnerability in age-related macular degeneration. *Invest Ophthalmol Vis Sci.* 2000;41(1):267-273.
29. Owsley C, Jackson GR, White M, Feist R, Edwards D. Delays in rod-mediated dark adaptation in early age-related maculopathy. *Ophthalmology.* 2001;108(7):1196-1202.
30. Greenstein VC, Thomas SR, Blaustein H, Koenig K, Carr RE. Effects of early diabetic retinopathy on rod system sensitivity. *Optom Vis Sci.* 1993;70(1):18-23.
31. Mainster MA. Violet and blue light blocking intraocular lenses: photoprotection versus photoreception. *Br J Ophthalmol.* 2006;90(6):784-792.
32. Mainster MA, Turner PL. Intraocular lens spectral filtering. In: Steinert RF, ed. *Cataract Surgery.* 3rd ed. London, England: Elsevier Ltd.
33. Asplund R, Lindblad BE. Sleep and sleepiness 1 and 9 months after cataract surgery. *Arch Gerontol Geriatr.* 2004;38(1):69-75.
34. Asplund R, Ejdervik Lindblad B. The development of sleep in persons undergoing cataract surgery. *Arch Gerontol Geriatr.* 2002;35(2):179-187.
35. Mainster MA. Intraocular lenses should block UV radiation and violet but not bluelight. *Arch Ophthalmol.* 2005;123(4):550-555.
36. Mainster MA, Sparrow JR. How much blue light should an IOL transmit? *Br J Ophthalmol.* 2003;87(12):1523-1529.

37. Meyers SM, Ostrovsky MA, Bonner RF. A model of spectral filtering to reduce photochemical damage in age-related macular degeneration. *Trans Am Ophthalmol Soc.* 2004;102:83-93; discussion 93-95.
38. Sutter FK, Menghini M, Barthelmes D, et al. Is pseudophakia a risk factor for neovascular age-related macular degeneration? *Invest Ophthalmol Vis Sci.* 2007;48(4):1472-1475.
39. Xu L, Li Y, Zheng Y, Jonas JB. Associated factors for age related maculopathy in the adult population in China: the Beijing eye study. *Br J Ophthalmol.* 2006;90(9):1087-1090. Epub 2006 Jun 14.
40. Montés-Micó R, Alió JL. Distance and near contrast sensitivity function after multifocal intraocular lens implantation. *J Cataract Refract Surg.* 2003;29(4):703-711.
41. Mester U, Hunold W, Wesendahl T, Kaymak H. Functional outcomes after implantation of Tecnis ZM900 and Array SA40 multifocal intraocular lenses. *J Cataract Refract Surg.* 2007;33(6):1033-1040.

Suggested Readings

Cionni RJ. Screening and counseling refractive IOL patients. In: Chang DF, ed. *Mastering Refractive IOLs. The Art and Science.* Thorofare, NJ: SLACK Incorporated; 2008.

Sokol S, Moskowitz A, Skarf B, Evans R, Molitch M, Senior B. Contrast sensitivity in diabetics with and without background retinopathy. *Arch Ophthalmol.* 1985;103(1):51-54.

Stavrou EP, Wood JM. Letter contrast sensitivity changes in early diabetic retinopathy. *Clin Exp Optom.* 2003;86(3):152-156.

9

Accommodative Intraocular Lenses

Lucio Buratto, MD; Stephen F. Brint, MD, FACS; and Domenico Boccuzzi, MD, PhD

Accommodative lenses are a potential solution for presbyopia. These lenses were developed to modify the patient's ability to focus; they theoretically use movements of the ciliary muscle that contracts during accommodation. There are basically 2 types of accommodative lenses: lenses with a single optic and lenses with 2 optics.

The Bausch + Lomb Crystalens and the Lenstec Tetraflex are lenses with a single optic; the group of lenses using 2 optics includes the Synchrony lens manufactured by AMO (Figure 9-1).

These lenses are accommodative through displacement of the z axis of the lens itself. However, the degree of accommodation differs from lens to lens. This factor (degree of accommodation) depends on the dioptric power of the moving lens. If we compare 2 Crystalens lenses, with equal excursion, the lens with the greater dioptric power will have greater accommodative power.

In lenses with "dual optic" technology such as the Synchrony, accommodative capacity is greater compared to lenses with a single optic, and it is always the same and repeatable. This second type of lens has an anterior optic of diameter 5.5 mm with a high positive spherical power (+32 D) that, in theory, is capable of accommodation of +2.5 D.

Compared to the multifocal diffractive (eg, Tecnis or ReSTOR), in theory this type of lens does not cause a reduction in contrast sensitivity or lead to the appearance of haloes or glare around light sources. However, they cannot produce the same near vision quality because of reduced accommodative excursion (max +1.5 D) possible with this type of lens.

Crystalens

One possible solution for correcting presbyopia is the accommodative Crystalens. These lenses were developed to attempt reproduction of the physiological process of accommodation, through a mechanism of variable geometry induced by the contraction of the ciliary muscle.

The first accommodative Crystalens was introduced in 2003—model AT-45. Unfortunately, because of the flexible nature of this lens and the reduced size of the optic (4.5 mm), it caused pathological contractions of the capsular bag, with an abnormal position of the lens inside the eye, changes in the refraction, and loss of accommodative ability. For these reasons, it was necessary to create a new platform and the Crystalens AT-50, known as "Five-Zero" was launched in November 2006 (Figure 9-2).

The latest model of the Crystalens is called HD. It is the logical evolution of the previous model, with technical characteristics that are very similar to the Five-Zero; it has a central button of diameter 1.5 mm; it is hyperprolate with negative spherical aberration that can create pseudo-accommodation, and it can also provide positive addition for near vision.

The Crystalens HD is an innovative development in the process of postoperative presbyopia, as its mechanism can imitate the physiological action of the natural lens eliminating haloes and glare that appear with refractive and diffractive multifocal lenses.

In January 2010, Bausch + Lomb released the latest Crystalens, the model AO (Aberration Zero).

Buratto L, Brint SF, Boccuzzi D.
Cataract Surgery and Intraocular Lenses (pp 73-78).

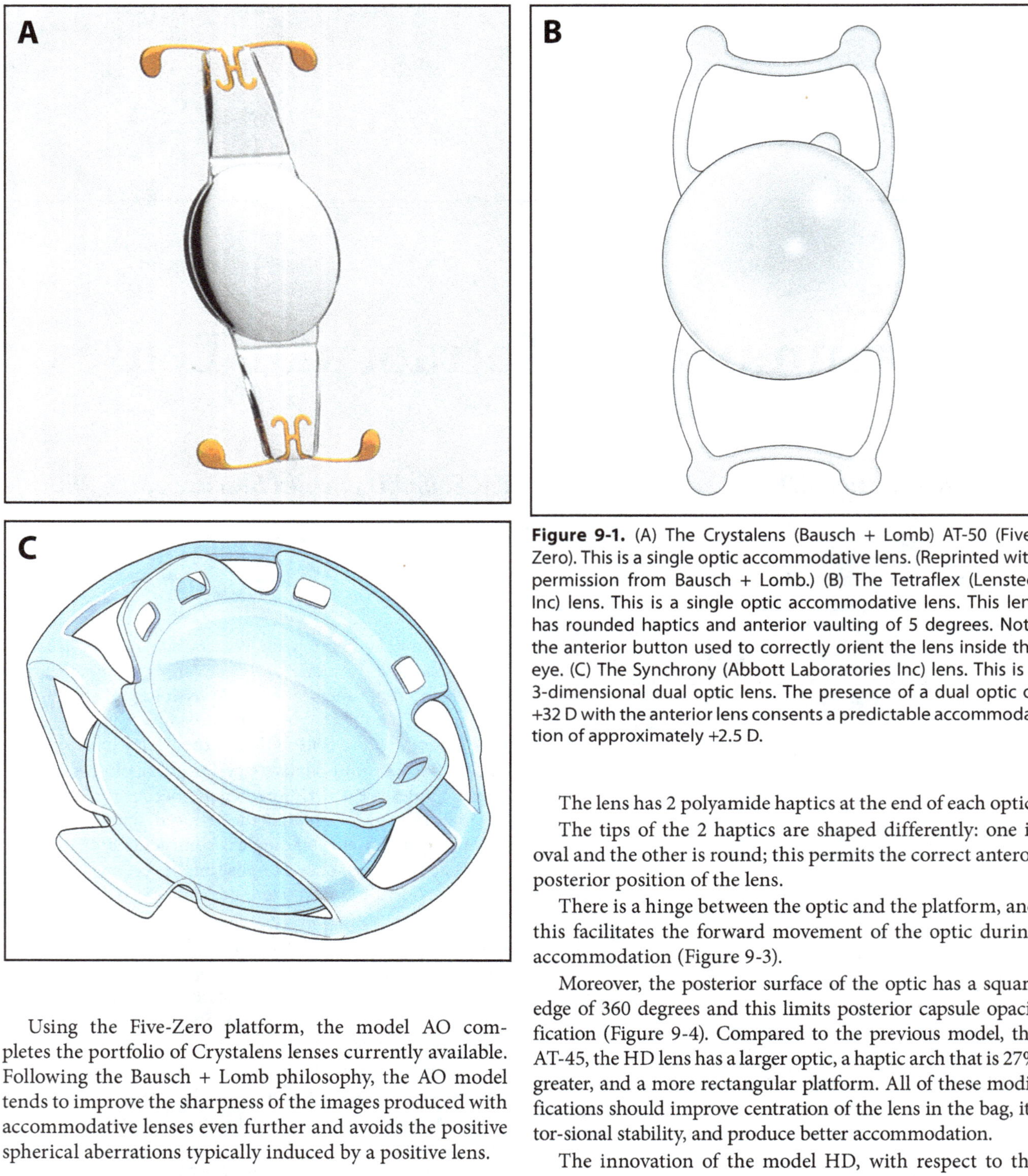

Figure 9-1. (A) The Crystalens (Bausch + Lomb) AT-50 (Five-Zero). This is a single optic accommodative lens. (Reprinted with permission from Bausch + Lomb.) (B) The Tetraflex (Lenstec, Inc) lens. This is a single optic accommodative lens. This lens has rounded haptics and anterior vaulting of 5 degrees. Note the anterior button used to correctly orient the lens inside the eye. (C) The Synchrony (Abbott Laboratories Inc) lens. This is a 3-dimensional dual optic lens. The presence of a dual optic of +32 D with the anterior lens consents a predictable accommodation of approximately +2.5 D.

Using the Five-Zero platform, the model AO completes the portfolio of Crystalens lenses currently available. Following the Bausch + Lomb philosophy, the AO model tends to improve the sharpness of the images produced with accommodative lenses even further and avoids the positive spherical aberrations typically induced by a positive lens.

Characteristics

The Crystalens HD and the AO are lenses produced using a third-generation silicone, called Biosil; this material has a high refractive index (1.427). The diameter of the optic is 5.0 mm, and the loop-loop distance is 11.5 mm for the HD 500 (range +17.0 to +33.0 D, step 0.5 D) and 120 mm for the HD 520 (range +10.0 to +16.5 D, step 0.5 D).

The lens has 2 polyamide haptics at the end of each optic.

The tips of the 2 haptics are shaped differently: one is oval and the other is round; this permits the correct antero-posterior position of the lens.

There is a hinge between the optic and the platform, and this facilitates the forward movement of the optic during accommodation (Figure 9-3).

Moreover, the posterior surface of the optic has a square edge of 360 degrees and this limits posterior capsule opacification (Figure 9-4). Compared to the previous model, the AT-45, the HD lens has a larger optic, a haptic arch that is 27% greater, and a more rectangular platform. All of these modifications should improve centration of the lens in the bag, its tor-sional stability, and produce better accommodation.

The innovation of the model HD, with respect to the previous Five-Zero version, is the presence of the hyperprolate central button of diameter 1.5 mm that acts as a positive spheric addition.

Under conditions of accommodative miosis, this polyspheric profile increases the negative spherical aberration, a powerful pseudoaccommodative factor.

According to the theories presented by Helmholz, Tscherning, and Schachar,[1] the contraction of the ciliary

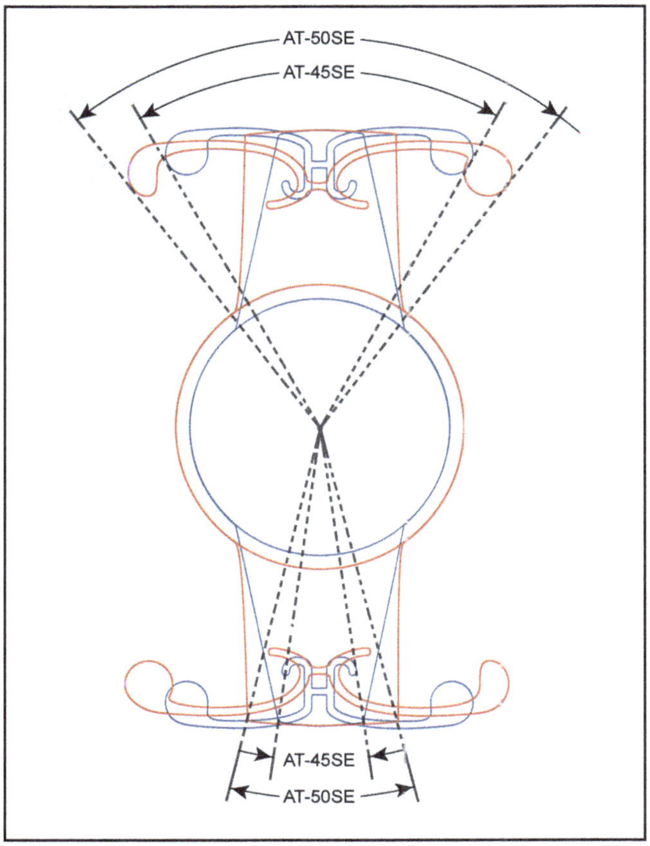

Figure 9-2. The photo illustrates the differences between the first model of the Crystalens (4.5) and the 5.0 platform. The first fundamental difference lies with the difference in the diameter of the optics that shifts from 4.5 to 5 mm. Beyond these measurements, even the span of the haptics is larger with a maximum diameter of 11.5 mm and an increase in the loop angle of 27%. All of these changes lead to a more stable lens position, and this results from 90% of the length of the junction plate of the haptics and 17% more contact surface between the optic of the lens, the junction plate, and the capsular bag.

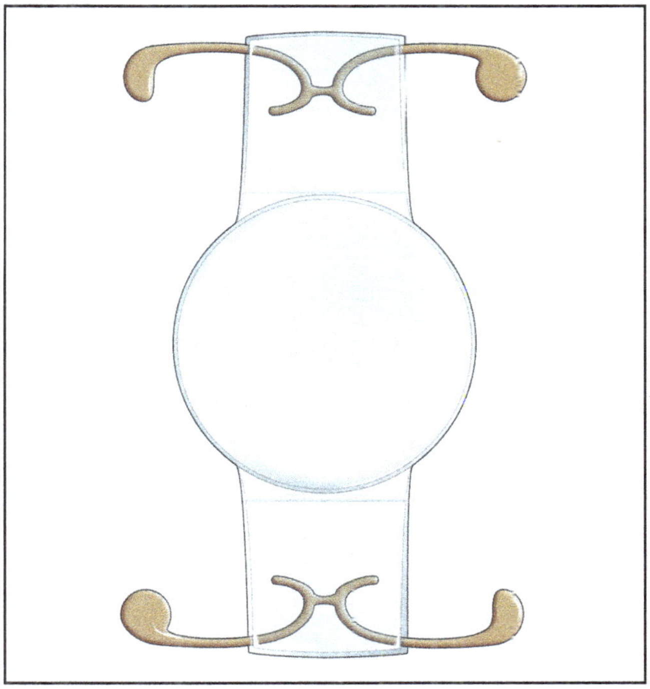

Figure 9-3. Crystalens 5.0. The tips of the 2 haptics have different shapes: one is oval and the other is round, and this facilitates the correct orientation of the lens inside the capsular bag.

muscle during accommodation causes the zonular fibers and the capsular bag to relax, allowing the lens to move forward. This movement produces the effect of accommodation because the effective power of the lens increases. Moreover, studies by Waltz[2] showed that during accommodation, the central optic of the lens is curved, increasing the accommodative effect of the lens.

Patient Selection

Candidate selection for implantation of the Crystalens is not difficult; however, there are some basic rules that must be followed to ensure a good postoperative outcome.

As with all the premium lenses that require a period of postoperative adaptation, it is essential that the surgeon and his or her assistants carefully explain the advantages and drawbacks of this lens.

Even under these circumstances, patients who have had ocular trauma, previous eye surgery, corneal pathologies, and macular degeneration are not ideal candidates for this type of lens.

Corneal astigmatism is an important limitation. Patients with preoperative corneal astigmatism greater than 1 D must be clearly informed that refractive laser surgery may be necessary to correct the residual astigmatism (to be performed some months later when the refraction is stable). The lens has recently been released in a toric version. Because of its design, this type of lens does not lead to the formation of haloes. However, patients with a large pupil diameter (>5.0 mm) under scotopic or photopic conditions may notice diffraction of the light at the flat edge of the lens (optic diameter of 5.0 mm.)

An evaluation of the patient's psychological status is essential for correct selection of the candidate. Patients who demonstrate obsessive or excessively perfectionist personality traits may not fully appreciate the benefits of the Crystalens implant. Moreover, it is essential that the surgeon explain to the patient that the lens can produce accommodation of approximately 1.5 D. This means that distance and intermediate vision should be excellent; however, reading small print will normally require spectacles.

Selection of the Power of the Intraocular Lens

Special attention must be paid to the selection of the lens power. First of all, the surgeon must perform accurate biometry, using the IOL Master (Carl Zeiss Meditec) or

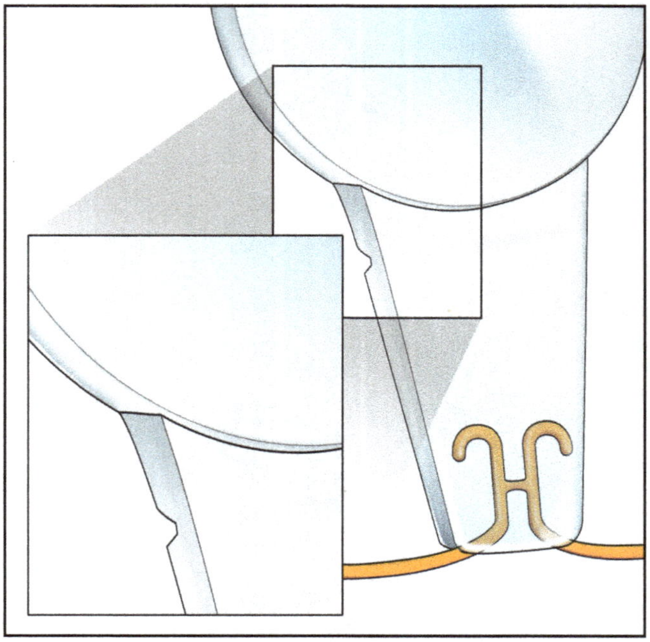

Figure 9-4. High-magnification image of the Crystalens showing the square-edge design of 360 degrees.

A-scan immersion biometry in patients for whom interferometric measurements do not provide reliable data because of the density of the cataract or dense posterior subcapsular opacities.

One strategy is to implant a lens attempting a residual refractive error of –0.50 D in the nondominant eye. The surgeon must check the postoperative refraction, and if he or she has been able to achieve this refractive result, he or she should implant a lens that will produce emmetropia in the fellow eye.

Small degrees of anisometropia will not compromise distance vision; fusion will be good, and intermediate and near vision will improve.

The decision to implant a lens in the nondominant eye first allows the surgeon to enhance the result in the case of unexpected refractive error, to produce good distance vision with the dominant eye, and to reduce the need for spectacles.

Synchrony

The accommodation of a single-optic accommodative intraocular lens (IOL) is based on the displacement of the optic along the z axis, in other words along the anteroposterior axis of the eye, and is directly proportional to the dioptric power of the displaced lens.

Synchrony is a foldable 1-piece silicone lens with 2 optics: an anterior mobile optic with a high positive power (+32.0 D), combined with hinges; and a fixed posterior lens with negative power that varies on the basis of the patient's biometry.

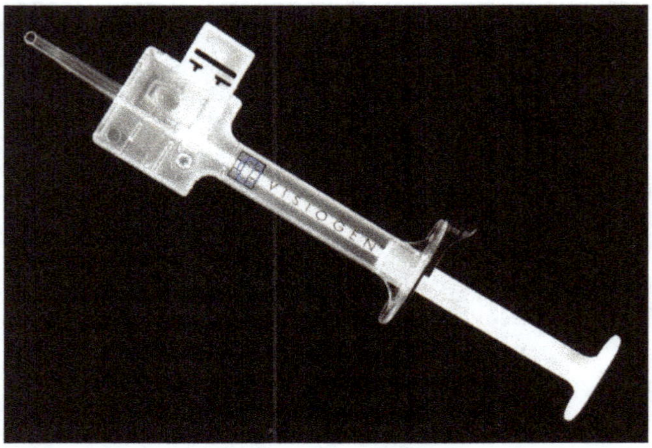

Figure 9-5. Preloaded injector for the Synchrony accommodative IOL. (Reprinted with permission from Ossma IL, Galvis A. Visiogen Synchrony—clinical pearls. In: Chang DF, ed. *Mastering Refractive IOLs: The Art and Science.* Thorofare, NJ: SLACK Incorporated; 2008.)

Once it has been implanted inside the capsular bag, the tension of the capsular bag determines the compression of the lens so that the 2 optics are close together. The compression of the 2 optics creates elastic energy in the joining hinges. Under accommodative stimulus, zonular relaxation will release the tension in the capsular bag, releasing the energy accumulated and permitting the forward displacement of the anterior optic. This process modifies the focal point of the lens and allows accommodation of up to 2.5 D.

The anterior optic of the lens is coupled with the aqueous and stretches the anterior bag; the openings facilitate the continuous passage of fluids and this avoids contact between the anterior capsule and the optic, leading to fibrosis.

Biocompatibility studies have demonstrated rare episodes of fibrosis and contraction of the capsular bag.

The lens is introduced into the eye using a preloaded injector through an incision measuring 3.7 mm. This eliminates manipulation of the lens and removes any risk of lens contamination (Figure 9-5).

Technical Features

Synchrony is a 1-piece silicone lens with 2 optics (n = 1.43); the diameter of the anterior optic is 5.5 mm with a power of +32.0 D, and the diameter of the posterior optic is 6.0 mm with a variable negative power. The 2 optics are connected by flexible hinges. The lens measures 9.8 mm on the horizontal axis and 9.5 mm on the vertical axis.

This lens also includes a series of features that have specific roles to allow the movement of the lens itself:

- Canals for the aqueous
- Posterior wings
- Separators
- Mobile haptics

The canals for the aqueous provide anterior support for the capsular bag, maintaining the anterior capsule under tension and encouraging liquid flow through the various openings in the lens. These avoid chafing and adhesion between the anterior capsule and the IOL. The posterior wings allow the IOL to be positioned correctly and compensate for any variations in the size of the capsular bag while avoiding decentration of the IOL.

The separators create the correct distance between the optics during emmetropia, avoiding adhesion between the 2 optics.

Finally, the mobile loops allow the system to open, allowing the right degree of separation between the optics.

The lens possesses the technical features of a Galilean optical system, with 2 optics: a fixed one with negative power and a mobile anterior one of known power +32.0 D. The combination of the 2 optics will magnify the images and produce accommodation of 2.5 D. The variation of the dioptric power (ΔDc) produced by the shift (Δs) is proportional to the dioptric power of the optic that moves (Dm).

$\Delta Dc = (Dm/13)\Delta s$

A shift of 0.78 mm induces accommodation of 2.5 D.[3-5]

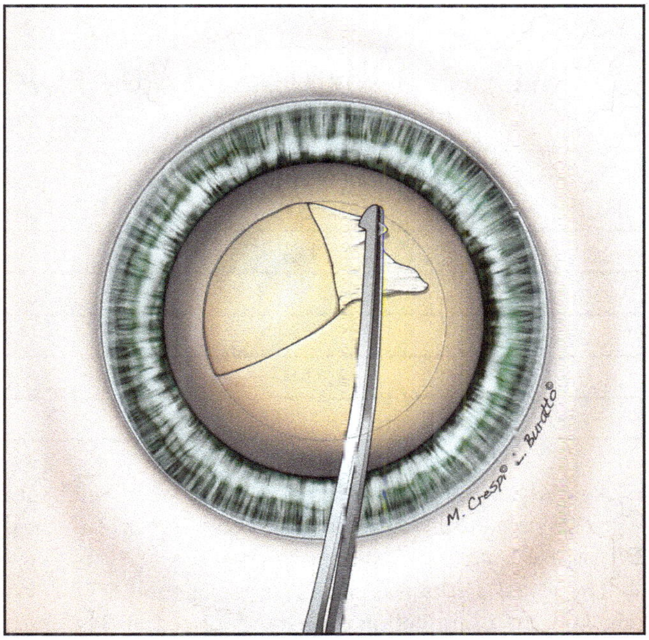

Figure 9-6. Continuous circular anterior rhexis, using a corneal marker as a guide.

Choice of Patient

The performance of the Synchrony lens is closely correlated with the patient's ability to use the ciliary muscle, and this results in movement of the anterior optic that modifies the focal point of the lens.

Consequently, patients with alterations of the zonular apparatus, pseudoexfoliation, Marfan's syndrome, homocystinuria, Weill-Marchesani, Ehlers-Danlos, sulphite oxidase deficiency, aniridia, traumatic cataract associated with zonular damage, etc, should be excluded from surgery. Moreover, as with other premium IOLs, the performance of the lenses is optimized when they are implanted bilaterally.

It should be pointed out that the mixing and matching option available with other types of premium multifocal lenses is not possible with the Synchrony. As will be explained later, the mechanism of action of the Synchrony is based on the combination of 2 lenses. The optical system, comparable to a Galilean telescope, can provide a degree of image magnification that may generate aniseikonia if implanted in combination with other "single-optic" IOLs.

Surgical Suggestions

For the Synchrony to maximize its characteristics, a series of events are essential during surgery.

- The rhexis must be well centered with a variable diameter of between 4.5 and 5.5 mm (Figure 9-6).
- The zonular apparatus must be perfectly functional (avoid implanting the lens when small dehiscences of the zonular apparatus are seen).
- The anterior and posterior capsules must be accurately cleaned.
- The posterior capsule must be intact.
- The lens must be fully unfolded in the capsular bag.
- All of the viscoelastic substance must be carefully removed.
- The lens should not be implanted in patients with high astigmatism.

An incision of 3.7 mm must be managed by the surgeon with the use of a suture to regulate and limit astigmatism. Where possible, the incision should be created along the steep axis.

The decision to implant a PC-IOL must be dictated by the need to improve the patient's visual performance, allowing independence from spectacles for distance, intermediate, and near vision. The disadvantage of the diffractive multifocal lenses is that they are dual focal; they provide good near and distance vision with intermediate vision that is not optimal. Patients implanted with this type of lens will often complain that they have visual problems at the computer. They have to change their position at the computer, by moving backward away from the screen or by sitting closer to it.

This problem can be solved if the patient uses a positive spectacle lens of approximately +1.50 D to approach the focal point of the distance lens and obtain optimal vision when seated at the computer.

The Synchrony Lens

The Synchrony has a different technology and can provide significantly better intermediate vision (50 to 80 cm) compared to multifocal lenses.

Table 9-1

Incidence of Haloes at 6 Months After Implantation With Four Different Presbyopia-Correcting Intraocular Lenses*

INCIDENCE	SYNCHRONY (N=31)	RESTOR (N=27)	REZOOM (N=28)	TECNIS MF (N=34)
Mild	2 (6.4%)	3 (11.1%)	5 (17.5%)	4 (11.8%)
Moderate	0	1 (3.7%)	0	2 (5.8%)
Severe	0	0	1 (3.5%)	0
Overall	2 (6.4%)	4 (14.8%)	6 (21%)	6 (17.6%)

*P=0.49 chi-square test.

A study was completed on 120 patients split into 4 groups (Synchrony, ReZoom, ReSTOR, Tecnis Multifocal Diffractive Lens).[6]

The visual acuity was measured using the EDTRS system and the illumination was standardized at 85 cd/m^2, measuring visual acuity at distances between 30 cm to 4 m.

Patients implanted with the Synchrony accommodative IOL showed the best intermediate visual acuity (between 50 and 80 cm) with statistically significant values.

The speed of photopic reading between the Synchrony accommodative IOL and the other multifocal IOLs was superimposable. Under mesopic conditions, on the other hand, speed was greater for the Synchrony and the Tecnis lenses compared to the ReZoom and the ReSTOR.[6]

Contrast Sensitivity

Because of their mode of action, the diffractive and refractive multifocal lenses cause a reduction in contrast sensitivity of at least 50%. This is not seen with accommodative lenses, as the incident light is focused simultaneously on a single visual target.

A comparative study between the Synchrony, the ReSTOR, and the Alcon SA60AT (monofocal) lenses demonstrated that the Synchrony and the monofocal Alcon lenses had the same contrast sensitivity; it was reduced in the group of patients implanted with the ReSTOR lens.

Haloes and Glare

Haloes and glare are additional drawbacks associated with the implantation of the multifocal lens.

Frequently, patients will be reluctant to accept implantation of a multifocal IOL because the surgeon has explained the possible risk of haloes around light sources. In reality, this phenomenon is extremely subjective and the potential degree of patient dissatisfaction cannot be measured preoperatively. A number of factors—both psychological and anatomical—can affect this phenomenon. Undoubtedly, one of the important factors that determines the appearance of haloes is pupil kinetics: large pupils will undoubtedly be affected more than small pupils!

In comparison to the accommodative lenses, the diffractive shape of the lens is less important; this is responsible for the formation of haloes and glare around the lights.

Regarding the Synchrony lens, the haloes and glare are caused by the 3-dimensional shape of the lens and optic of diameter of 5.5 mm.

The incidence of haloes with Synchrony has been estimated at approximately 6.4% compared to incidences ranging between 14.8% and 21% with different multifocal technologies (Table 9-1).

Conclusion

When the Synchrony lens is implanted in both eyes, approximately 83% of patients enjoy independence from spectacles for distance, intermediate, and near vision.

Basically the Synchrony lens has a lower reduction in contrast sensitivity and formation of haloes that are characteristics of diffractive and refractive multifocal lenses.

References

1. Schachar RA, Bax AJ. Mechanism of human accommodation as analyzed by nonlinear finite element analysis. *Ann Ophthalmol.* 2001;33(2):103-112.
2. Waltz KL. Crystalens—what is the mechanism. *Mastering Refractive IOLs: The Art and Science.* Thorofare, NJ: SLACK Incorporated; 2008:186-188.
3. Mc Leod SD, Vargas LG, Portney V, Ting A. Synchrony dual-optic accommodating intraocular lens. *J Refract Surg.* 2007;33:37-46.
4. Smith WJ. Basic optical devices. In: Fischer RE, Smith WJ, eds. *Modern Optical Engineering: The Design and Optical Systems.* 2nd ed. New York, NY: McGraw-Hill; 1990:235-239.
5. Mc Leod SD. Optical principles, biomechanics, and initial clinical performance of a dual-optic accommodating intraocular lens. *Trans Am Ophthalmol Soc.* 2006;104:437-452.
6. Ossma IL, Galvis A. Binocular performance after implantation of multifocal and dual optic accommodating intraocular lens implantation. Presented in part at *The Annual Meeting European Society of Cataract and Refractive Surgery.* Stockholm, September 2007.

10

Mix and Match

Lucio Buratto, MD; Stephen F. Brint, MD, FACS; and Domenico Boccuzzi, MD, PhD

The surgeon elects to implant a multifocal lens to eliminate or at least decrease the use of spectacles. It is not always a success because no currently available lens can ensure good distance, near, and intermediate vision under all light conditions.

Refractive lenses (eg, the ReZoom) offer 3 focal points—distance, near, and intermediate. However, these lenses are pupil dependent, meaning that their action works well only in patients with good pupil kinetics. However, in these patients, the reduction in contrast sensitivity caused by these lenses is associated with poor vision under low light and dysphotopsias, in association with numerous focal points.

The diffractive lenses—ReSTOR (Alcon), AT LISA (Zeiss), ZMB00 (AMO)—differ from the previous ones as they have a different mechanism of action; under all lighting conditions and with any degree of pupil dilatation, they simultaneously split the light into a portion for distance and for near with different amounts for each type of lens. Diffractive lenses differ from refractive lenses in that they are dual or bifocal lenses with 2 focal points, one for distance and a second for near vision, with the focal distance dependent on the amount of addition of the lens. This innovation was deliberately developed for 3 main reasons:

1. To make the lens independent of pupil diameter
2. To reduce to minimum haloes associated with the simultaneous presence of multiple focal points
3. To avoid excessive light dispersion between the various focal points, a phenomenon that greatly reduces contrast sensitivity

Neither of these 2 lens types, therefore, can produce "optimal vision" under all lighting conditions; consequently, at the end of 2003, surgeons considered the possibility of combining 2 lenses, to use the characteristics of each one and offer good distance, intermediate, and near vision.

At that time, the diffractive lens available was the ReSTOR, and the refractive lenses available were the ReZoom and the Array. They caused haloes when implanted in both eyes; however, they provided good intermediate vision.

The Mix and Match procedure involved using different lenses to reduce to a minimum patient discomfort and improve vision under almost all conditions.

The trend was to combine a diffractive and a refractive lens. Typically, a diffractive lens was implanted in the dominant eye, allowing good distance vision and good near vision. In the nondominant eye, a refractive lens was typically implanted to improve intermediate vision. The refractive lens produced good intermediate vision; moreover, haloes were less obvious because the 3 focal points were perceived with less intensity when the lens was implanted in the nondominant eye.

This technique that involved the combination of 2 different lenses, a refractive and a diffractive, has been abandoned for a number of reasons:

- Currently, refractive lenses have limited success and surgeons are implanting them less frequently. This is because of their pupil-dependent mechanism of action, meaning that they are not suitable for all patients. Moreover, the fact that they have 3 focal points means that they cause glare and haloes, phenomena that are

Buratto L, Brint SF, Boccuzzi D.
Cataract Surgery and Intraocular Lenses (pp 79-81).

poorly tolerated, and the reduction in contrast sensitivity does not translate into good visual performance.

- The latest generation of diffractive lenses, with a pupil-independent mechanism, have less addition for near vision and discrete intermediate vision, due to depth of focus of the near image. Moreover, they are more tolerated by patients because they result in less dysphotopsia.
- Finally, surgeons came to the conclusion that 2 eyes that can see are clearly better than one. This phenomenon is known as *binocular summation*. Everyone knows that patients with monovision find reading easier when the fellow eye of the distance lens has been corrected for reading. When a diffractive lens (ReSTOR) and a refractive lens (Array or ReZoom) are implanted, a mismatch is created at the near focal vision and this interferes with the process of binocular summation at near. Patients with this choice will perceive the asymmetry. It is as though a sort of monovision has been created and this may be tolerated by the patient. However, introduction of multifocal lenses was developed because monovision was not well tolerated by all patients.

Mix and Match Today

The concept of Mix and Match arose from the need to combine different types of lenses with different mechanisms to try to fill the refractive gap left by a certain type of lens.

The current array of multifocal lenses includes well-known diffractive lenses, accommodative lenses (dual-optic and single-optic), and the more recent zonal lenses. The only combination viable at present is the association of a single optic accommodative lens (a Crystalens) and a diffractive lens (Alcon, AMO, or Zeiss). No other combination is possible, as other lenses would induce aniseikonia or mismatch of the images, interfering with vision without any advantage gained.

The objective was always to provide good distance vision and good quality intermediate and near vision. Two Crystalens implants provide good intermediate vision with poor near vision; the diffractive implants do not provide good intermediate vision, but give good-quality near vision.

This sounds very similar to monovision; both lenses produce excellent distance vision and differ only in terms of intermediate near vision.

The approach to this method of combining 2 types of lenses must begin with the patient's need for near and intermediate vision without requiring corrective lenses.

Mix and Match Quick Start

This type of surgery with premium intraocular lens (IOL) implants is based on an analysis of the patient's requirements and understanding the reasons he or she desires this choice.

First, for a correct Mix and Match, the surgeon must determine the dominant eye and implant the Crystalens in this eye. This lens produces excellent distance vision (because it is a "mobile" monofocal) not associated with a reduction in contrast sensitivity, haloes, or dysphotopsia and produces acceptable intermediate vision. The surgeon should implant this lens and aim to achieve emmetropia while simultaneously eliminating astigmatism. As the toric component was recently introduced, with preoperative astigmatism, it is necessary to plan refractive surgery with excimer laser to correct the residual cylinder or use the newer toric version. The nondominant eye should be implanted with a diffractive lens (Tecnis ZMB00, Zeiss AT LISA, or Alcon ReSTOR). The surgeon must pay attention to some factors when choosing between these 3 lenses. Firstly, he or she must check for corneal astigmatism. Currently, only the Alcon ReSTOR and the Zeiss AT LISA lenses are able to correct cylinder, while Tecnis will soon launch a toric multifocal lens. Moreover, it is essential to evaluate pupil kinetics and the visual needs the patient has for near vision. The ReSTOR is an apodized diffractive-refractive lens that has a near vision component that varies depending on the pupil diameter. Currently, the version D3 is being withdrawn; thus, the surgeon can consider implanting a D1 lens with an additional +3 D for near vision (not excessive); the visual proportion depends on the pupil diameter (small pupil, distribution 50-50).

A large photopic pupil is the only contraindication for implantation of the ReSTOR lens as this interferes with the action of the lens itself.

The Zeiss AT LISA is a full diffractive lens that has a distance-near distribution of 65%-35%, with an addition of +3.75 D.

The addition for near vision tends to compensate decreased contrast sensitivity that the lens provides for reading. Unfortunately, this type of lens does not provide good near vision with monocular implants.

The third choice is the Tecnis, a full diffractive lens with a uniform split (50-50) of distance-near visual amounts, with an addition of +4 D. It is undeniably the best for producing good near vision with a monocular implant, and now that it is available as a toric version, it can also correct any corneal astigmatism.

It should be pointed out that for distance vision, even though the 2 lenses are different, their visual performance can be summated; however, for near vision, each of the 2 lenses seems to work in mini-monovision for intermediate-near vision. This is why it is essential to correct even small degrees of astigmatism.

Can Mix and Match Be Performed With Monofocal Lenses?

Opting for monovision is a solution for near and distance vision, albeit a simplistic one. If the patient's preoperative refraction in one eye is good for distance vision and in the other eye it is good for near vision, continuing this should be considered to be effective. There will be no need to induce neuroadaptation, as the patient is already used to this.

The same applies if a myopic patient has already had cataract surgery in the first eye (with the implantation of a monofocal IOL), with emmetropia and good adaptation to monovision. Neuroadaptation will have occurred already.

A second situation is when the patient, already having had a cataract procedure with implantation of a monofocal IOL and good uncorrected distance vision, has special requirements for near vision and for intermediate vision.

Under these circumstances, the surgeon can implant an accommodative IOL in the second eye, aiming for a slightly myopic visual result. A monofocal IOL should be implanted in the dominant eye, and the accommodative lens implanted in the fellow eye. The residual myopia will provide good intermediate and good near vision in the nondominant eye with a slight loss of perfect distance vision.

A third possible solution applies to the patient who has had a cataract procedure in one eye with the implantation of a monofocal IOL. Distance vision is good; however, the patient also requires good intermediate and near vision without corrective spectacles. A multifocal lens can also be implanted in the fellow eye. If the patient spends prolonged periods at the computer, seated at an intermediate distance with minor reading requirements, and good pupil kinetics, the ReZoom could prove to be an optimal choice.

If the patient requires good intermediate vision when there are poor pupil kinetics, the surgeon should opt for a diffractive IOL; under these circumstances, the choice should be the ReSTOR with a +3 D addition for near vision. This version of the ReSTOR will produce good pupil-independent intermediate vision and fairly good near vision. The AT LISA may also provide a good solution under these circumstances.

If the patient requires good near vision, the surgeon should opt for the Tecnis ZMB00 or the ReSTOR +4 D. These lenses provide good near vision with poor intermediate vision.

Suggested Readings

Pepose JS. Mixing versus matching IOLs. *Cataract Refract Surg Today.* 2007;August:65-67.

Woodhams JT. Combining the Crystalens and the AcrySof ReSTOR IOLs. *Cataract Refract Surg Today.* 2007;August:53-55.

11

Refractive Cataract Surgery

Lucio Buratto, MD; Stephen F. Brint, MD, FACS; and Domenico Boccuzzi, MD, PhD

In view of what has been discussed, it is seen that scientific progress and techniques have developed in the field of cataract surgery and it has become easier to understand how patient expectations of the past no longer apply to those of the present.

In the past, the patient would have been satisfied with the recovery of vision, and accept that he or she would still require thick spectacle lenses; in today's world, the patient not only expects visual recovery but also a complete elimination of the need for spectacles to correct any refractive errors and possibly for near vision.

This is now possible due to ongoing research in the field of cataract surgery.

Currently, cataract surgery is no longer considered to be a procedure to restore some degree of vision in patients on the verge of total blindness; this surgery is now an opportunity for correcting visual and refractive errors, improving the quality of the patient's vision, and greatly improving his or her quality of life.

All of this is possible due to newer and safer phaco equipment. These instruments allow surgical procedures to be performed through increasingly small incisions; biometry and new formulas provide very accurate information for increasingly reliable calculations of intraocular lens (IOL) power; topography allows extremely precise measurement of corneal astigmatism, important information when planning incisions used in surgeries; the latest generation of IOLs can correct spherical errors, cylinder, and reduce optical (usually spherical) aberrations; and finally, the use of the new femtolasers will soon be widespread and will allow the creation of perfect incisions and a precisely centered rhexis of the desired diameter.

Over the past decades, and particularly in the past 5 years, surgical techniques and the approach to surgery have been completely revolutionized.

All these procedures are now possible but not always straightforward.

With the implantation of a presbyopia-correcting IOL, the surgeon must theoretically aim for emmetropia (if this was the desired objective); however, it is not always possible to achieve this desired result for a number of reasons:

- There may be a biometry error caused by imprecise measurement of the axial length; this occurs largely with posterior subcapsular cataracts or because of alterations in the posterior pole of the eye.
- There may be a biometry error due to imprecise calculation of Ks (the mean K value measured by biometry is not always reliable). It is essential that the surgeon compare these measurements with those obtained from topography and also take into consideration any irregular astigmatism. This is particularly important in the decision to implant a multifocal toric IOL. It should be remembered that any error in the calculation of the K value will have a directly proportional 1:1 effect on the calculation of the IOL; an error in the calculation of K of 0.5 D will correspond to a 0.5 D residual error.
- The wrong choice of formula for the calculation of the IOL. The calculation should not be based on the application of a single formula; the surgeon should always compare the results of several formulas to check

Buratto L, Brint SF, Boccuzzi D.
Cataract Surgery and Intraocular Lenses (pp 83-89).

agreement of the results. For myopic eyes, the surgeon should use the Holladay and the Haigis formulas. For hyperopic eyes, he or she should use the Hoffer Q.

- Previous refractive surgery procedures (myopic or hyperopic). It is worth noting that there there are numerous formulas that allow the minimization of the residual refractive error in eyes with previous myopic refractive surgery; however, there is no such formula available for hyperopic eyes, and consequently the calculation is only empirical!
- There is also the effect of factors such as abnormalities in the size of the capsular bag (that will lead to errors in the calculation of the effective lens position [(ELP)] with a risk of residual hyperopia of up to 2 D).

This can occur when the lens is positioned in a more posterior position than expected, altering the IOL power calculated by the formulas.

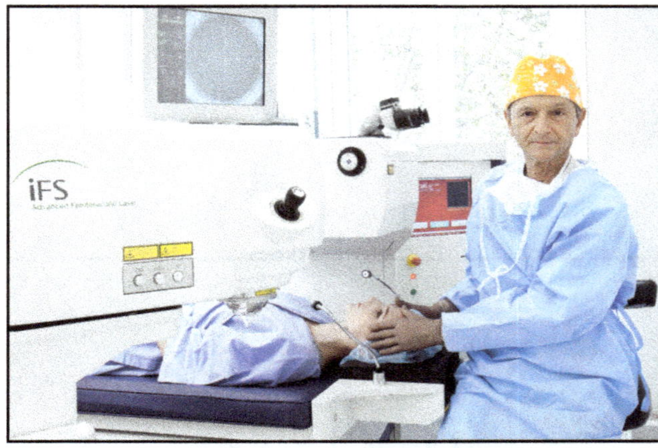

Figure 11-1. The risk of residual refractive is not acceptable for patients implanted with a premium IOL. For this reason, it is necessary to offer the patient a laser vision correction package that allows the correction of any residual defect using a laser procedure.

Biometry Errors: Correction Methods

A refractive error following the implantation of an IOL will be obvious soon after surgery and almost always during the first postoperative exam. The importance of the problem must be calculated on the basis of the refractive error and patient's expectations.

Patients who have undergone previous surgery to improve their refractive errors are more sensitive to this type of complication.

Under these circumstances, one should measure the residual refractive error and any decision regarding corrective treatment should be postponed until surgery has been performed in the fellow eye and after having examined the results of the binocular vision.

Sometimes, mild errors, particularly if they involve the nondominant eye, will have limited importance in binocular vision and can be ignored.

The postoperative complication of an incorrect IOL may be an indication for secondary surgery with a laser technique, a piggyback IOL, or lens exchange.

The refractive error may be based on an error of calculation, a flaw in the manufacture of the IOL, or incorrect positioning of the IOL; however, it is due to a condition of the eye that does not allow correct collection of information that is used to calculate the refractive error.

This situation is frequently seen in patients post keratorefractive surgery (eg, radial keratotomy, photorefractive keratectomy [PRK], LASIK); it is also seen in patients post lamellar or perforating keratoplasty or in patients with severe myopia and alterations of the posterior pole.[1,2]

Alterations in the post corneal surgery corneal curvature will influence the accuracy of the IOL power and can translate into a significant refractive error.

Generally speaking, eyes having had myopic corneal surgery are prone to a hyperopic refractive error; vice versa, eyes that have been steepened to correct a hyperopic error may show a myopic shift.

Bioptics

In refractive cataract surgery, when the surgical objective is to create a precise refractive error, it is essential to inform the patient on the possibility of a laser vision correction "fine-tuning" package. This offers the patient a complete package that may include a refractive laser treatment. The patient must be informed that the target result can sometimes only be achieved with a second refractive surgery to fine-tune or perfect the outcome (Figure 11-1).[3-5]

In the majority of cases, the 2 objectives are emmetropia with the implantation of a presbyopia-correcting IOL, and a residual myopic refraction that will allow patients to read comfortably or perform activities at near, without the need for spectacles.

This means complete elimination (or compensation) of the spherical errors, and more importantly, the cylinder, responsible for the loss of visual quality.

The decision for any treatment should always be postponed until after the implantation of an IOL in the fellow eye. In many cases, when the refractive error is small, binocular compensation will tend to minimize the problem, resulting in good patient satisfaction.

Refractive stability is essential before laser treatment for the correction of residual refractive errors can be performed. Consequently, the surgeon must wait 1 to 3 months after surgery—the time required for perfect closure of the surgical incisions.

In the rare cases in which bioptics is scheduled along with the cataract procedure, the flap with the femtolaser (or with the microkeratome) may be created prior to surgery;

the flap should be lifted and closed until the refractive treatment is performed post cataract procedure. The flap requires high levels of suction and creating it before the cataract procedure is recommended because the surgical incisions can open under high negative pressure (suction).

Bioptics may be necessary under some specific circumstances, for example:

- Posterior subcapsular cataracts with imprecise calculation of the IOL
- Residual cylinder defects that cannot be completely corrected with toric IOLs (eg, astigmatism greater than 3 D and the need to implant a ReSTOR Toric that does not cover these cylinder values)
- A risk of spherical or sphere-cylindrical errors for patients with severe myopia or severe hyperopia implanted with multifocal IOLs that do not allow such values

Moreover, a series of examinations are essential.

Firstly, the surgeon must ensure that corneal thickness is suitable for a refractive treatment. LASIK or better still iLASIK with the femtosecond laser is the elective technique. If the cornea is thin, it is possible to use PRK; however, this can cause considerable discomfort for the patient initially and rehabilitation times are considerably longer. This may also disappoint the patient. As in all laser procedures, it is necessary that topography is performed to exclude pathologies such as keratoconus or pellucid marginal degeneration and avoid the risk of postoperative ectasia (Figures 11-2 and 11-3).

The eye must be examined carefully; blepharitis and poorly positioned eyelids must be treated, to avoid dry eye syndrome, keratitis, and keratopathies from malocclusion; all of the indications and the contraindications of the standard LASIK procedure must be followed.

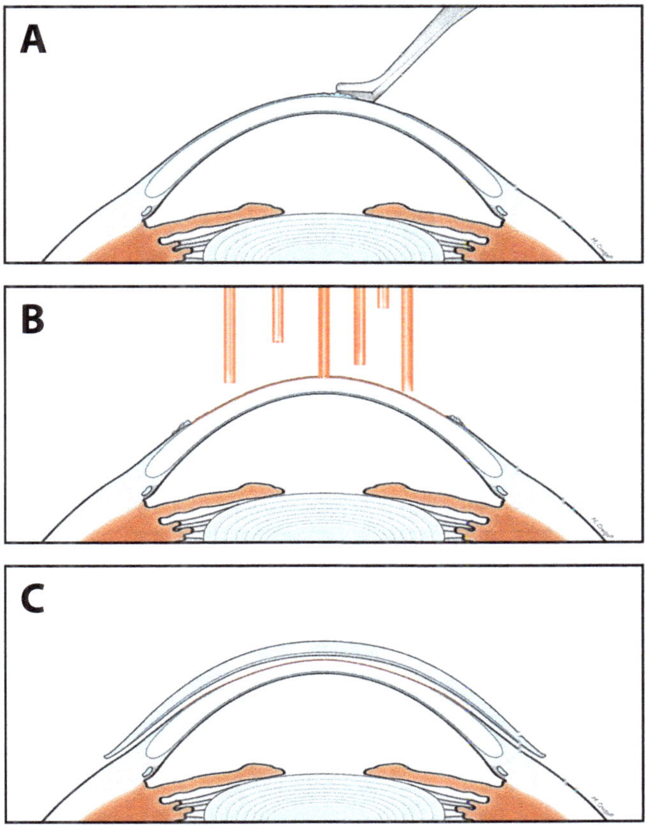

Figure 11-2. PRK method. Following the de-epithelialization (A), the surgeon performs a laser treatment on the anterior stromal surface (B). At the end of the procedure, the eye is protected with contact lens (C) that the surgeon will remove 4 or 5 days after surgery, depending on the degree of corneal re-epithelialization.

Guidelines for a Laser Refractive Procedure in Pseudophakic Eyes

1. The surgeon should wait between 1 and 3 months from cataract surgery and removal of the sutures. This interval is necessary to ensure stable refraction.
2. Dry eye syndrome that may appear following cataract surgery must be treated.
3. The posterior capsule must be clear.
4. The surgeon must perform appropriate preoperative tests to confirm that the laser procedure will result in an improvement in uncorrected visual acuity of at least 2 Snellen lines.
5. Corneal topography should demonstrate the absence of corneal pathologies and defects that could lead to ectasia and other problems.
6. The surgeon must ensure that pachymetry is sufficient and appropriate for the planned treatment.
7. The cornea must be transparent with an endothelial cell count of at least 1800 cell/ mm^2.
8. The fundus should be normal, and the intraccular pressure should be within normal limits.
9. The patient should not have any eye surgery procedures between the cataract operation and the laser treatment.

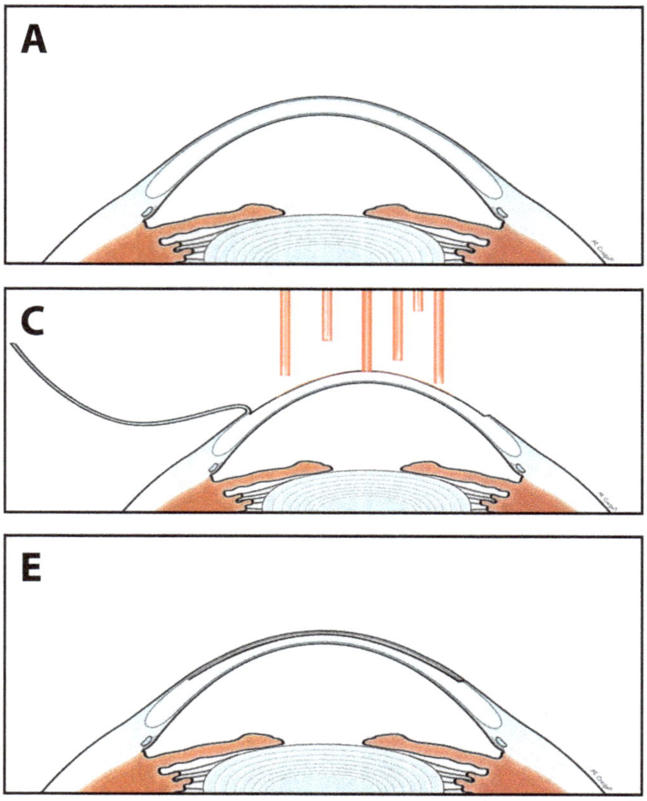

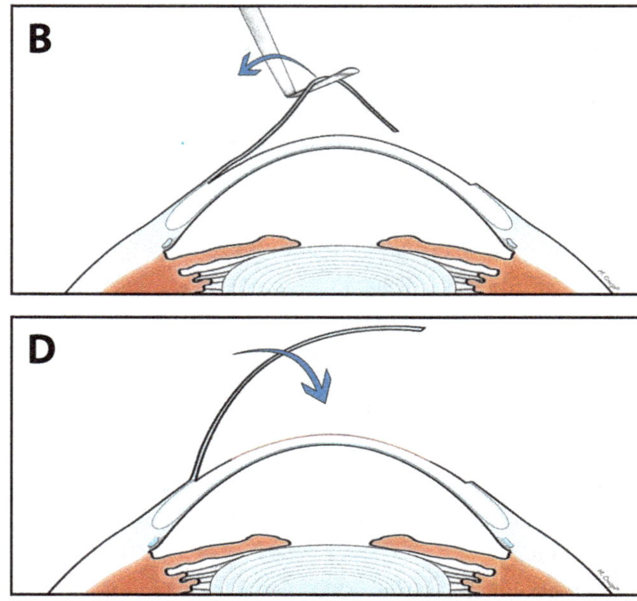

Figure 11-3. LASIK–iLASIK methods. (A, B) Irrespective of whether the cut is performed with a surgical blade (microkeratome) or using a laser (femtosecond laser), the surgeon creates a corneal flap consisting of epithelium and part of the stroma (generally 110 µm, but this figure is variable). (C) The surgeon performs the corrective laser treatment for myopia and astigmatism on the residual stroma. (D, E) At the end of the procedure, the flap is repositioned. The advantages of this procedure are the shorter postoperative recovery time and the very low degree of associated pain and irritation.

If laser correction of the refractive error occurs months or years after an implant, the surgeon must carefully examine the eye for any opacity of the posterior capsule as this can interfere with aberrometry and precise refraction (Figure 11-4). So with partial or total opacity, the surgeon should use the yttrium-aluminum-garnet (YAG) laser.

With excimer laser treatment, when there are residual bilateral errors, it is preferable to treat both eyes in the same session to reduce stress for the patient (who will undergo one procedure instead of 2); this will also avoid an excessive number of postops, reducing the time required for postoperative medical treatment.

Piggyback

Residual refractive errors can also be corrected by implanting a piggyback IOL. This option should be considered with caution for a number of reasons.

If multifocal lenses are implanted, the superimposition of a second lens will reduce contrast sensitivity further; this will have already decreased through the use of the multifocal lenses. It may also limit the excursions of the optic of accommodative lenses.

In any case, any decentration of the piggyback lens with respect to the lens implanted in the bag would induce higher-order aberrations because of lenses shifting.

If it is not possible to exchange the lens that was previously implanted because of partial rhexis escape, posterior capsular rhexis, fragile zonules, cystoid macular edema that appears after the first procedure, a long time interval between the primary implant, and the potential exchange, the surgeon should select a specific piggyback lens and not use an acrylic 3-piece lens for implantation in the posterior chamber. This is because piggyback lenses have been designed with a posterior meniscus that fits into the anterior convex surface of the lens. Moreover, the overall diameter of these lenses (including the haptics) is larger than the diameter of traditional lenses for bag implantation; this improves the centration. Finally, the lenses are produced in a hydrophilic acrylic material that is different from the hydrophobic acrylic lenses used for the vast majority of lenses for implantation in the bag (this will improve the compatibility between the 2 lenses).

Three-piece lenses for implantation in the bag are designed with a biconvex shape (meaning that both the anterior and the posterior surfaces are convex); the posterior convexity will automatically position itself in an eccentric position with respect to the first lens, as the anterior surface is also convex. Moreover, greater degrees of decentration (ie, beyond the pupil margin) create formation of higher-order aberrations (eg, coma, which under these circumstances can reach high levels), further compromising the refractive result (Figure 11-5).

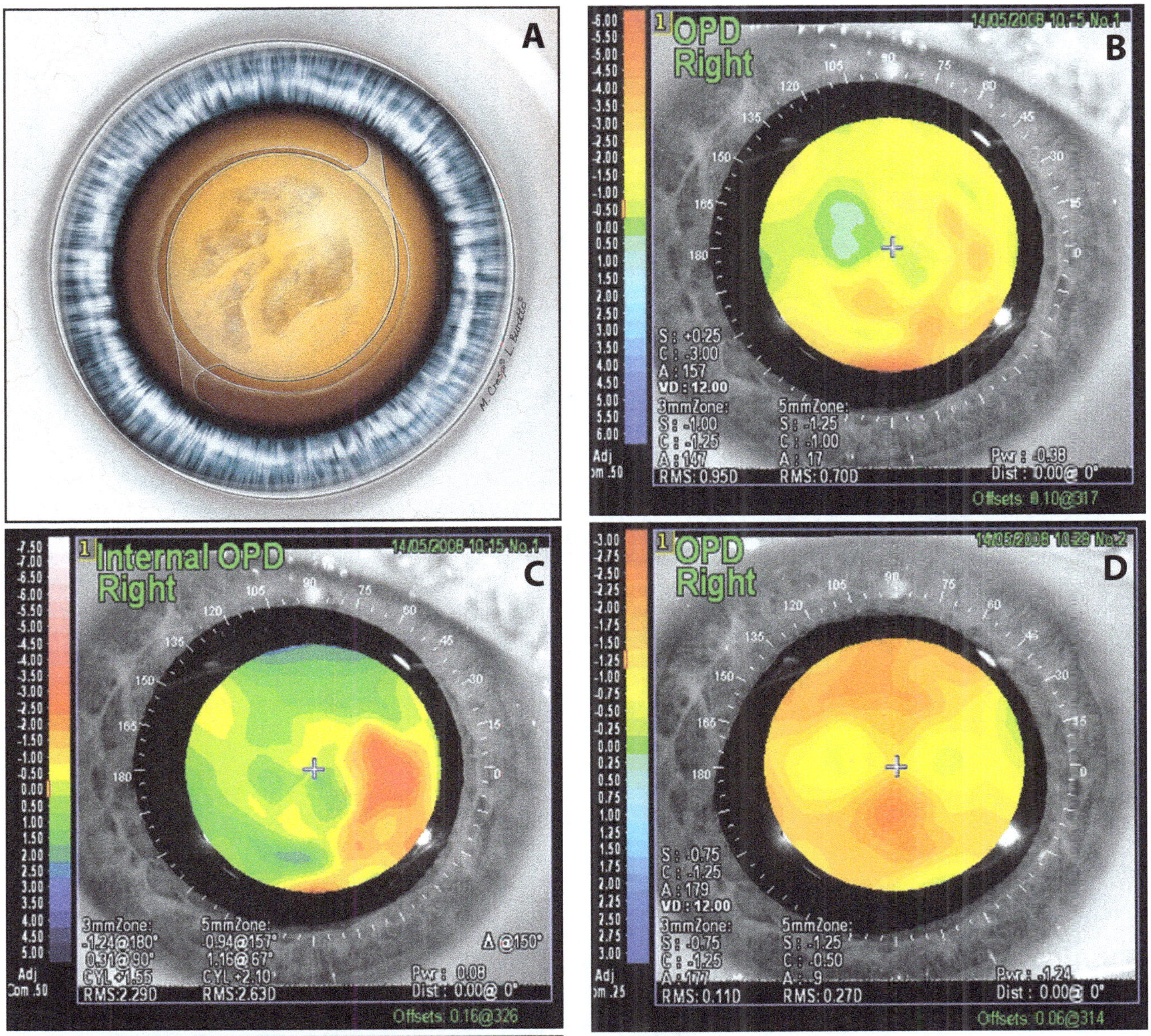

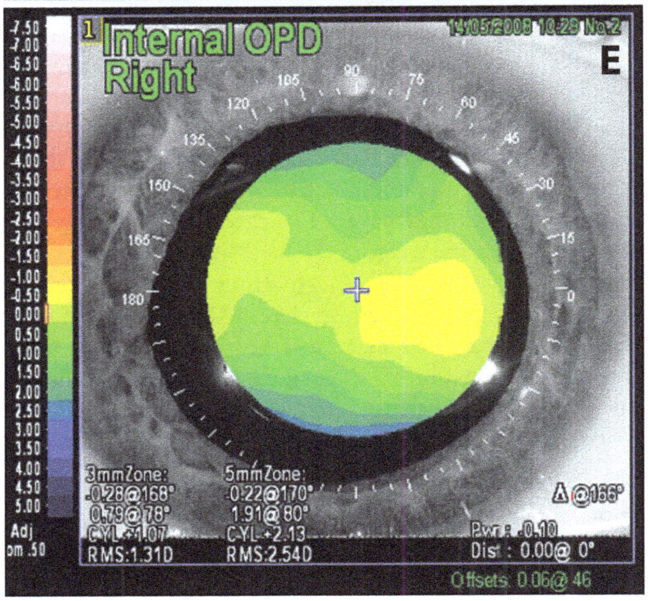

Figure 11-4. (A) Secondary opacity of the posterior capsule reduces the transparency of the optic media. (B) The total aberrometry and (C) the internal aberrometry in a patient affected with a secondary cataract. Opacification of the capsule can lead to the appearance of false astigmatism and important deformation of the wavefront. (D) The total and (E) internal aberrometry in the same patient following the YAG laser capsulotomy procedure. Between the pre- and postoperative situations there has been an important change in the refraction with a reduction in the astigmatism, induced by secondary opacities of the capsule. (Figures B-E are reprinted with permission from Dr. V. Orfeo.)

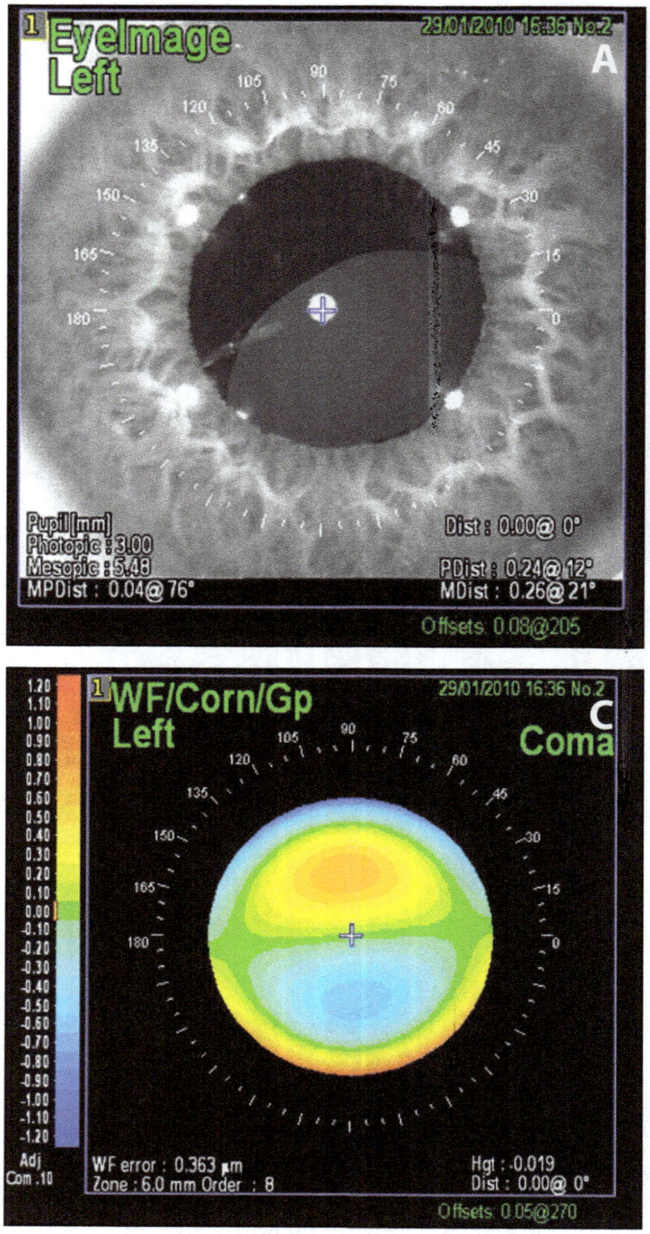

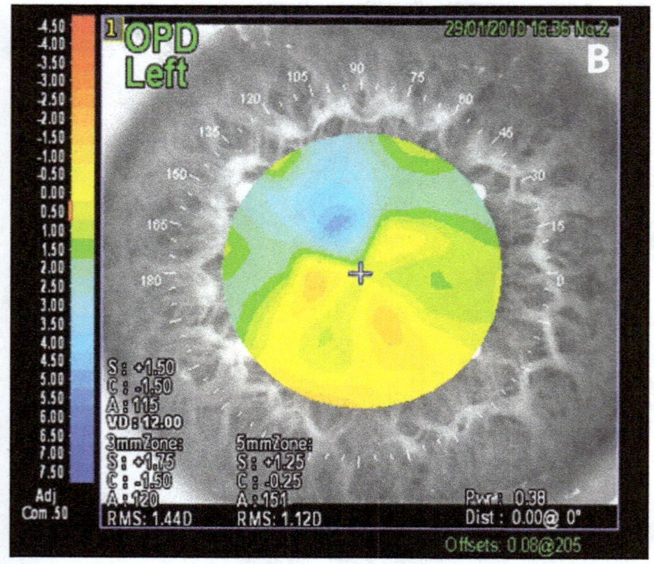

Figure 11-5. (A) Three-piece lens, model AR40E positioned piggyback in the sulcus. Note how the lens has decentered in the sulcus and luxates into the inferotemporal sector. (B) The OPD refractive reference (Nidek OPD Scan II) of the previous image. It is possible to observe the difference in refraction (indicated by the different colors) between the points not covered by the lenses and the points where the 2 lenses overlap. (C) Image of the OPD Scan showing significant coma caused by the luxation of the IOL. (Reprinted with permission from Dr. V. Orfeo.)

Finally, methods to calculate the power of the piggyback lenses are inaccurate; the refractive result is not always the same and there is the risk that the problem will not be resolved.

Piggyback Lenses

Rayner is one of the oldest manufacturing companies of IOLs. It may actually be the first as it manufactured the first IOL for Sir Harold Ridley.

This British company produces piggyback lenses, the Sulcoflex, which were developed for implantation in the sulcus and designed to adapt to the presence of a first IOL in the eye. The design of these lenses is different from traditional posterior chamber IOLs. They are 1-piece lenses of hydrophilic acrylic with a convex-concave shape that will assume a position in relation to the convexity of the first lens. They have a larger optic (6.50 mm), with an overall diameter of 14 mm. The haptics also have an unusual shape as the outer edges are undulated to provide greater adhesion and stability and they have a 10-degree angle with respect to the optic plane (Figure 11-6). They are made using Rayacryl, a copolymer of 2-hydroxy-ethylmethacrylate (HEMA) and methyl-methacrylate (MMA) with ethylene glycole dimethacrylate as a cross-linking agent, due to its greater biocompatibility, greater degree of adaptability to the optical structures present in the eye, and finally, its greater transparency and resistance to treatment with the YAG laser.

There are 3 types of Sulcoflex lenses: aspheric, toric, and multifocal with refractive technology, or rather, the presence of concentric optic zones.

Calculation of the Power of the Piggyback IOL to Be Implanted

In 1993, Holladay described a method for calculating lens powers for pseudophakic and aphakic lenses, independent of axial length.[6]

If severe ametropia appears following the implantation of an IOL, the Vergence Formula is extremely useful for the calculation of the optic power that must be added or subtracted. This formula works well for phakic and aphakic eyes.

The power of the IOL to be implanted is calculated according to the following formula:

$$IOL_e = \frac{1336}{\dfrac{1336}{\dfrac{1000}{\dfrac{1000}{PreRx} - V} + K_o} - ELP_o} - \frac{1336}{\dfrac{1336}{\dfrac{1000}{\dfrac{1000}{DPostRx} - V} + K_o} - ELP_o}$$

ELP_o = effective lens position

K_o = net corneal power

IOL_e = IOL power

V = vertex distance

PreRx = preoperative refraction

DPostRx = desired postoperative refraction

The effective lens position (ELP_0) is the distance between the first and second principal corneal planes. The keratometric power of the cornea (K_k) is converted into the net optic power (K_0) as follows: $K_0 = K_k * 0.98765431$. For example, if the keratometric power (K_k) is 44.50 D, then K_0 will be 44.50 D * 0.98765431 = 43.95.

The net optic power of the cornea (K_0) will therefore be 43.95.

The ELP_0 (the distance of the lens from the principal corneal plane) should be calculated as follows.

Capsular bag depends on the characteristics of the lens. It is preferable to use the ACD constant supplied by the manufacturer. Sulcus with a fixation suture: subtract 0.25 mm from the ACD for IOLs with haptics having a 10-degree angle with respect to the plane. Anterior chamber: use the ACD parameters supplied by the manufacturer of the IOL; this should be between 2.95 and 3.50 mm.

For the vertex, use 12 mm for the lenses and 13.75 mm for the phoropter.

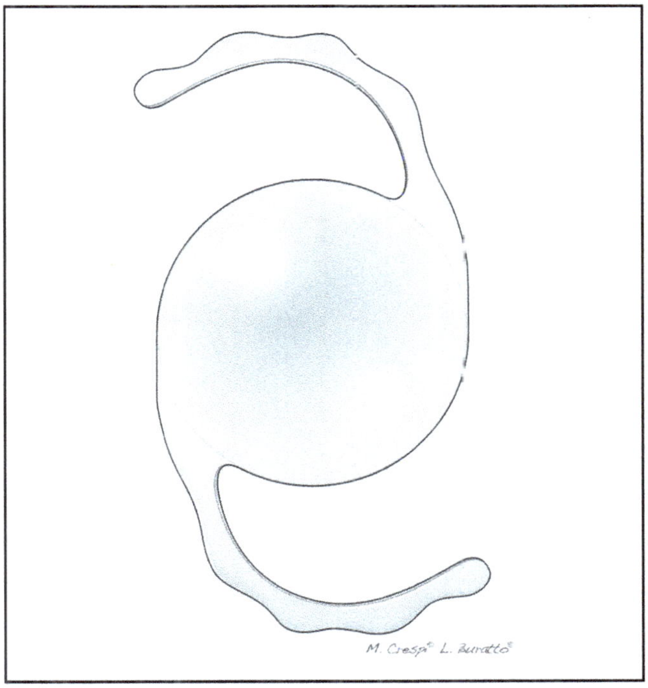

Figure 11-6. A piggyback lens for implantation in the sulcus, the Rayner Sulcoflex. The characteristics of this lens have been studied specifically for implantation in the sulcus and can be used as piggyback lenses. The greater diameter of the haptics, the undulated shape of the outside edge, the shape of the optic meniscus, and the diameter of the optic (6.5 mm) are ideal for the correct implantation in the sulcus and to avoid decentration of the lens.

References

1. Mesa-Gutiérrez JC, Ruiz-Lapuente C. Intraocular lens power calculation after corneal photorefractive surgery. Literature review. *Arch Soc Esp Oftalmol.* 2009;84(6):283-292.
2. Kalyani SD, Kim A, Ladas JG. Intraocular lens power calculation after corneal refractive surgery. *Curr Opin Ophthalmol.* 2008;19(4):357-362.
3. Gunvant P, Ablamowicz A, Gollamudi S. Predicting the necessity of LASIK enhancement after cataract surgery in patients with multifocal IOL implantation. *Clin Ophthalmol.* 2011;5:1281-1285. Epub 2011 Sep 8.
4. Macsai MS, Fontes BM. Refractive enhancement following presbyopia-correcting intraocular lens implantation. *Curr Opin Ophthalmol.* 2008;19(1):18-21.
5. Leccisotti A. Bioptics: where do things stand? *Curr Opin Ophthalmol.* 2006;17(4):399-405.
6. Holladay JT. Refractive power calculations for intraocular lenses in the phakic eye. *Am J Ophthalmol.* 1993;116:63-66.

Suggested Reading

Jin GJ, Merkley KH, Crandall AS, Jones YJ. Laser in situ keratomileusis versus lens-based surgery for correcting residual refractive error after cataract surgery. *J Cataract Refract Surg.* 2008;34(4):562-569.

12

Intraocular Lens Exchange

Lucio Buratto, MD; Stephen F. Brint, MD, FACS; and Domenico Boccuzzi, MD, PhD

With a high degree of ametropia, or if it is not possible to correct the refractive error with the excimer laser (because a laser is not available or for a number of other reasons), the intraocular lens (IOL) must be exchanged. This procedure is a good way to correct residual refractive errors post cataract surgery and should be used when it is not possible to use any other simpler or more straightforward alternative.

A paper published in 2008 showed how IOL exchange is a procedure that is as safe and as effective as the laser (LASIK), even though the success rate (residual refractive error of between ±0.5 D) is 81% compared to 92% achieved with LASIK.[1]

It is important to remember that lasers allow the surgeon to eliminate even small amounts of residual cylinder, which could not otherwise be corrected with standard IOLs.

The surgeon should discuss the decision to explant the IOL with the patient and perform the procedure as soon as clinical conditions of the eye permit. Preferably, this should be within 2 weeks from surgery, although explantation procedures performed at a later date do not necessarily carry any increased risk.

When there is suspicion of an undesired result, the surgeon should measure the refraction on the first day postoperative, and again after 1 week (this should be part of the routine postoperative exams). He or she should decide whether it is necessary to intervene surgically to replace the IOL. The exchange of the IOL is straightforward during the first 2 to 3 postoperative weeks, before any capsular fibrosis develops.

The appearance of late-onset ametropia, particularly myopia, may be the result of capsular contraction that results in an anterior shift of the optic. This phenomenon appears more frequently in eyes in which the anterior rhexis has a diameter larger than the diameter of the optic of the IOL, or when a 3-piece round edge IOL has been implanted. This situation may also dictate exchange of the IOL. However, if there is severe capsular fibrosis that may compromise successful exchange of the IOL, the surgeon may opt for a piggyback implantation or a corneal refractive surgery procedure (photorefractive keratectomy [PRK] or LASIK).

In addition to biometry errors, IOL exchange may be necessary because of the following reasons:

- A decentered IOL
- An opacified IOL
- A damaged IOL
- A considerable amount of glistening
- Intolerance to haloes and glare induced by multifocal IOLs
- When all other methods for correcting the error have been excluded (LASIK/iLASIK, PRK, piggyback IOL)

Surgical Technique

The technique used to explant the IOL is associated with its material and the shape of the lens. Rigid polymethylmethacrylate (PMMA) lenses require a large incision (up to 7 mm) with obvious effects on corneal astigmatism; with foldable acrylic IOLs, the dimensions of the incisions are considerably smaller. Corneal incisions of just 3 to 4 mm are usually sufficient for this procedure and are self-sealing,

Buratto L, Brint SF, Boccuzzi D.
Cataract Surgery and Intraocular Lenses (pp 91-94).

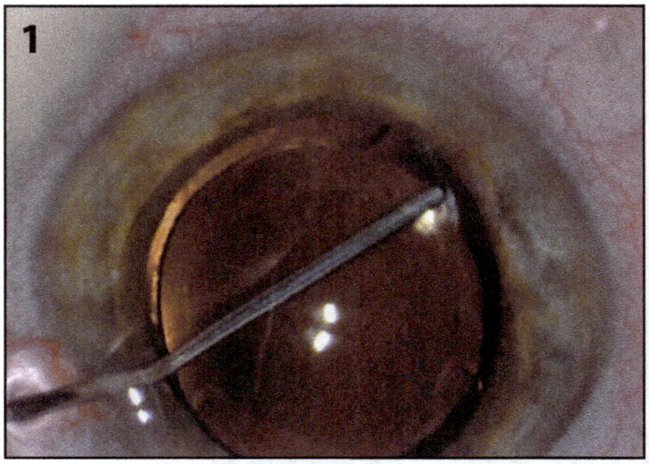

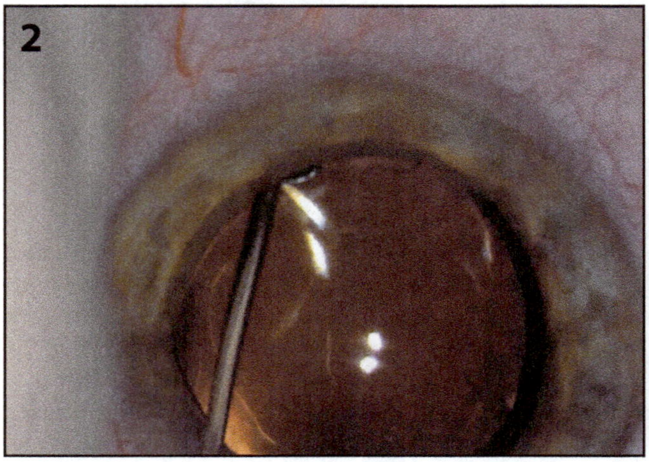

Figures 12-1 and 12-2. Following the creation of the access incision (2.75 mm) in clear cornea, the IOL is detached using a viscoelastic cannula and injecting the VES to raise the IOL from the capsule. (Reprinted with permission from Dr. V. Orfeo.)

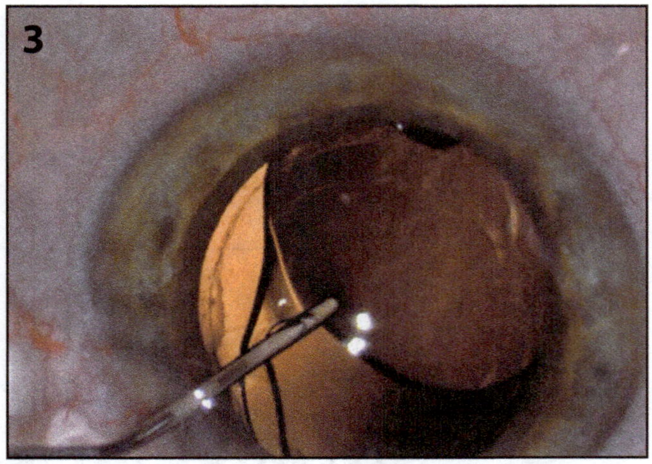

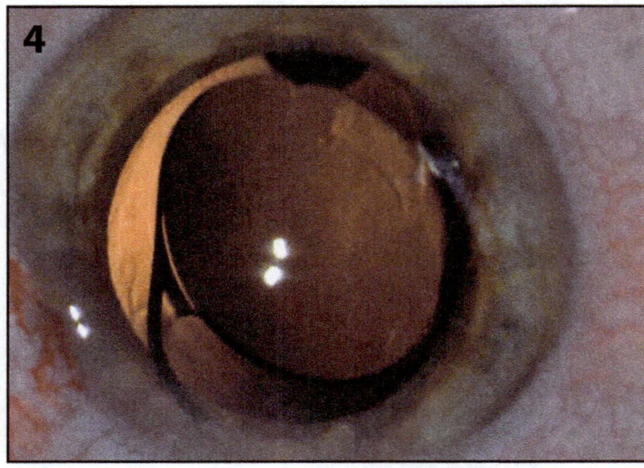

Figures 12-3 and 12-4. The lens is mobilized delicately and exits the bag, luxating in the sulcus. (Reprinted with permission from Dr. V. Orfeo.)

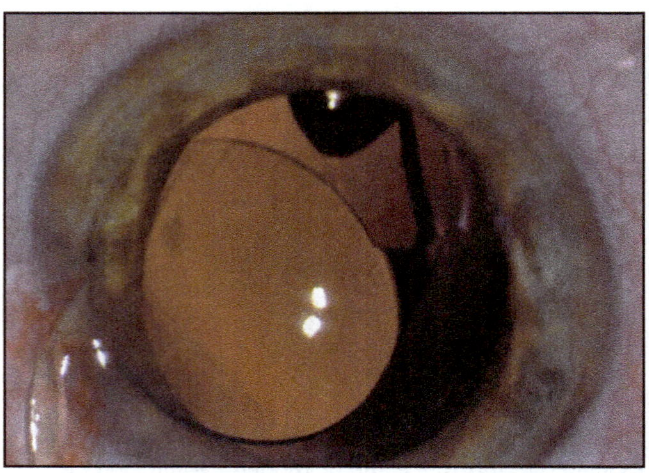

Figure 12-5. A McPherson forceps is used to extrude the haptic from the main entrance. (Reprinted with permission from Dr. V. Orfeo.)

rarely requiring sutures. They have little influence on postoperative astigmatism.

Again with this type of surgery, it is essential to respect the ocular tissues and pay maximum attention to the corneal endothelium, the iris, and the zonules. A dispersive viscoelastic substance (VES) is ideal for maintaining the spaces, even though excessive inflation of the anterior chamber may accentuate capsular rupture or tear the zonules.

During the first step of surgery in IOL removal, it is important to achieve good mobilization of the lens, detaching it from possible adhesions to the capsular bag. The material of the IOL and the shape of the haptics play an important role in the outcome of this step.

It is advisable to perform a viscodissection of the anterior and posterior capsules and delicately inject VES below the anterior rhexis. If this is tightly adhered, the surgeon can assist with a 25-gauge needle and detach the anterior capsule from the anterior face of the lens optic (Figures 12-1 through 12-12).

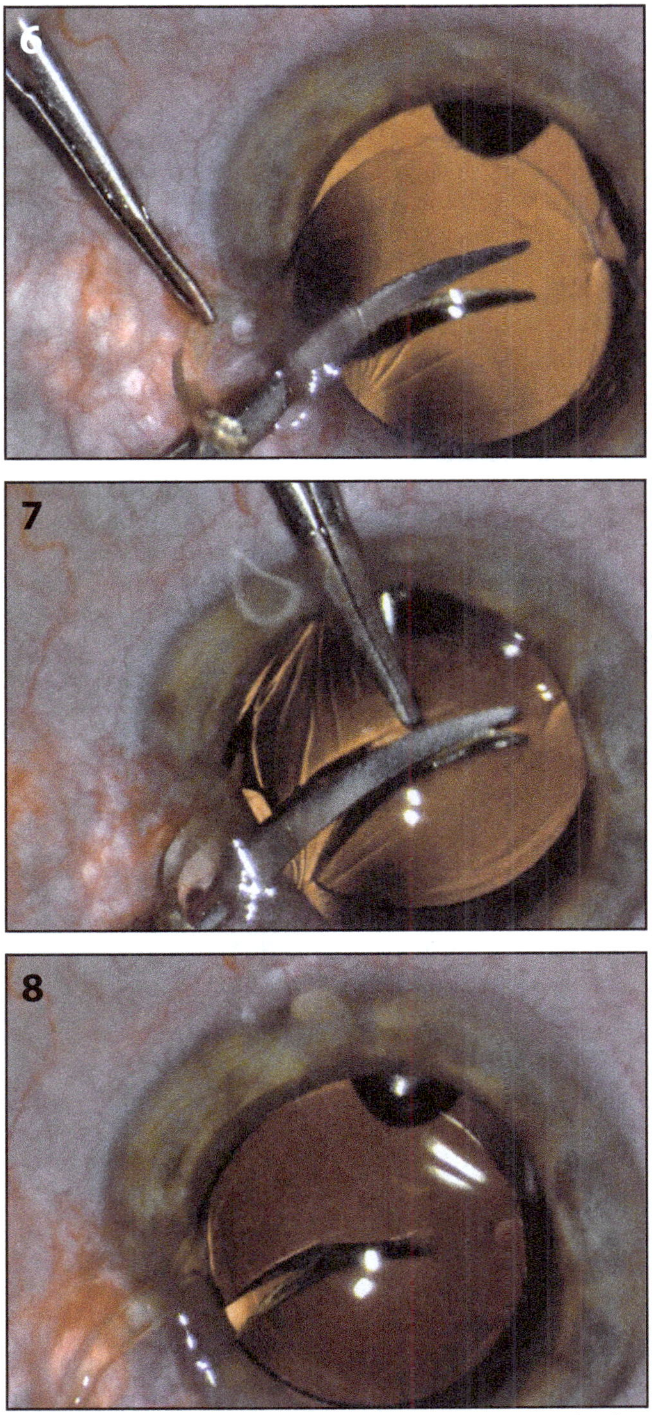

Figures 12-6, 12-7, and 12-8. Holding the loop with the forceps, the surgeon introduces Vannas scissors to cut the IOL. It is not necessary to cut the IOL completely; however, the surgeon must split the optic into 2 halves. (Reprinted with permission from Dr. V. Orfeo.)

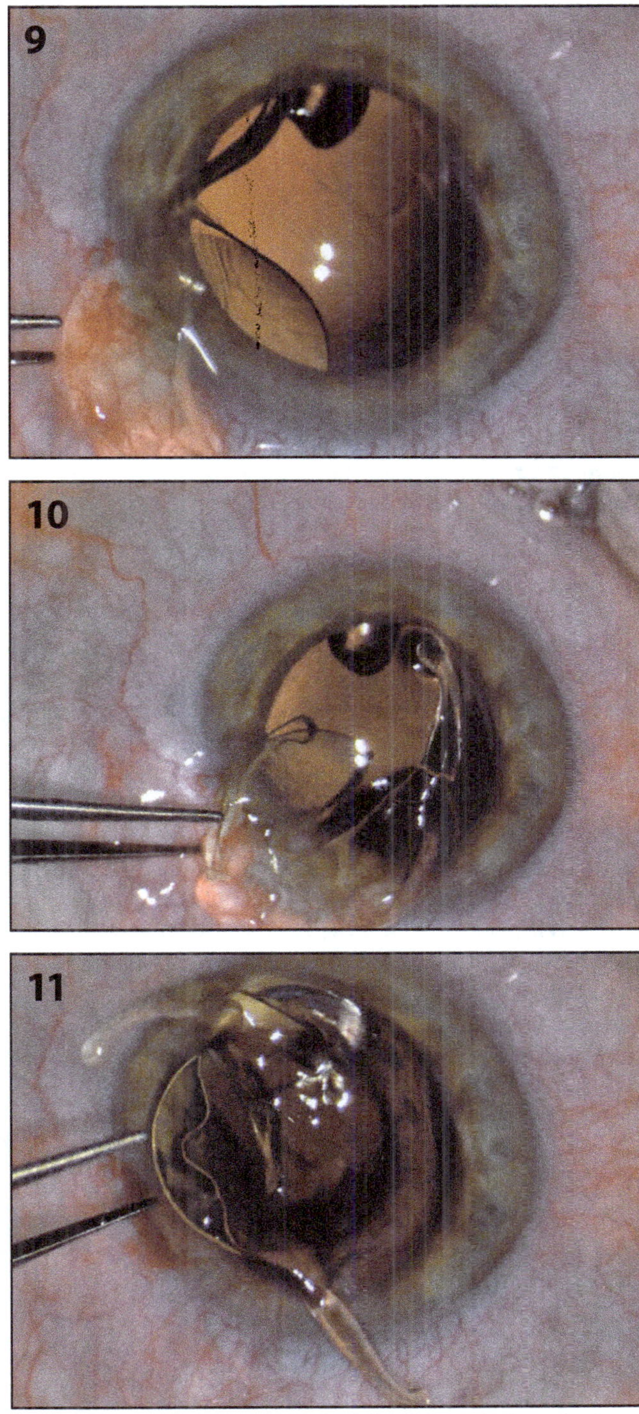

Figures 12-9, 12-10, and 12-11. The IOL splits into 2 pieces, exits through the incision, and rotates in an counterclockwise direction. (Reprinted with permission from Dr. V. Orfeo.)

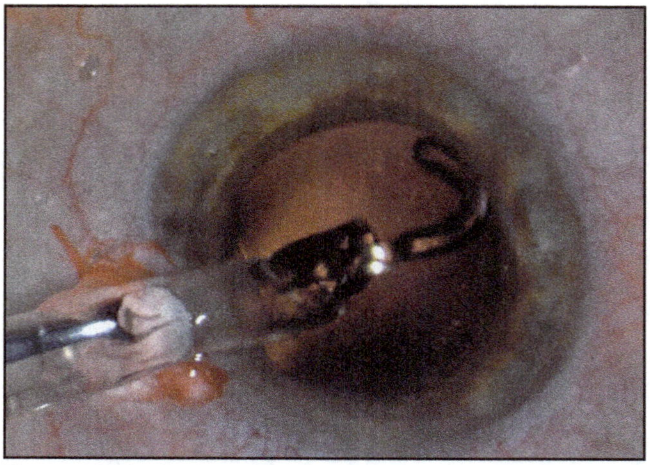

Figure 12-12. At this point the surgeon can inject a VES and implant a new IOL. (Reprinted with permission from Dr. V. Orfeo.)

With phimosis of the anterior capsule, the rhexis should be enlarged and the IOL mobilized.

Once the foldable lens has been detached from the capsular bag, it is possible to remove the lens by cutting it completely or partially or by folding it over on itself.

In the first 2 cases (complete or partial cutting), the surgeon grasps one of the 2 haptics and pulls it out through the corneal incision; then, holding the lens steady using the haptic or grasping the optic itself with a toothed forceps, special scissors are used to cut the IOL in a number of points. With partial (as opposed to total) section of the IOL, it is possible to pull half of the lens out through the incision. Then, by rotating it in a clockwise direction (respecting the orientation of the haptics that could otherwise become trapped in the ocular tissues), the surgeon can also remove the left half of the lens.

The IOL can also be folded inside the anterior chamber and removed intact. This maneuver is not possible with silicone IOLs because this material is very slippery and difficult to manage. However, it is suitable with acrylic IOLs; the maneuver involves the use of a dispersive VES injected into the anterior chamber.

In order to fold the lens inside the anterior chamber, the surgeon must use suitable forceps to hold the IOL, with a blunt instrument acting as a fulcrum for folding the lens. The forceps arms must be positioned on the optic of the IOL; the blunt instrument, introduced through a side access positioned at 180 degrees from the main incision, must be positioned below the entire length of the IOL. The folding movement must be performed by exerting gentle downward pressure with the arms of the forceps while exerting gentle counterpressure with the other instrument. When the surgeon begins to fold the lens, it is necessary to remove the blunt instrument before this procedure has been completed to avoid it becoming trapped in the lens. With the lens folded in this way, it can be removed through the main incision with forceps.

If there is excessive fibrosis of the IOL haptics, when it is impossible to mobilize the lens without rupturing the zonules, the surgeon should cut the haptics and remove the optic of the lens. This problem may arise with C-shaped haptics, with IOLs that have plate haptics with large central openings (that will encourage perfect adhesion of the anterior and posterior capsules), and with the haptics of the Crystalens.

Reference

1. Jin GJ, Merkley KH, Crandal AS, Jones YJ. Laser in situ keratomileusis versus lens-based surgery for correcting residual refractive error after cataract surgery. *J Cataract Refract Surg.* 2008;34(4):562-569.

Suggested Readings

Osher RH. Late reopening of the capsular bag. *Video J Cataract Refract Surg.* 1993;9(1).

Snyder ME, Osher RH. Refractive IOL exchange: indications and techniques. In: *Mastering Refractive IOL: The Art and Science.* Thorofare, NJ: SLACK Incorporated; 2008:831-834.

13

Correction of Astigmatism

Lucio Buratto, MD; Stephen F. Brint, MD, FACS; and Domenico Boccuzzi, MD, PhD

Until the development of toric lenses, the correction of astigmatism during cataract surgery was performed using incisional methods that were neither reliable nor precise. The initial difficulty included the position selected for the main incision for the cataract procedure; it had to be oriented along the steep axis. Another problem involved creation of limbal relaxing incisions or astigmatic keratotomies. There were numerous variables, and consequently, it was difficult to standardize the procedure (depth and width of the incisions, optic zone, patient's age).

These are acceptable methods but not always precise and unquestionably responsible for the appearance of some postoperative problems such as dyslachrymia and foreign body sensation. These methods did not always completely eliminate the astigmatism; moreover, their use was limited to a small number of diopters.

In a study by Ferrer-Blasco et al, published in the *Journal of Cataract & Refractive Surgery* in 2009,[1] on 4540 eyes, post cataract surgery, the findings were as follows:

- 87% of the eyes examined had astigmatism
- In 64% of cases, the value was between 0.25 and 1.25 D
- In 22% of cases, the value was 1.5 D or more

In other words, one person in 5 had astigmatism of 1.5 D or greater, and the quality of his or her vision was poor with the effects of the uncorrected astigmatism (the visual quality of severe astigmatism is not always optimal with spectacle or contact lens correction).

The implantation of a toric intraocular lens (IOL) allows the resolution of the problem in a more physiological manner, eliminating the corneal cylindrical component.[2-5]

The introduction of the latest generation of toric lenses has overcome significant initial resistance regarding their efficacy and rotational stability. As a result, failures reported for the initial lenses (inappropriate lens material and design) led to initial prejudice against current toric lenses, which are actually extremely reliable. The rotational stability of the earlier lenses was not good and the lenses did not maintain their position in the eye. The papers published and mentioned in the references stated that every degree of displacement from the correct axis leads to a reduction of approximately 3% of the refractive effect. Misalignment of up to 5 degrees is acceptable and will still allow a good refractive effect. A shift greater than 10 degrees can lead to oblique astigmatism and may necessitate repositioning of the lens.

With the surgeon's confidence in these lenses, they are currently the best and most physiologic option for correcting astigmatism.

Topography, keratometry, and aberrometry are essential in the decision to implant a toric IOL, for the determination of the type of astigmatism (regular, asymmetric) (Figures 13-1 and 13-2), to define the precise positioning axis (total corneal astigmatism considers any coma component that has a refractive effect on the cylinder) (Figures 13-3 and 13-4), and to exclude keratoconus and pellucid marginal degeneration (Figure 13-5).

When planning the correct IOL power for implantation, the surgeon must remember that he or she has to mark the desired axis with the patient in an erect position to avoid torsion of the eye and it must be extremely precise; the axis for positioning a toric lens, on the steepest corneal axis, will be affected by variations of the incision site and

Buratto L, Brint SF, Boccuzzi D.
Cataract Surgery and Intraocular Lenses (pp 95-97).

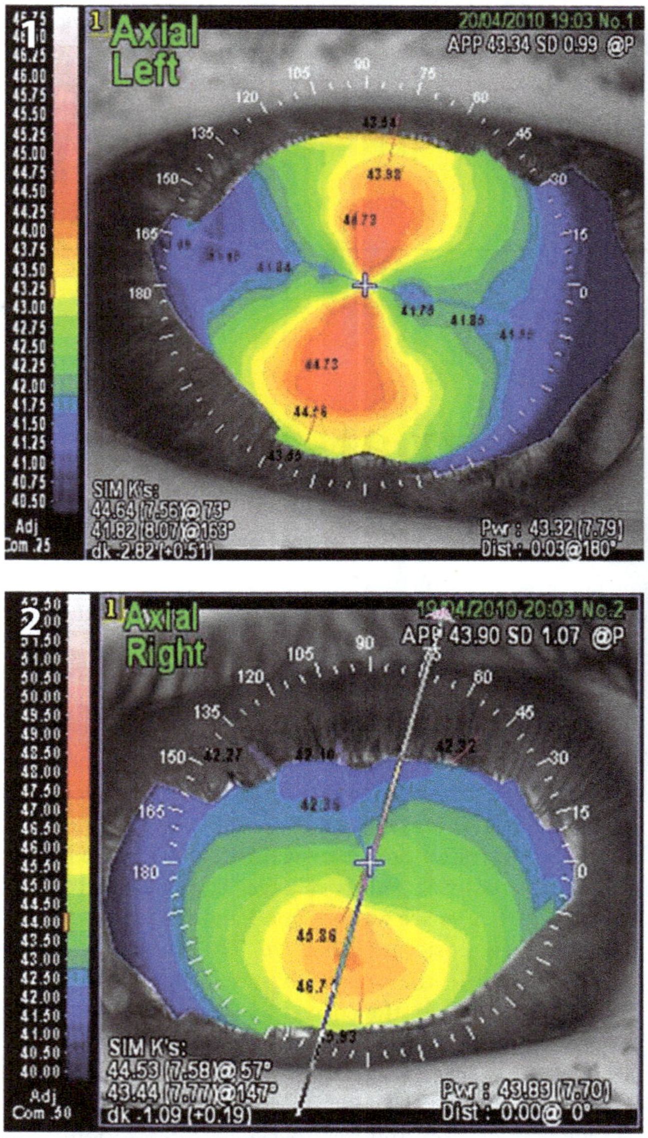

Figures 13-1 and 13-2. These images present regular symmetrical and irregular astigmatism. (Reprinted with permission from Dr. V. Orfeo and Dr. D. Boccuzzi.)

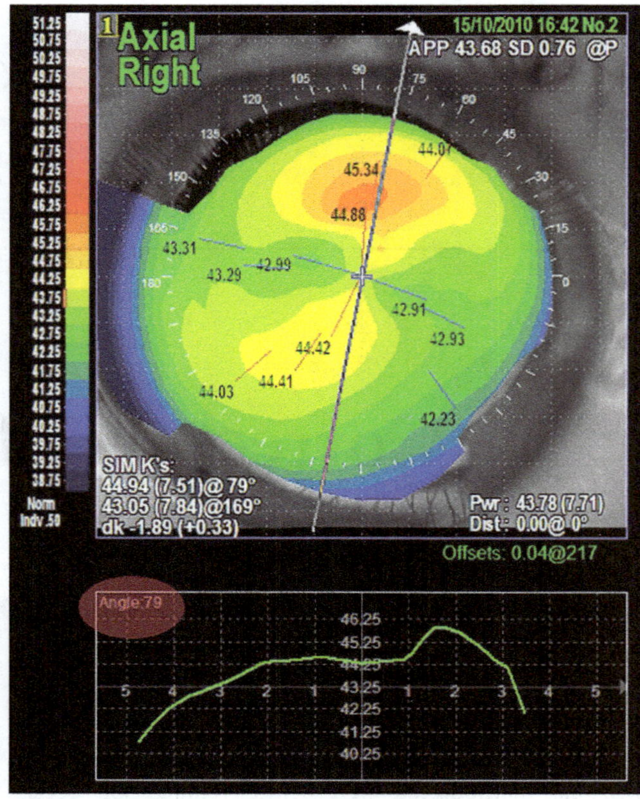

Figure 13-3. Topographic image of asymmetrical astigmatism with the axes of greatest curvature indicated by sim K positioned at 79 degrees. (Reprinted with permission from Dr. V. Orfeo and Dr. D. Boccuzzi.)

size. Consequently, this should be standardized as much as possible.[6]

With the implantation of a toric IOL, the astigmatic patient will have the following possibilities:

- Eliminating or reducing residual cylinder
- Improving uncorrected distance vision
- Increasing independence from spectacles for distance vision

In expert hands, these lenses produce exceptional results, and they are free from side effects, with the exception of an incorrect position in the eye or possible postoperative rotation. Their popularity depends on cost, the surgeon's commitment, and the patient's desire for treatment.

Toric lens technology has been extended to include multifocal lenses and the use of multifocals has increased.

The cylinder and multifocal components of the lens are corrected on the 2 separate sides of the lens and the combination of the 2 corrections produces an excellent result.

The correction of even small degrees of astigmatism (more than 0.75 D) will optimize the outcome, and the residual refractive error will be minimal. In the past, the methods used to correct astigmatism in patients implanted with a multifocal lens produced imprecise results; moreover, even when the refractive result was acceptable, it was altered by higher-order aberrations (coma, trefoil) that would further reduce the contrast sensitivity that had already been compromised by the multifocal factors.[7]

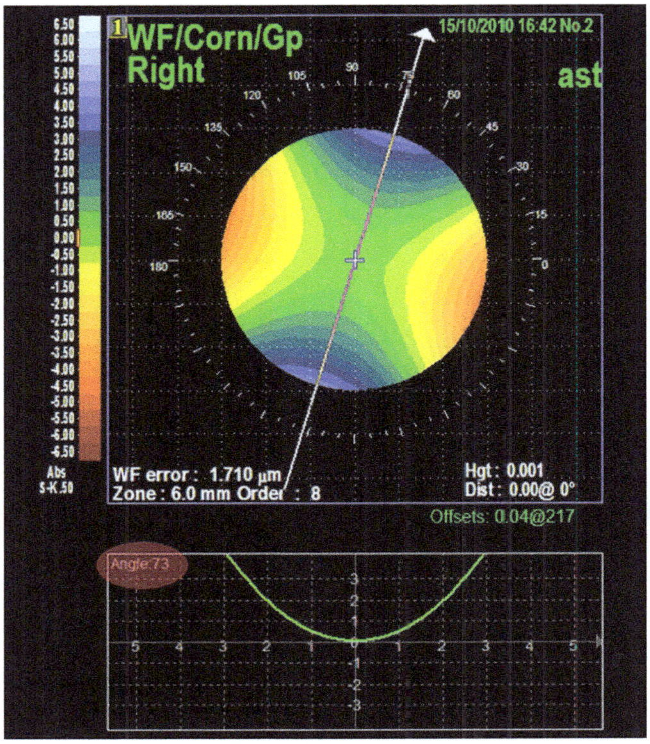

Figure 13-4. An aberrometric image of the corneal astigmatism (low-order aberration) that highlights the aberrometric axis localized at 73 degrees. The aberrometric axis identified corresponds to the most refractive axis and positioning axis for the toric IOL. (Reprinted with permission from Dr. V. Orfeo and Dr. D. Boccuzzi.)

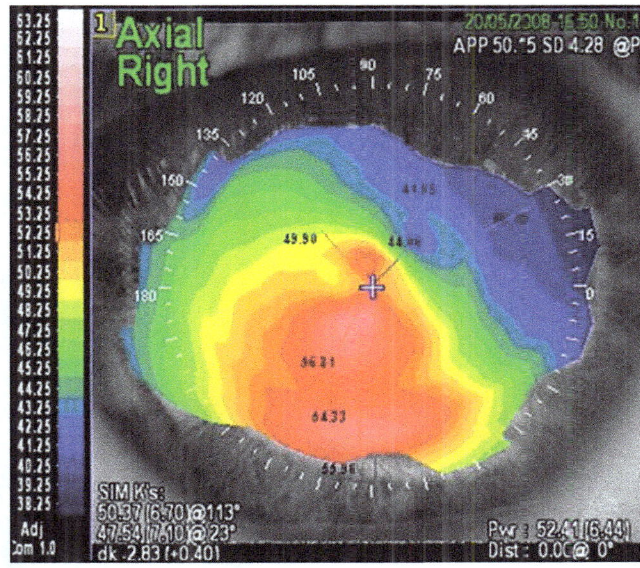

Figure 13-5. Topographic image that presents a pattern typical of keratoconus. (Reprinted with permission from Dr. V. Orfeo and Dr. D. Boccuzzi.)

References

1. Ferrer-Blasco T, Montés-Micó R, Peixoto-de-Matos SC, González-Méijome JM, Cerviño A. Prevalence of corneal astigmatism before cataract surgery. *J Cataract Refract Surg.* 2009;35(1):70-75.
2. Bachernegg A, Rückl T, Riha W, Grabner G, Dexl AK. Rotational stability and visual outcome after implantation of a new toric intraocular lens for the correction of corneal astigmatism during cataract surgery. *J Cataract Refract Surg.* 2013;39(9):1390-1398. doi: 10.1016/j.jcrs.2013.03.033. Epub 2013 Jul 2.
3. Vicković IP, Loncar VL, Mandić Z, Iveković R, Herman JS, Sesar. A Toric intraocular lens implantation for astigmatism correction in cataract surgery. *Acta Clin Croat.* 2012;51(2):293-297.
4. Sheppard AL, Wolffsohn JS, Bhatt U, Hoffmann PC, Scheider A, Hütz WW, Shah S. Clinical outcomes after implantation of a new hydrophobic acrylic toric IOL during routine cataract surgery. *J Cataract Refract Surg.* 2013;39(1):41-47. doi: 10.1016/j.jcrs.2012.08.055. Epub 2012 Nov 14.
5. Levy P. [Toric IOL's]. *J Fr Ophtalmol.* 2012;35(3):220-225. doi: 10.1016/j.jfo.2011.09.006. Epub 2012 Jan 17.
6. Cha D, Kang SY, Kim SH, Song JS, Kim HM. New axis-marking method for a toric intraocular lens: mapping method. *J Refract Surg.* 2011;27(5):375-379. doi: 10.3928/1081597X-20101005-01. Epub 2010 Oct 15.
7. Frieling-Reuss EH. Comparative analysis of the visual and refractive outcomes of an aspheric diffractive intraocular lens with and without toricity. *J Cataract Refract Surg.* 2013;39(10):1485-1493. doi: 10.1016/j.jcrs.2013.04.034.

14

Vision Quality

Lucio Buratto, MD; Stephen F. Brint, MD, FACS; and Domenico Boccuzzi, MD, PhD

The primary objective of cataract surgery is visual rehabilitation. This means offering cataract patients the possibility of their vision being restored to the level before the cataract developed as long as there are no other pathologies. This improvement aims for improved interaction with the surroundings—driving, reading, watching television, and the like—all those situations that may be difficult or impossible because of the cataract. Intraocular lenses (IOLs) in general, and in particular the premium IOLs and presbyopic-correcting IOLs, restore the patient's vision and simultaneously give him or her the possibility of being almost totally independent of spectacles where distance and near vision are concerned. When a patient returns for follow-up following cataract surgery and visual acuity is measured, he or she may be pleased with the excellent visual result; however, surgeons do not always evaluate the visual performance of their patients. Achieving 10/10 vision or better does not always provide patient satisfaction. The surgeon should evaluate both visual quantity and visual quality. This means developing parameters that are not exclusively based on the patient's ability to read small print in the surgeon's office, but whether the patient is comfortable with everyday activities—working at the computer, night driving, reading a newspaper, or simply sending a text message on his or her mobile phone. His or her ability to perform these and many other everyday activities are the real expression of how successful the surgery has been and how satisfied the patient is now that he or she is independent of spectacles.

It is not easy to express a universal parameter for the evaluation of visual quality, and examining the patient with lengthy tests may not always be useful and productive; however, these procedures may be useful in improving the surgery.

Surgeons require a test that evaluates the patient's visual performance in an objective and repeatable manner. For this reason, simulators were introduced attempting to reproduce all of the most frequent everyday tasks—reading a text message, the price of an item, and the dashboard or driving.

All these tests simulate a series of everyday situations and evaluate the patient's vision and, under some circumstances, the adaptation time and the comprehension of what he or she is doing. When a patient can read a single tiny letter, it does not necessarily mean that he or she can read a full article and understand the meaning of what is written.

One of these tests is the EYEVISPOD (Pietro Giardini, Nicola Hauranieh PGB srl), which is a tablet PC with a software package that can reproduce the most common everyday activities (eg, reading a newspaper, the dashboard in a car, or a textbook). The software can calculate the near vision and the intermediate vision by calculating the defocus curve. It can evaluate visual quality, reading speed, and comprehension of what has been read. It therefore allows evaluation of visual quality, standardization of the results, and allowing a comparison between these parameters from pre- and postoperative and between the different types of IOLs implanted. There is also a section dedicated to classification and quantification of dysphotoptic phenomena, a parameter useful for understanding the source of any patient discomfort.

Buratto L, Brint SF, Boccuzzi D.
Cataract Surgery and Intraocular Lenses (pp 99-118).

What Factors Influence Visual Quality?

A perfect surgical procedure does not always result in a perfect outcome. Visual quality is influenced by numerous factors, apart from the surgical manuevers. The corneal surface, the quality of lacrimal film, and the presence of vitreal and retinal abnormalities are all factors that can totally or partially degrade the optimal surgical procedure. The same applies to the presence or the onset of strabismus or the loss of binocular vision.

These factors play an essential role in the economic importance of a surgical procedure and are elements that must be carefully evaluated particularly prior to the implantation of a multifocal IOL.

Importantly, severe dry eye syndrome, macular dystrophy, maculopathy, and retinal and optic nerve abnormalities are all exclusion criteria for implantation of a multifocal IOL and are also conditions responsible for the deterioration of visual quality.

Under some circumstances, however, the surgeon may be faced with problems that appear after surgery, and consequently, there is a need for careful evaluation and early implementation of treatments selected specifically to improve the patient's visual potential.

As described in the previous chapters, the factors responsible for visual quality can be refractive or neurological. The combination of modulation transfer function (MTF) and neural transfer function (NTF) can express the contrast sensitivity function (CSF), which affects visual performance.[1]

$$CSF = MTF \times NTF$$

The term *MTF* is not restricted to the concept of transparency of the optical system, but extends to include the broader process of transmission of light, or better still, the purity of this type of signal.

In other words, if a perfectly transparent IOL has been badly positioned and decentered or tilted, it will not be able to correctly transmit the visual signal that is dispersed through higher-order aberrations (HOA), and these will be perceived as visual disturbances.

The same applies to the process of signal transmission from the retina to the optic pathways and the cerebral decodification areas.

Reduced Visual Quality: Surgical Reasons

Unfortunately, there are many surgical phenomena that can lead to a reduction in vision and can compromise the refractive result possible with a premium IOL.

The following sections will examine the most frequent surgical complications and the possible effects in terms of visual quality.

Rupture of the Capsule

Rupture of the capsule is an unpleasant event for any surgeon, and even when managed correctly, it can lead to a series of complications such as retinal tears, retinal detachment, cystoid macular edema, and a greater risk of endophthalmitis due to the rupture of the posterior capsule barrier.

With a small central posterior capsular rupture, the surgeon may convert the tear into a posterior rhexis (posterior continuous curvilinear capsulorrhexis) with implantation of an IOL in the bag.

In all other cases, it is necessary to implant a 3-piece acrylic IOL in the sulcus. A silicone lens should never be implanted in case of a retinal detachment for which a silicone oil tamponade may be used, as the interface created will seriously compromise visual quality. At any rate, a silicone lens is more difficult to implant when the capsule is open and these lenses are more likely to shift from their central position when implanted in the sulcus.

This means that the implantation of a premium IOL (toric, multifocal, or accommodative) should be avoided. This is an even greater problem if this is the patient's second eye and the first eye was previously successfully implanted with a premium IOL. The only exception is the ReZoom, which is a 3-piece acrylic hydrophobic multifocal IOL that can be implanted in the sulcus. Under these circumstances, the surgeon must adjust the power of the IOL if this is implanted entirely in the sulcus.

One-piece acrylic IOLs must be avoided because, when implanted in the sulcus, they may cause iris chafing, pigment dispersion, iris defects, uveitis, and glaucoma.[2,3]

When the rhexis is centered, the capsule can be used, the haptics are positioned in the sulcus, and the optic is placed beneath the rhexis.[4]

This approach permits good centration of the IOL with no adjustment of the dioptric power. However, when the surgeon cannot use this approach for other reasons, including small or decentered rhexis or rhexis escape, he or she must implant the IOL in the sulcus. Under these conditions, the surgeon must adjust the power of the IOL to be implanted, in an attempt to achieve the same residual refraction desired.

- For powers between +15.0 and +23.0 D, the power of the IOL for implantation in the sulcus must be reduced by 1.0 D.
- For IOLs of powers below +15.0 D, it is sufficient to reduce the power by 0.5 D.
- For powers in excess of +23.0 D, the lens power should be reduced by 1.5 D.[5]

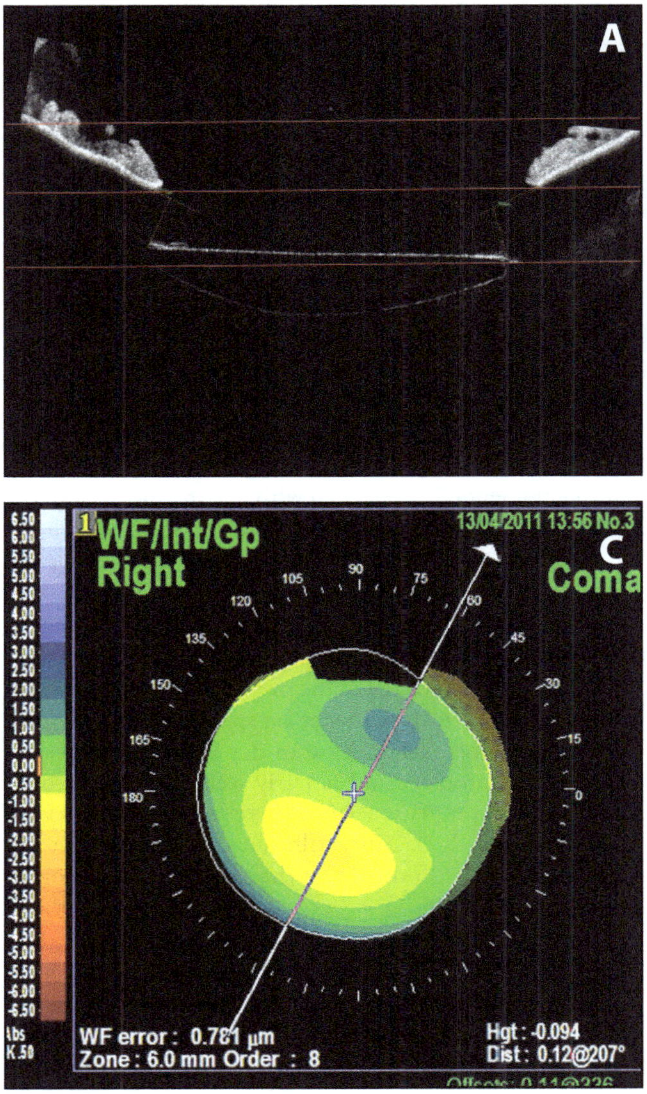

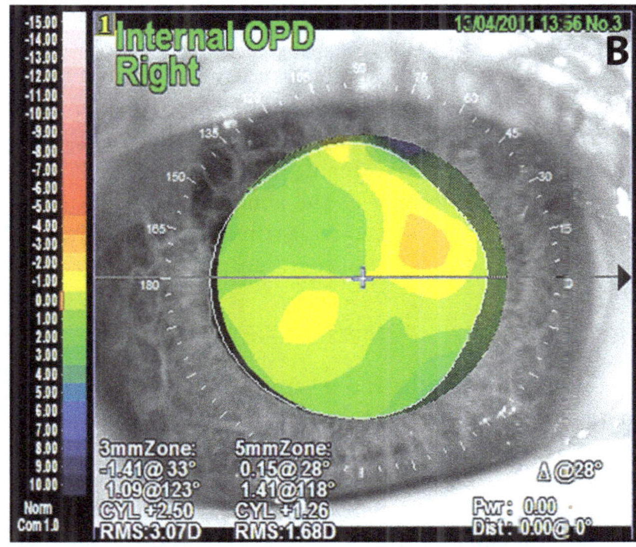

Figure 14-1. Optical coherence tomography (OCT) of a toric lens, positioned in the capsular bag with a slightly decentered rhexis. (A) The rhexis does not rest symmetrically on the edge of the lens and will cause mild tilting of the lens itself. This tilting creates (B) asymmetrical internal astigmatism and (C) coma demonstrated with internal aberrometry. Repositioning the lens inside the bag will be sufficient to normalize the clinical picture, eliminate the asymmetry of the internal astigmatism, and remove the coma. (Reprinted with permission from Dr. V. Orfeo and Dr. D. Boccuzzi.)

Under this situation, the refractive result will be even less predictable, with a reduction in the visual quality.

Malpositioning of the Intraocular Lens

Any errors in the positioning of the IOL will be responsible for alterations in visual quality. A decentered rhexis, asymmetrical retraction of the capsular bag, or phimosis of the anterior capsule can cause deterioration of the MTF. Even incorrect positioning of the lens in the capsular bag with just one haptic in the sulcus will lead to decentration and tilt of the IOL with reduction in the visual quality. If there is severe decentration, coma will appear due to misalignment between the corneal axis and the lens axis (Figure 14-1).

For example, a 20-D IOL that is luxated or tilted will lead to astigmatism of 1 D if the tilt is 5 degrees.

Tilt of 10 degrees will induce astigmatism of 2 D, and tilt of 30 degrees will induce astigmatism of 5 D.

Decentration of the IOL can occur when, following capsular rupture, the lens is positioned in the sulcus. A "standard" 3-piece IOL, with a maximum haptic diameter of 13 mm, can decenter if implanted in the sulcus. This is more likely to happen in myopic patients who have a "larger eye," with diameters that can reach 14 to 15 mm.

This phenomenon can also appear when the haptics erode a portion of the zonules, or penetrate an area that is free of zonular fibers and slide into the vitreous, dislocating the IOL; the lens will tend to position with the optic on the edge of the zonules

Oblique Cuts

Creation of the corneal incision is one of the most important steps for a good outcome. In the previous chapters, we discussed how the incision can have an important effect on the refractive result of surgery and how the creation of a longer or shorter tunnel can be used.

However, the creation of oblique cuts—in which the blade cuts the corneal layers asymmetrically (eg, one edge of the incision is in the limbus and the opposite area is in clear cornea)—can create irregular astigmatism and coma, particularly trefoil, that will alter the MTF with a deterioration in visual quality (Figure 14-2). This phenomenon occurs because of the abnormal distribution of corneal traction forces that are distributed over a plane that is oblique and not tangential to the cornea.

Incorrect Suture Placement

Sutures placed at the end of surgery to close the corneal tunnel or to fine-tune the astigmatism may deform the corneal surface with alteration of the visual quality. Sutures that are excessively tight or in an oblique and not a centripetal position can lead to abnormalities in the corneal curvature and this can alter visual quality. Sutures that have been placed incorrectly should be removed as quickly as possible.

Wound Burns

This is now a very rare occurrence because of major technological developments in modern phacoemulsification machines. Nevertheless, despite this being a rare occurrence, the wound may be burned by older pieces of equipment that are still being used, when the cornea is particularly hard, or when a high viscosity type of viscoelastic substance ([VES] such as Healon 5) is used.

The problem can also occur when the tunnel is unusually long and with prolonged surgical times. The corneal retraction will be abnormal and there will be problems closing the corneal incision with an inevitable induction of high astigmatism.

Endothelial Decompensation

Successful "perfect" surgery will not always result in an excellent visual result. Sometimes, even when the surgery has an optimal outcome, there may be persistent corneal edema; and if there is significant endothelial decompensation, there may be irreversible bullous keratopathy.

Careful preoperative examination of the patient is essential to assess the surgical risks and to dispel the widespread belief that cataract surgery is a short straightforward procedure.

Slit-lamp examination, endothelial cell count, and pachymetry are essential prior to proceeding. With guttata or manifest Fuchs' endothelial dystrophy, the surgeon must inform the patient of the high risk of postoperative corneal decompensation. A chondroitin sulfate (CDS) VES can be used to improve adhesion to the corneal endothelium; enriched balanced salt solution (BSS plus) can be used to minimize endothelial trauma; and phaco equipment can be used as it emits very low ultrasound energy. For example, Alcon's OZIL system with intelligent phaco can preclude the use of classical ultrasound and can be used exclusively to release the tip of the handpiece when occluded. Even using lower parameters of vacuum, the flow will make an important contribution to reducing turbulence in the anterior chamber and avoid unnecessary endothelial trauma.

Reduced Visual Quality: Dry Eye

Dry-eye syndrome is a multifactorial pathology of the lacrimal film and the eye's surface that is reported as discomfort in the eye, visual disturbances, or instability of the lacrimal film with potential damage to the eye's surface. This phenomenon is associated with hyperosmolarity of the lacrimal film and inflammation of the eye's surface. This is the definition of dry eye issued by the International Dry Eye Workshop. On its own, chronic dry eye is not a contraindication to cataract surgery.

Problems with the lacrimal film are important, particularly in patients interested in the implantation of a premium IOL to reduce their dependence on spectacles. Fortunately, for many patients, an increase in dry eye after surgery is not a serious problem and is fairly well tolerated in both visual and symptomatic terms. Nevertheless, patients with disturbances of the lacrimal film must be treated prior to surgery and fully informed that the symptoms may worsen after the procedure.

During the evaluation process, it is essential to consider both ocular abnormalities and the presence of correlated systemic pathologies that could exacerbate the symptoms. These conditions include Stevens-Johnson syndrome, systemic lupus erythematosus, Sjögren's syndrome, rheumatoid arthritis, sarcoidosis, etc (Table 14-1).

For the oculo-palpebral pathologies, it is advisable to examine the quantity of lacrimal film, the volume of the lacrimal meniscus and the effect of striations, and to pay attention to the shape of the eyelid rim; the surgeon should also check dysfunctions of the meibomian glands, the presence of blepharitis, and the formation of collars around the base of the eyelashes. Eyelid malocclusion may be a sign of recurring inflammation and be responsible for greater evaporation of the lacrimal film itself. Similarly, alterations of the meibomian glands and the presence of chronic blepharitis are signs of a lacrimal film lacking the lipid component. Lipids slow down the evaporation of the aqueous component in the tears.

The absence of lipids leads to excessive evaporation and excessive osmolarity of the tears. This means a lower volume of tears, an increase in burning and foreign body sensations, chronic inflammation, and deterioration in visual quality (Table 14-2).

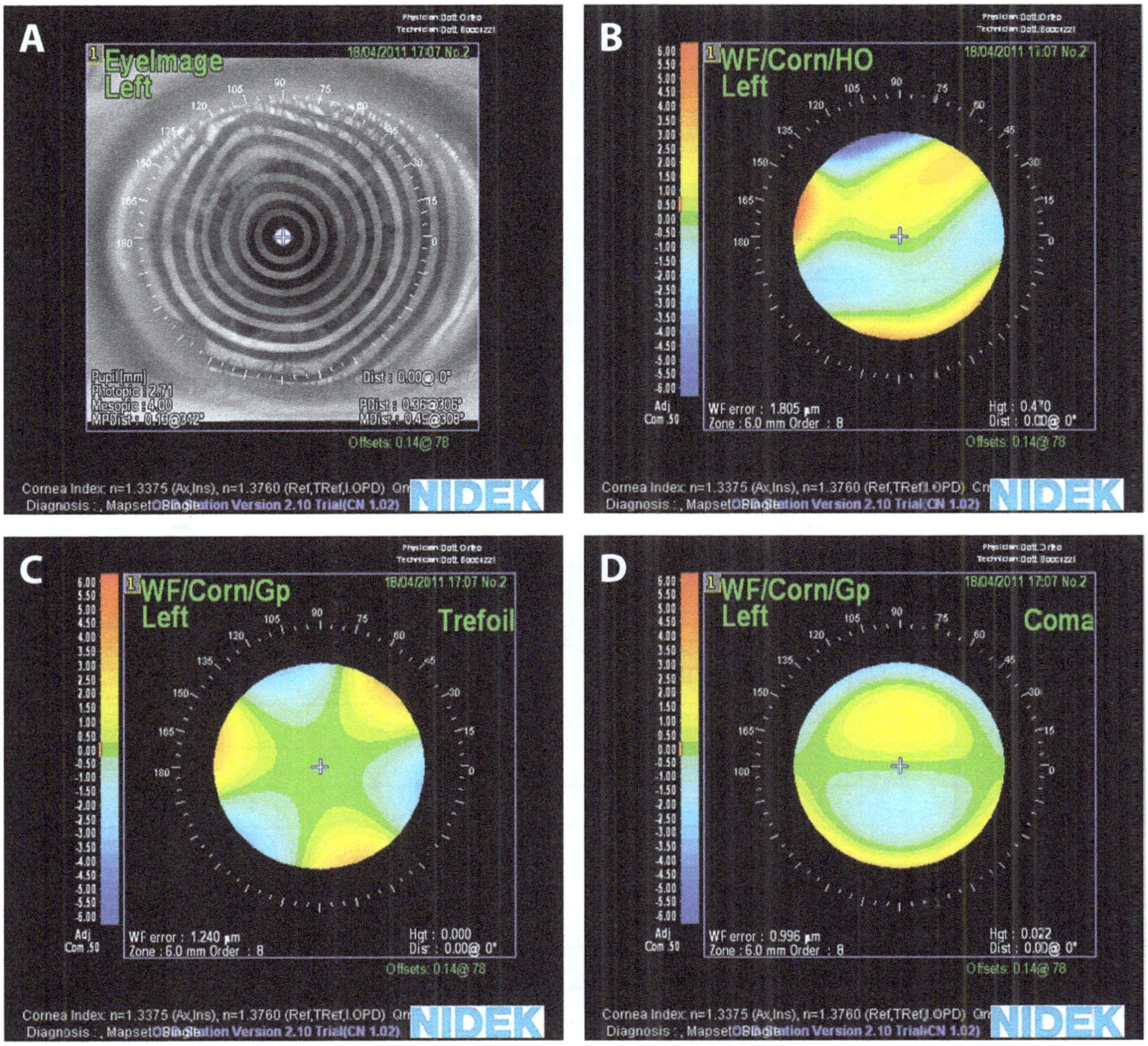

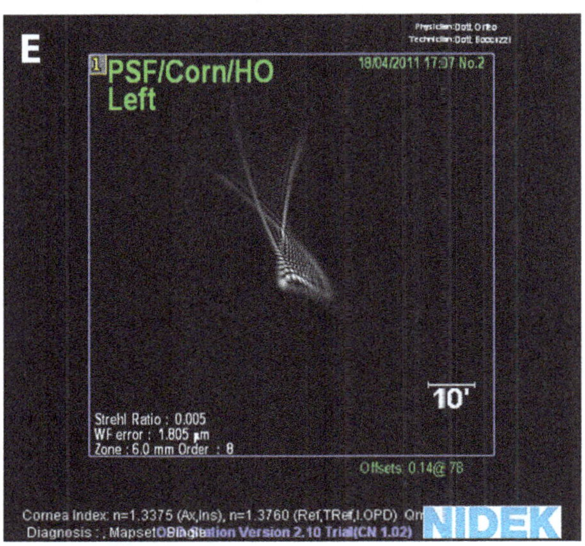

Figure 14-2. (A) In the keratoscopic image, the deformation of the Placido disks induced with the creation of an oblique incision can be observed. This deformation causes (B) the appearance of HOA with an increase in (C) trefoil and (D) coma. (E) All of this will lead to an alteration in the MTF with important deformation in point spread function. (Reprinted with permission from Dr. V. Orfeo and Dr. D. Boccuzzi.)

Table 14-1

Dry Eye Pertinent Medical History

SYSTEMIC PATHOLOGY	SYMPTOMS	MEDICATIONS
Systemic lupus erythematosus	Contact lens intolerance	Antidepressants
Steven-Johnson syndrome	Foreign body sensation	Antihistamines
Environmental allergies	Fluctuation of vision	Antihypertensives
Neurological pathology	Redness	
Sjögren's syndrome		
Rheumatoid arthritis		
Acne rosacea		
Sarcoidosis		
Menopause		
Ocular cicatricial pemphigoid		

Table 14-2

Dry Eye Preoperative Clinical Evaluation

OCULAR SURFACE	SYSTEMIC
Punctate epithelial keratopathy	Dental and peridontal disease (Sjögren's)
Meibomian gland inspissation	Rhinophyma
Tear meniscus/Schirmer's	
Eyelid collarette formation	
Conjunctival pleating	
Exposure/ectropion	
Conjunctival tylosis	
Hyperosmolarity	
Palpebral fissure	
Telangiectasia	
Tear break-up time	

Reduced Visual Quality: Anatomical-Functional Alterations

Anatomical alterations can cause deterioration in visual quality, limiting or compromising the final result. These changes mean that it may not be possible to implant a premium IOL in the eye.

Keratoconus or marginal pellucid degeneration can lead to HOA that may compromise the visual quality and the final refractive result.

It has already been stated that keratoconus is a contraindication for surgical correction of refractive errors to allow a good refractive outcome.

Due to corneal collapse, keratoconus (Figures 14-3 and 14-4) will induce characteristic HOA, called *coma* (Z3 -1; +1) (Figure 14-5); this will lead to a misalignment of the wavefront. The analysis of the point spread function illustrates the formation of a tail around the light spot in the shape of comet (Figure 14-6). By definition, this aberration cannot be corrected with lenses and the resulting refraction is associated with moderate/severe astigmatism.

Even in the presence of a debilitating pathology such as keratoconus, the surgeon should evaluate the error carefully and decide if and when a toric lens, for example, should

What Causes Dry Eye?

Following cataract surgery, post surgical imbalance of the lacrimal film may be due to irregularity of the eye's surface or an incision of the nerve plexus.

Dry eye syndrome post cataract surgery can appear in patients already having an existing pathology; symptoms may worsen in previously healthy patients who had no evidence of symptoms prior to surgery (approximately 10% of patients).

What is responsible for the appearance of the symptoms? Do any modifiable risk factors exist?

How can we prevent the appearance of the symptoms and reduce their duration?

Postoperative medical treatment and preoperative preparation procedures also make an important contribution.

Contributing factors in the appearance or exacerbation of the symptoms include the site and shape of the incision, the amount of time the eye is exposed to the microscope's light, the duration of the surgery, an existing dry eye syndrome, and the presence of any systemic pathologies such as diabetes, collagen diseases, or other autoimmune diseases that are co-responsible for alterations of the lacrimal film.

A second area of interest is the effect the incision has on the corneal nerves. The long branches of the ciliary nerve (the sensitive nerve of the cornea) penetrate the limbus at 3 and 9 o'clock. The fibers of the fifth cranial nerve, through the nasociliary plexus, reach the corneal limbus through the long ciliary nerves.

Approximately 70 to 80 radial branches originate in the peripheral cornea and run through the anterior corneal stroma. The nerve trunks extend from this area and fold orthogonally to proceed to the surface to form the sub-basal plexus. The intraepithelial nerve endings originate in the sub-basal nerve plexus. When the corneal nerve endings are damaged, the scarring process is abnormal; there is increased epithelial permeability and reduced metabolic activity. Corneal nerves have a role in the corneal epithelial repair processes and the creation of lacrimal secretion.

In the medial and lateral corneal sectors that are normally exposed, there is greater sensitivity than the other 2 sectors, normally covered by the eyelids.[2]

Studies on patients having LASIK demonstrated that when the flap hinge is superior, both the lateral nerve trunks are cut (at 3 and 9 o'clock).

Vice versa, when the hinge is created in a nasal or lateral position, at least one of the 2 nerve trunks is preserved, with a better outcome in terms of sensitivity (and postoperative recovery).[3]

There is a difference in cataract surgery as the incision is considerably smaller despite the fact it is full thickness. The effect of denervation is different in the 2 surgeries. Based on new models of corneal innervation,[6] the interruption of the long ciliary nerve fibers in the temporo-superior region is responsible for reduced corneal sensitivity in the central region (because some of the fibers may extend as far as the central part of the cornea).

It could be suggested that the reduction in the corneal reflex is the element responsible for a reduction in the blink rate with the following:

- A reduction in lacrimal film formation
- A reduction in tear break-up time
- An increase in the amount of evaporation
- Reduction in the tear film turnover rate

In normal patients, decompensation of the system leads to a reduction in the corneal blink reflex and the secretion of the basal tear film, which induces a reduction in the aqueous component of the tears. This phenomenon induces excessive osmolarity of the tear film and the activation of compensation by the main lacrimal glands. This is one reason why many patients complain of tearing after surgery.

In patients with dry eye syndrome, the system has no reserves and the hypoesthesia resulting from surgery induces an increase in excessive evaporation with a consequent chronic damage to the corneo-conjunctival structures (goblet cells, alteration of the epithelial microvilli) and a chronic inflammatory process.

Diabetic patients have a greater risk of developing dry eye syndrome, or their pre-existing condition may deteriorate postoperatively. This is seen through the neuropathy that alters the secretory processes of the lacrimal glands with a consequent alteration in the quality and quantity of the tears.

Finally, preservatives contained in postoperative eye drops can lead to a deterioration in symptoms and in the clinical picture, compromising the glycocalyx of the precorneal lacrimal film. Consequently, the surgeon should use preservative-free eye drops, as these will protect the eye's surface and should always include artificial tears that will compensate any alterations in the tear film itself.

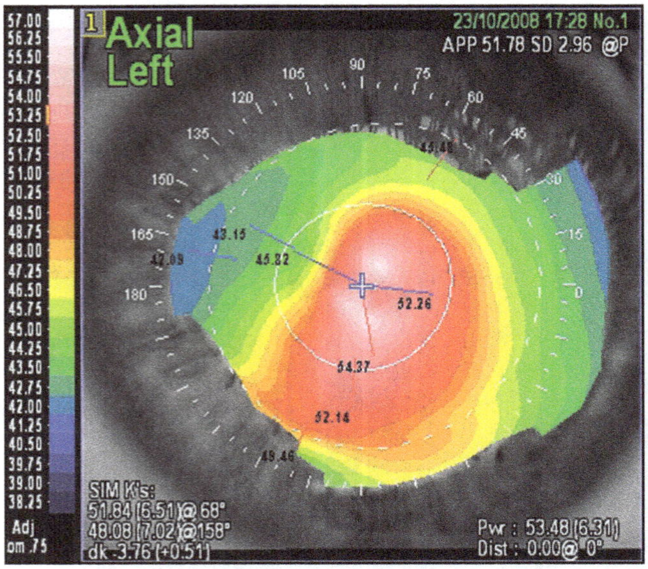

Figure 14-3. Topographical image of keratoconus. (Reprinted with permission from Dr. V. Orfeo and Dr. D. Boccuzzi.)

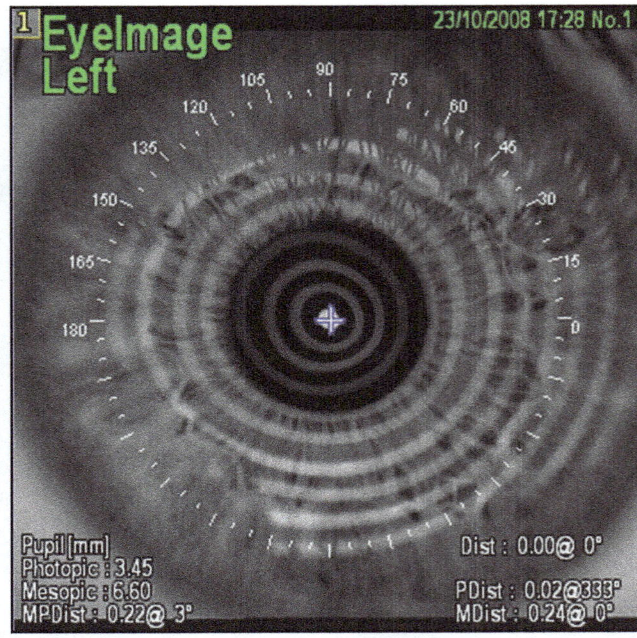

Figure 14-4. Image showing a cornea affected by keratoconus, with the projection of the Placido rings. It is possible to show the distortion of the rings induced by the deformed cornea. (Reprinted with permission from Dr. V. Orfeo and Dr. D. Boccuzzi.)

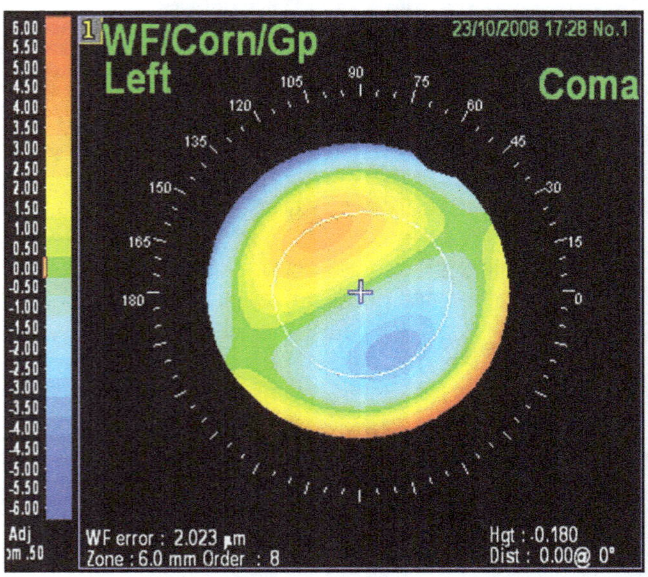

Figure 14-5. The aberrometric analysis of the eye indicates the presence of coma induced by keratoconus. (Reprinted with permission from Dr. V. Orfeo and Dr. D. Boccuzzi.)

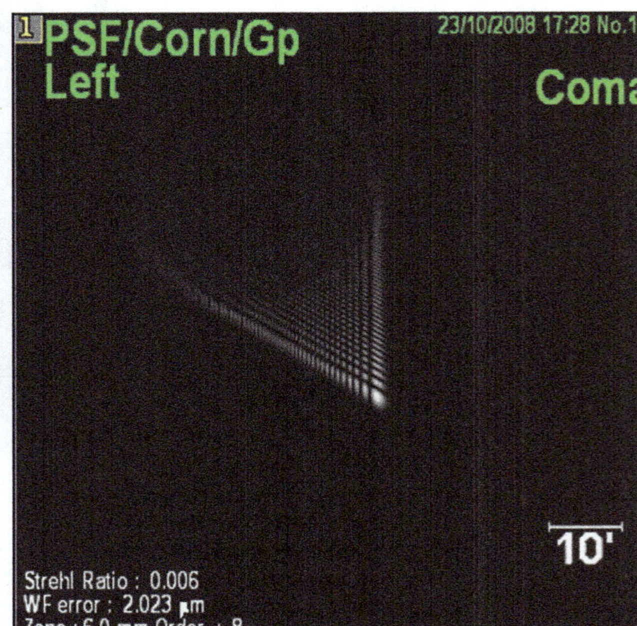

Figure 14-6. The analysis of point spread function highlights the "comet" deformation of a punctiform light source, induced by keratoconus. (Reprinted with permission from Dr. V. Orfeo and Dr. D. Boccuzzi.)

be implanted to partially correct the astigmatism induced. With low-grade keratoconus (stages 1 to 2), with alterations that are stable in time and astigmatism that is not excessively asymmetric or irregular, in patients who are over 50, the implantation of a toric IOL can be somewhat beneficial to the overall functional result. Even though this type of lens cannot correct the HOA induced by the corneal collapse, it will be able to provide a better correction of the low-order aberrations induced by coma (astigmatism) compared to eyeglasses. After a toric IOL's implant, however, it is not possible to use a contact lens to improve quality of vision.[7]

Aniridia

Aniridia is a severe anatomical functional alteration that can severely compromise the patient's visual quality. This can be described as partial or total lack of iris formation

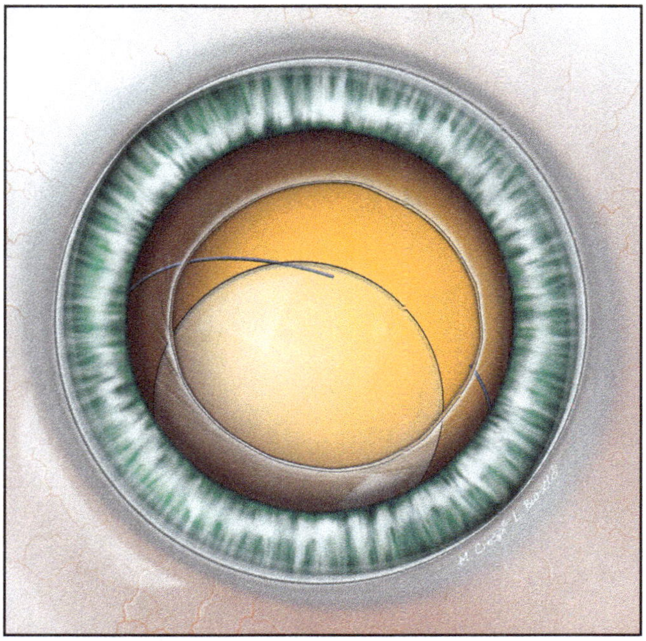

Figure 14-7. Inferior decentration of the IOL. Sunset syndrome.

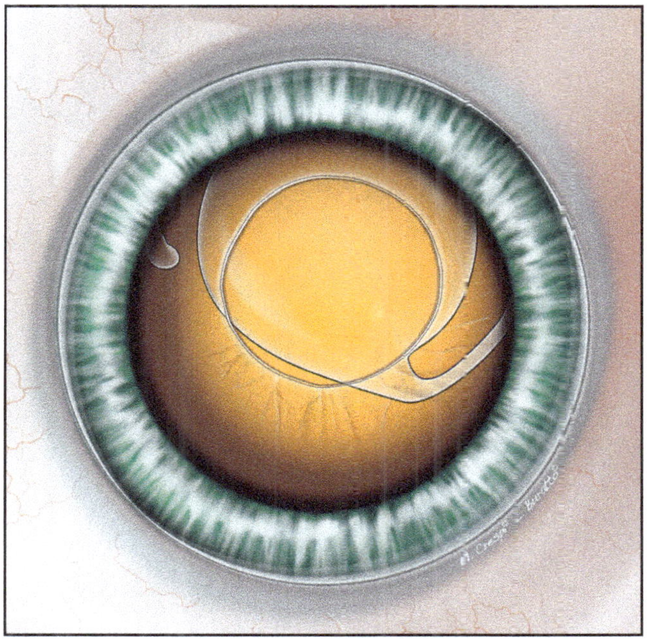

Figure 14-8. Superior decentration of the IOL. Sunrise syndrome.

and can also be associated with glaucoma, cataract, corneal opacity, and foveal hypoplasia. This alteration is due to the PAX6 gene present on chromosome 11 and can be hereditary or associated with de novo mutation. In this group of patients, vision is very poor and may be associated with nystagmus. In these cases, cataract surgery may be an opportunity for inserting an IOL with opaque sectors or segments for the creation of an artificial iris and reduce the glare and dysphotopsia associated with this pathology.

Iris Coloboma

Iris coloboma is responsible for significant sight reduction. Congenital iris coloboma may be associated with alterations of the choroid, the retina, and the optic nerve.

With small exclusively iris defects, vision will not be affected. However, this may prevent implantation of multifocal lenses. Under these circumstances, cataract surgery is an opportunity to insert an IOL with opaque segments that can "bridge" the iris defect.

The same applies to post-surgical or post-trauma colobomas or coloboma of other origins.

Abnormalities With the Position of an Intraocular Lens (Centration, Optics, etc)

IOLs play an essential role in the vision of the patient post cataract surgery and make an important contribution to visual quality.

The IOL implanted can affect astigmatism, the multifocal component, or correction of corneal spherical aberration. In other words, the type of IOL implanted will significantly alter the quality of the patient's refractive result.

We will evaluate a standard 1-piece IOL with a nonaspheric optic. The refractive result will depend on the residual refractive error of the patient and the amount of astigmatism present will determine the need for spectacles for distance vision. When the size of the standard pupil is not large, the refractive result will be acceptable with good patient satisfaction.

If the pupil is large, the choice of an aspheric IOL will make a significant improvement in visual quality, particularly at night (eg, when driving). As previously mentioned, the approaches to correction of positive spherical corneal aberration developed by various companies are different; however, all of the lenses provide excellent visual results.

With severe decentration of the IOL, particularly if the optic is not in the pupillary field during physiological mydriasis, the patient will perceive visual disturbances, predominantly the presence of coma (induced by decentration of the lens and by the appearance of peripheral portions of the IOL in the visual axis), and finally, dysphotopsia caused by the edge of the lens and aberrations created by portions of the pupil not "covered" by the IOL.

A large decentration of the IOL is a major problem, irrespective of the type of lens (Figures 14-7 and 14-8); however, with small amounts of decentration, the implantation of an aberration-free implant will offer a better refractive result than both normal spherical lenses and lenses with negative spherical (hyperspherical) aberration. This occurs because,

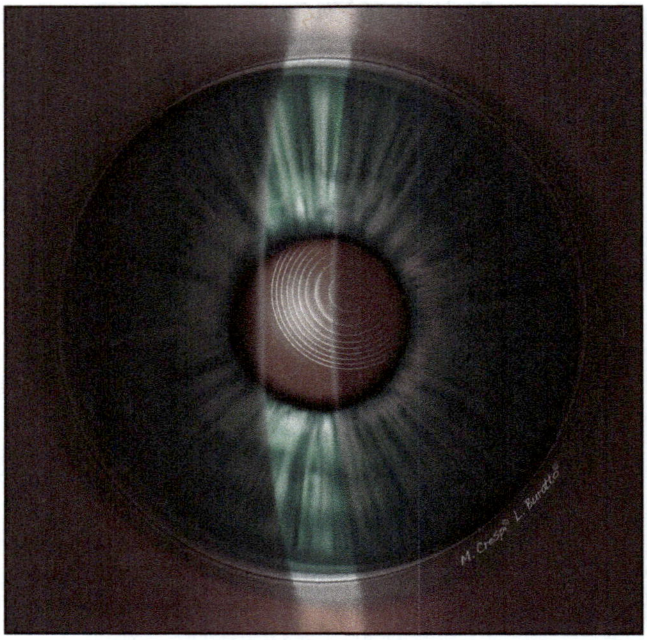

Figure 14-9. Decentration of a diffractive multifocal IOL (ReSTOR) highlighted under the slit lamp.

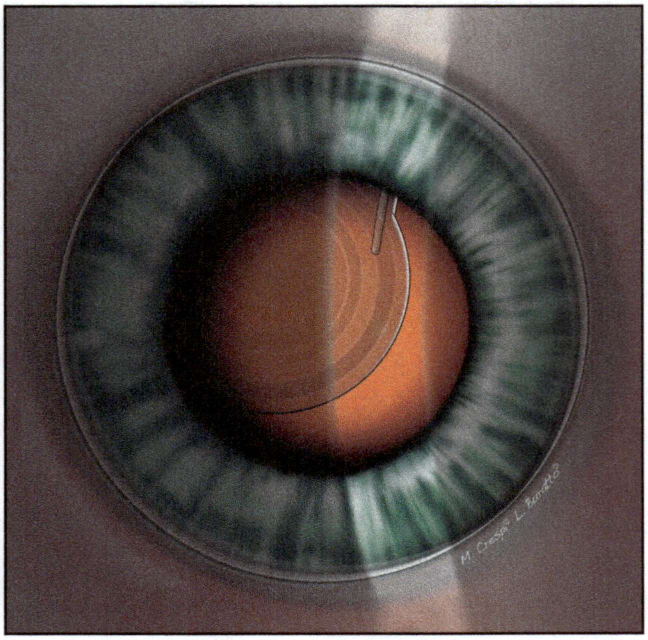

Figure 14-10. Symptomatic decentration of a refractive multifocal IOL. Array, in silicone (Advanced Medical Optics).

with normal lenses and hyperspherical lenses, any decentration leads to formation of coma.

When corneal sphericity is combined with a hyperaspheric IOL, the optical center of the cornea and the IOL should coincide to avoid the risk of coma. However, the eye is not a well-centered visual system because the visual axis and the optical axis do not coincide. When an IOL is centered in the capsular bag, it is possible that it will not be centered on the visual axis and this induces a small amount of coma that can be added to or subtracted from the physiological coma of the cornea. Consequently, we can conclude that hyperaspheric IOLs and normal spherical IOLs can lead to coma. With decentrations of larger amounts, the aberrations induced by hyperaspheric IOLs can exceed those of normal spherical IOLs that in turn are greater than those induced by neutral spheric IOLs.[8,9]

Decentration of the IOL is responsible for significant decreases in visual quality with multifocal IOLs and toric lenses. For correct performance, multifocal lenses (diffractive lenses and refractive lenses) require perfect centration on the visual axis.

Any abnormal positioning of this type of lens will jeopardize a good surgical outcome, with haloes and glare and a loss in multifocal component (Figures 14-9 and 14-10).

Finally, the performance of toric IOLs can be greatly affected by decentration. It is extremely unlikely that a decentered IOL will maintain the orientation intended by the surgeon. With decentration or rotation of a toric IOL, the risk is that the rotation will exceed the tolerance by 5 degrees, with induction of oblique astigmatism that will severely compromise visual quality.

Because of their mechanism of action, even decentration of accommodative IOLs can compromise the optimal functional outcome of the surgical procedure. Accommodative IOLs such as the Crystalens, with a 5-mm optic, must be centered "within" the rhexis without overlapping it except at the hinge portion; it will be greatly affected by decentration, with the appearance of haloes or glare; the expected accommodation may also be compromised (Figure 14-11).

Other factors that can lead to a reduction in visual quality are the presence of small scratches on the optic of the lens, caused by incorrect handling of the lens. This is more significant if these optical alterations are more central, and particularly crucial with multifocal lenses.

Even a decentered capsulorrhexis can change the correct position of the lens in the bag and alter its correct alignment.

Alterations of the Transparency of the Posterior Capsule

Secondary opacification of the posterior capsule cannot be ignored as one of the causes for reduction in visual quality. Even though the square edge of the latest generation of IOLs has been designed to avoid cell migration, posterior capsule opacification (PCO) still occurs today and can greatly affect visual quality.

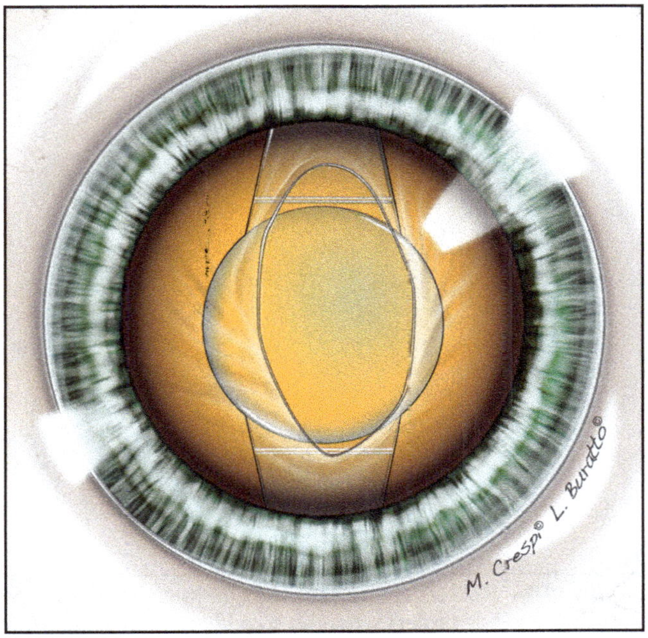

Figure 14-11. Decentration of the Crystalens caused by the contraction of the capsular bag. The Crystalens has a small optic, and even small degrees of decentration can lead to dysphotopsias and compromise the lens movements responsible for accommodation.

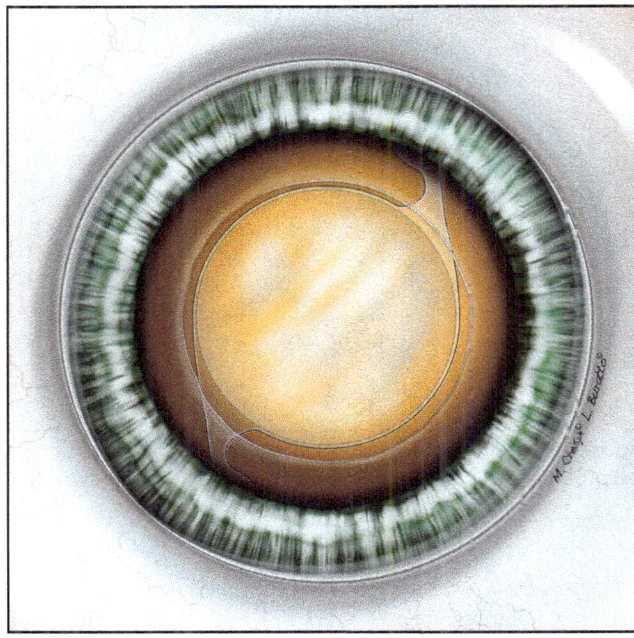

Figure 14-12. Image showing PCO.

Posterior Capsule Opacification

PCO is one of the most frequent complications following cataract surgery. This is seen in approximately 50% of patients within 2 or 3 years after surgery. It is caused by the presence of epithelial cells in the capsular bag that then proliferate, migrate, and are transformed into myofibroblasts. These lead to small retractions and deformations of the posterior capsule. Cell proliferation and the formation of Elschnig pearls alter the transparency of the optical media, altering the MTF and exponentially reducing visual quality (Figures 14-12 and 14-13).

Actually, small dense areas of cells in asymmetrical positions on the posterior surface of the lens can "defocus the light rays" because of a change in the refractive index and can create small "comas" with the consequent onset of astigmatism. It is important to consider that even modest alterations in transparency of the capsule can reduce visual function because they cause a reduction in MTF. Under these circumstances, patients with multifocal lenses may detect the decrease because of the reduced contrast sensitivity caused by the lens itself.

The Nd:YAG laser can be used to treat secondary opacity of the capsule. This treatment allows the transparency of the media to be restored in patients with opacity of the posterior capsule. However, this must be performed with maximum attention and precise location. It is important to carefully regulate laser power, laser defocus posteriorly with respect to the target direction and the point at which the laser treatment is performed. Errors may lead to the formation of micro cracks in the optic of the lens induced by thermal and acoustic shock generated by the laser.

Central spots can cause visual disturbances that will be perceived by the patient.

Vitreous

Mobile vitreous bodies, also known as *floaters*, are deposits in a variety of sizes, shapes, consistencies, refractive index, and motility inside the eye's vitreous, a substance that is normally transparent. In young people, the vitreous is perfectly transparent; however, as the person ages, some dishomogeneous areas gradually develop. The mobile vitreous bodies generally derive from degenerative processes of the vitreous body. This perception of flies in flight is also known as *miodesopsias* or *mouches volantes* (from the French). The floaters are perceived by the patient because of the shadows they project when they are hit by a beam of light, or alternately due to the diffractive processes they generate. They can appear alone or in groups in the visual field. They normally appear as spots, threads, or web-like structures that float in front of the patient's eye. These floaters exist inside the eye; they are not optical illusions but real endoptic phenomena (Figure 14-14).

The mobile vitreous bodies are suspended in the vitreous and normally follow the direction of the eye movements. When the patient notices them, his or her initial instinct will be to try to look at them directly; however, this will be difficult as the movement associated with looking at the floater will generate pressure that will shift the floater in the same direction as the eye's movement, allowing them to persist in a peripheral zone of the visual field. The behavior

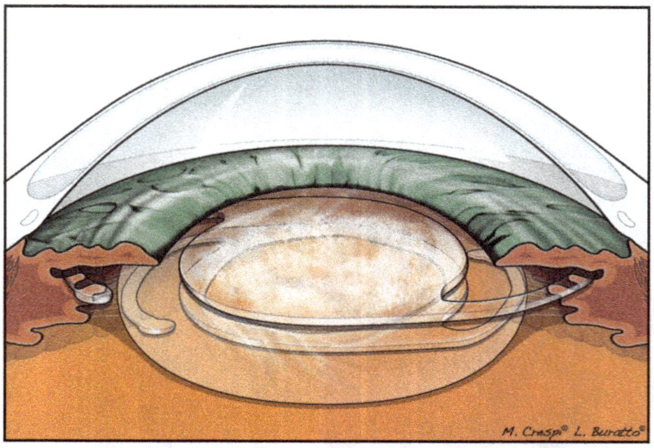

Figure 14-13. An image showing interlenticular opacification or cell proliferation between the 2 IOLs positioned in piggyback.

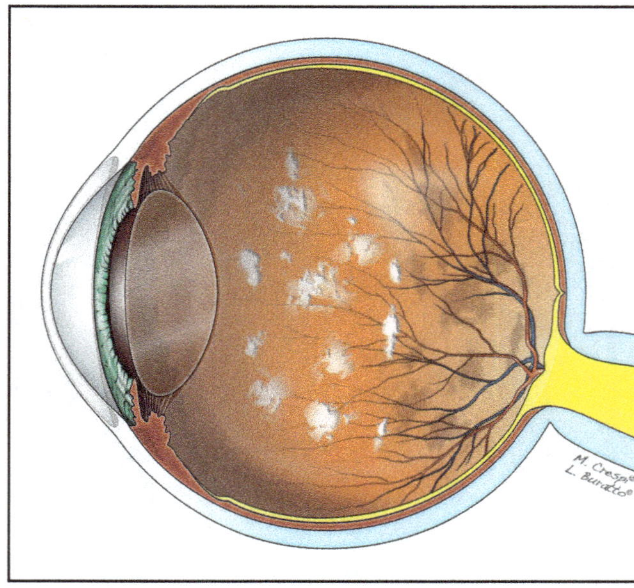

Figure 14-14. Floaters are perceived by the patient because of the shadows they project when hit by a light beam or through the diffractive processes they generate. They can appear as single entities or in groups.

of floaters resembles small flying insects, hence their name mouches volantes. The floaters are not always visible but will be more evident under specific lighting conditions, and when they are positioned in front of the visual field, they project their shadow onto the retina. When they are located in a peripheral position, and under conditions of poor lighting, neuroadaptation process "makes them invisible." They will be clearly perceptible under strong lighting conditions with extremely homogeneous backgrounds—for example, when the patient looks at a clear blue sky or a brightly lit white wall. This type of pathology is largely due to fibrillary degeneration of the vitreous and the aggregation of protein residues that have formed over the years and are trapped in the vitreous itself. They do not affect elderly people alone but can affect younger people, particularly with myopia. Frequently, the patient's observance of floaters is more apparent following cataract surgery. The replacement of the cataractous lens with an artificial lens will lead to a distinct improvement in contrast sensitivity, with a subsequent increase in the perception of the floater. The patient may report that he or she had not noticed them previously or, if he or she had, they were unobtrusive. Because the floaters will be more evident postoperatively, the patient may consider them to be a complication of the surgery. The floaters can capture and refract the light and temporarily blur the patient's vision until they shift into a different area inside the eye. When the floaters are small, the visual adaptation process will adjust to this situation and they will eventually be ignored. However, for patients with severe miodesopsias, it is almost impossible to completely ignore the large masses present in the visual field. Nevertheless, the floaters will not have a permanent effect on the visual quality and vision will generally be good.

Asteroid Hyalosis

In some patients, there may be a monocular formation of dense vitreous entities, similar to grains of sand. These are calcium precipitates and insoluble lipid compounds associated with the hyaluronic acid network. These alterations are called *asteroid vitreopathy* or *hyalosis*. The condition is typical of adults, in patients over 60 years of age, in a 2:1 male/female ratio. Asteroid hyalosis is a degenerative process caused by thickening of the lipids and precipitation of calcium inside the vitreous body. The reasons for the formation are still not clear. It may be due to aging of the collagen or depolarization of the hyaluronic acid. The numerous yellowish-white grains (of diameter between 0.01 and 0.1 mm) move with the eye's movements; there will also be a series of after movements; their density is variable and they float in the vitreous body. Despite rarely being perceived by the patient, the ophthalmologist may find that they obstruct his or her examination of the fundus. This clinical condition is not associated with an increase in the frequency of retinal detachment or refractive errors. In the White population, asteroid hyalosis has a prevalence of 1% to 2%, seen bilaterally in approximately 10% of cases. As mentioned previously, asteroid hyalosis is a benign condition that is often associated with diabetes, high blood pressure, dyslipidemia, and arteriosclerosis; it is rarely responsible for a significant reduction in visual quality. With very dense alterations of the vitreous that are positioned anteriorly (behind the lens), vision can be reduced significantly. In this case, a vitrectomy may be necessary to restore physiologic vitreous transparency. This pathology is

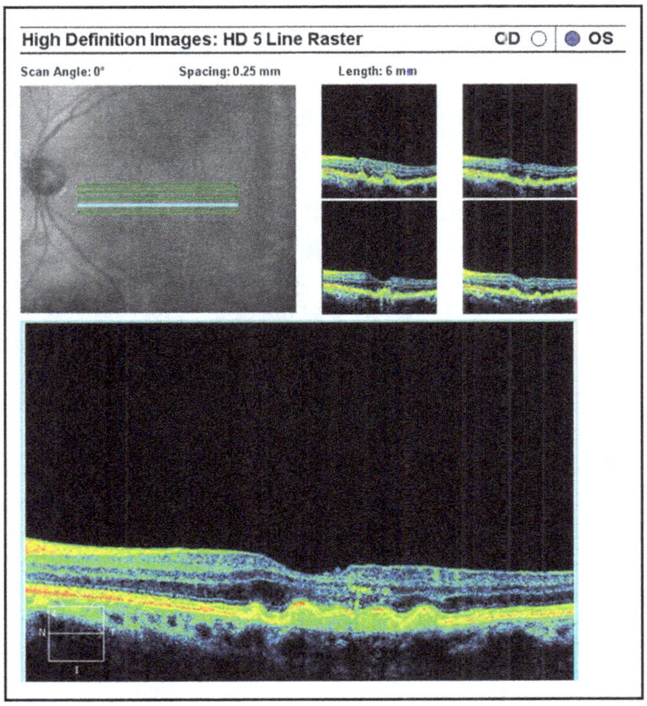

Figure 14-15. OCT image of a patient affected by hard drusen localized in a retrofoveal position, with alterations in the reflectivity and the profile of the retinal pigment epithelium. (Reprinted with permission from Dr. V. Orfeo and Dr. D. Boccuzzi.)

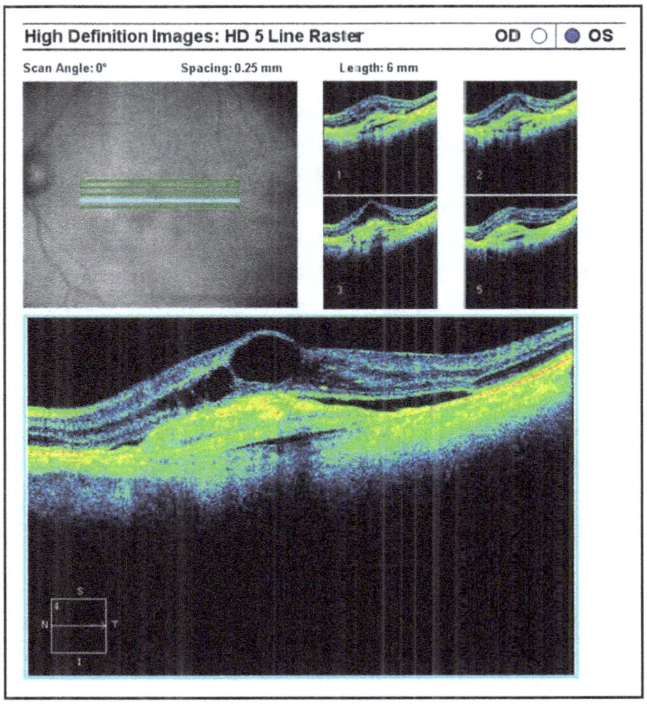

Figure 14-16. OCT image of a patient with age-related macular degeneration with active choroidal neovascularization. The image shows the neovascular membrane as a hyper-reflecting area next to the retinal pigment epithelium, the detachment of the neuroepithelium, and the intraneuroretinal hyporeflecting cystic edema. (Reprinted with permission from Dr. V. Orfeo and Dr. D. Boccuzzi.)

not always responsible for visual problems that are serious enough to severely compromise the quality of vision.

A retrospective study on patients operated for cataract and requiring vitreoretinal surgery (20 gauge) to treat vision disturbances associated with vitreous abnormalities showed that only 17% were associated with asteroid hyalosis and a concomitant posterior detachment of the vitreous. This indicates that this condition is rarely correlated to a reduction in visual quality. It should be emphasized that the implantation of a multifocal lens is not indicated for patients with this type of vitreous abnormality; this type of lens could increase reduction in contrast sensitivity that has already been compromised to some degree with this type of abnormality.

Scintillating Synchysis

This vitreous abnormality is also called *spinteropia*, *lightning vision*, or the *gold waters of Gdansk*; it is a visual disturbance caused by deposits of cholesterol crystals in the vitreous.

The amino acids leukine and tyrosine and calcium phosphate can also lead to the formation of crystals in the vitreous, which results in a rare and usually monocular disturbance that may be confused with asteroid hyalosis. The altered vision normally appears after bleeding or inflammation of the vitreous, and no specific cause has been identified.

The role of the ophthalmologist is extremely important in cases of asteroid hyalosis and synchysis scintillans; he or she must inform patients of the postoperative consequences of cataract surgery.

Actually, as mentioned for floaters, the perception of this disturbance may increase following the removal of the cataract. This type of pathology is an important contraindication to the implantation of multifocal lenses, as this type of lens could lead to further deterioration in the patient's visual quality.

In more complicated cases, a vitrectomy may be necessary to eliminate the numerous vitreous opacities and improve visual quality.

Macula and Posterior Pole

Alterations of the macula play an important role in the reduction of the eye's visual performance. The surgeon must, therefore, perform careful preoperative exams, even with secondary examinations such as OCT and fluorescein angiography, to exclude the presence of pathology, such as macular degeneration, an epiretinal membrane, or exudative maculopathy in diabetic patients (Figures 14-15 and 14-16). Precise evaluation of these pathologies is essential when implantation of a presbyopic-correcting IOL is being considered.

As explained previously in detail, multifocal lenses (with exclusion of accommodative lenses) are responsible for reduction in contrast sensitivity, a parameter that has already decreased due to the mechanism of the multifocal lenses. For this reason, with alterations of the macula (hard drusen, soft drusen, alterations of the retinal pigment epithelium, geographic atrophy), an epiretinal membrane, or in patients with diabetic retinopathy, the implantation of an multifocal IOL is not recommended.

The only option under these circumstances is the implantation of an accommodative IOL that will not cause a reduction in contrast sensitivity or deterioration in visual quality. The reason for this is that these lenses prevent an additional reduction in contrast sensitivity in case of evolution of the macular pathology, avoiding early problems with vision.

With maculopathy, the loss of visual acuity and contrast sensitivity may prevent the patient from performing everyday routine activities, such as recognizing faces, moving around, reading, and driving, and this causes a serious loss in the patient's quality of life.

A 25% reduction in contrast sensitivity can significantly reduce visibility with night driving and reaction times.

A 50% reduction in contrast sensitivity and visual acuity in patients over 65 years of age is associated with a 3- to 5-fold probability that the patient will have problems with routine tasks, irrespective of the loss of visual acuity.

A reduction of 90% in contrast sensitivity is a criterion for visual debilitation.

With normal vision, on the other hand, a 10-fold reduction in contrast sensitivity will only be responsible for a 2-fold reduction in reading ability. Finally, walking involves the low spatial frequencies and is not compromised by implantation of multifocal lenses.

Contrast sensitivity testing can demonstrate reductions in visual performance that would not normally be detected with measurements of visual acuity. Surgeons are also aware that age-related macular degeneration produces a reduction in contrast sensitivity, even in the initial phases, and as age-related macular degeneration progresses, the contrast sensitivity drops. This is similar to patients with diabetic retinopathy. Contrast sensitivity declines in diabetic patients compared to healthy patients and in diabetics with retinopathy compared to diabetics without retinopathy.[1]

Under these circumstances, the surgeon should explain to the patient that implantation of a monofocal IOL will result in better visual performance that will last for a longer period of time; as it does not cause a deterioration in the MTF associated with the multifocal component of the lens, it will not contribute to a reduction in the total visual performance (CSF). The probable visual deterioration that occurs over the years will be exclusively due to the reduction in the neural component (NTF) and will not be associated with the presence of a multifocal lens.

The uniform reduction of 6 Db (50%) of sensitivity caused by implantation of a multifocal lens is fairly well tolerated in healthy patients with no macular problems.

However, when it is combined with a reduction in neuro-retinal sensitivity (eg, 6 Db) induced in a patient with maculopathy, the additive effect of the 2 abnormalities will create a theoretical reduction in contrast sensitivity of 12 Db (4 logarithmic units or a 75% reduction).

The patient's visual quality and performance is, therefore, severely compromised and his or her everyday routine activities will probably be affected.

Patients with maculopathy can benefit from cataract surgery even when their visual acuity does not improve. The loss of contrast sensitivity caused by the cataract will be additive with the macular abnormalities. In this way, implantation of a monofocal IOL can improve visual performance in intermediate light frequencies, even when changes in the macula have completely compromised the vision of the higher frequencies (fine details).[10,11] The implantation of an aspheric IOL, with a higher MTF (or rather the greater capacity to transfer images to the retina), should provide greater visual improvement.[12,13]

Optic Nerve

Alterations of the optic nerve and the visual system in general are responsible for reduction in visual acuity.

When the surgeon is planning cataract surgery, the tests that quantify functional aspects of the visual system, such as measurement of vision and contrast sensitivity, are unable to express a real parameter that can reproduce the health status of the neuroretinal system. This happens because when the MTF is compromised—a situation caused by presence of a cataract—it is responsible for the reduction of visual function.

For this reason, in the evaluation of postoperative recovery and particularly when the surgeon has planned implantation of a multifocal IOL, they should base their decisions on the patient's clinical history to exclude pathologies of the optic nerve and on the results of the instrumental investigations that will exclude alterations of the thickness of the peripapillary nerve fibers (retinal nerve fiber layer thickness). As mentioned previously for macular function, responsible for reduction in contrast sensitivity, even pathologies of the optic nerve/central nervous system complex can compromise the results expected from cataract surgery.

Glaucoma or a history of optical neuritis should encourage the surgeon to pay maximum instrumental attention to the performance of the optic nerve. The OCT examination, which is extremely useful in the evaluation of the structure of the macula, will also prove to be of help in determining the condition of the optic nerve.

Measurement of Contrast Sensitivity

Measurement of contrast sensitivity is an essential examination for understanding the performance capacity of the patient's neurovisual system. Under uniform illumination, the patient is asked to distinguish characters or the orientation of a black-grayscale sinusoidal grid that is progressively more blurred against the backdrop.[1] This type of examination can measure the capacity of the visual system to distinguish the photometric contrast, that is the difference between the luminosity in 2 adjacent zones. It is measured as the ratio between the luminosity of 2 areas and their total (CIE method), also defined as the contrast of Michelson or modulation.[1]

The most frequent tests used to measure contrast sensitivity are the Pelli-Robson (PR)[2] and the Vision Contrast Test System (VCTS), or the more evolved version, the Functional Acuity Contrast Test (FACT) (Figures 14-17 and 14-18).

The Pelli-Robson test measures contrast sensitivity using letters of identical dimensions in which the contrast diminishes progressively from line to line.[3]

The luminance of the grids is distributed by square waves, and the value is noted as a logarithm. The plate is made of plastic, and on the back, there are other letters ordered in a different sequence to prevent the patient memorizing the format. The test consists of Sloan characters: 16 groups of 3 letters of equal size and legibility. The contrast for each group of 3 varies by 0.15 logarithmic units.

At the top of the test, there is almost 100% contrast, and at the bottom, the contrast is 0.5% (the final group of 3). The Pelli-Robson test measures the contrast sensitivity at high spatial frequencies 3 to 6 c/g.

On the other hand, the FACT, developed by Arthur P. Ginsburg, often allows the measurement of early loss of visual capacity with a more sensitive measurement compared to the Snellen visual acuity test.[3,4] FACT provides an accurate measurement of visual ability over a range of dimensions and contrasts that mimic normal conditions. It tests the patient's capacity to detect the presence and orientation of a grid in each of the 9 cells on the 5 lines of the test plate.

The patient is asked to indicate the orientation of the last grid on each line and the results are represented graphically on a curve of contrast sensitivity that allows the identification of the contrast threshold.[3,4]

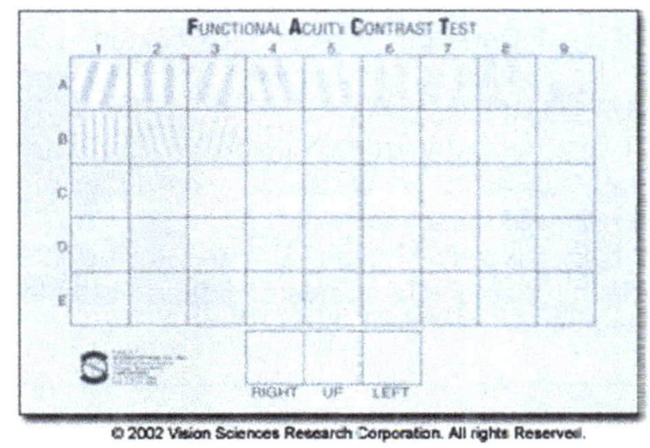

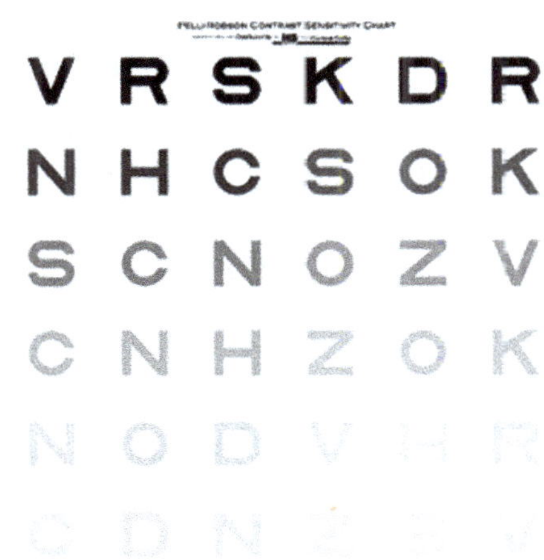

Figures 14-17 and 14-18. FACT and Pelli-Robson tests to measure contrast sensitivity.

The study of a patient's perception of contrast sensitivity is used widely in neuro-ophthalmology in the diagnosis of some subacute pathologies such as optic neuritis, multiple sclerosis, some optical pathologies, and some pathologies of the central nervous system such as Parkinson's and Alzheimer's diseases.[5-8] In some pathologies, there may be a reduction in contrast sensitivity but not in visual acuity; the progression of these pathologies can be monitored and the effects of the treatment evaluated with straightforward measurement of contrast sensitivity.

References

1. Contrast sensitivity charts. http://www.contrastsensitivity.net/csc.html
2. Johnson AT, Dooly CR, Simpson CR. Generating the snellen chart by computer. *Comput Methods Programs Biomed.* 1998;57:161–166.
3. FACT Test di Contrasto dell'Acuità Funzionale. Disponibile online da: http://www.coivision.com/index.php?ma in page=page&id=2&chapter=0.
4. Regan D, Silver R, Murray TJ. Visual acuity and contrast sensitivity in multiple sclerosis. Hidden visual loss. *Brain.* 1977;100:563-579.
5. Storch RL, Bodis-Wollner I. Overview of contrast sensitivity and neuro-ophthalmologic disease. In: Nadler MP, Miller D, Nadler DJ, eds. *Glare and Contrast Sensitivity for Clinicians.* New York, NY: Springer-Verlag; 1990:85-112.
6. Bodis-Wollner I, Diamond SP. The measurement of spatial contrast sensitivity in cases of blurred vision associated with cerebral lesions. *Brain.* 1976;99:695-710.
7. Regan D, Neima D. Low contrast letter chart in early diabetic retinopathy, ocular hypertension, glaucoma and Parkinson's disease. *Br J Ophthalmol.* 1981;68:885-889.
8. Cronin-Colomb A, Rizzo JF, Corkin S, et al. Visual function in Alzheimer's disease and normal aging. *Ann NY Acad Sci.* 1991;640:28-35.

A reduction in the retinal nerve fiber layer thickness (the peripapillary nerve fibers) is a clear sign of an alteration of nerve performance. A visual field can provide invaluable information, not only on the presence of pathology, but also on its evolution. Other examinations that are frequently used for monitoring alterations of the optic nerve are the GDX and the Heidelberg Retina Tomograph (HRT) tests.

GDX uses a laser emission that has been polarized to measure the thickness of the peripapillary nerve fibers. GDX directs the laser beam through the nerve fibers, and the light is split into 2 parallel rays that travel at different speeds. The change of speed of the laser caused by the transition through the nerve fibers is directly proportional to the thickness of the nerve fibers. A software algorithm can subtract the thickness of the vessel thickness to calculate the definitive thickness.

HRT, on the other hand, is a laser ophthalmoscope with confocal scanning. A laser beam can scan the retina in approximately 24 milliseconds, capturing retinal images at different depths, starting from the retinal surface. The union of the various profiles scanned can create a 3-dimensional map of the retinal surface analyzed. Analysis of the scans can determine thickness of the nerve fibers. Patients with glaucoma will have reduced contrast sensitivity and reduction in visual function under conditions of mesopic light, and these parameters may be present even before a reduction in the visual field has been documented. Reduction in contrast sensitivity is one of the optical functions that will be damaged early by glaucoma and is proportional to the evolution of the pathology.

It is well known that multifocal IOLs with splitting technology (refractive and diffractive) cause a reduction in contrast sensitivity, especially under mesopic conditions, affecting near vision as opposed to distance vision.

There is not a lot of information available in the literature regarding the use of multifocal lenses in glaucoma patients; nevertheless, their use in selected cases with stable vision and without a compromised visual field will result in good visual performance.

There is no doubt that aspheric IOLs with a higher MTF are preferable in these patients, even though multifocal IOLs can be implanted in carefully selected glaucomatous patients, with good results.

The surgeon must select the patients carefully, including only cases with excellent pharmacological control of intraocular pressure and with early-stage defects, with visual field parameters stable for at least 1 year.

Any patient with serious damage or progressive deterioration of the visual field and an IOP that is not well controlled must not be implanted with this type of lens. Examination of the visual field in glaucoma patients with a multifocal lens implant requires special attention; these patients will require near vision correction during the examination (despite the presence of the multifocal lenses). This will allow the surgeon to evaluate the contrast sensitivity of the distance focus, which generally receives a greater portion of light distribution.

Moreover, the surgeon may detect changes, a modest reduction in the threshold value of the visual field. He or she must anticipate a possible reduction (eg, 1 or 2 dB) in the grayscale, in the total deviation, and in the mean deviation for the standard computerized perimetry measurement.

Accommodative lenses differ from multifocal lenses in that they do not affect contrast sensitivity and may be a good alternative in patients with glaucoma.

Binocular Vision

Binocular vision is an extremely important consideration in cataract surgery and affects the type of IOL selected for implantation. In the pre-multifocal IOL era, when surgeons attempted to produce a pseudomultifocal result with monovision, binocular vision was altered. The development of multifocal lenses with different functions and different add levels for near/intermediate vision inevitably led surgeons to experiment with Mix and Match to improve visual performance at all distances.

When considering combinations of lenses with different mechanisms of action, the surgeon must decide which parameters can be safely sacrificed. Perfect binocular vision (eyes corrected with the same lenses and with the same residual refraction) involves a reduction in focal depth, and spectacles will inevitably be required under some circumstances (even when multifocal lenses have been implanted). Perfect vision at all distances requires compromise in terms of binocular vision and near distance binocular summation. This will result in a loss of stereopsis and slower reading speed.

Binocular summation is the name given to the phenomenon that allows better visual performance, at both distance and near vision, when both eyes are focused on the same target. A symmetrical stimulus on both eyes offers visual performance superior to the perception of the stimulus with just one eye. This means that both the Mix and Match approach and mini monovision proposed to increase the focal depth of the Crystalens are compromises that will alter binocular vision, particularly where near vision is concerned.

With monovision, the patient uses one eye for distance vision and the other eye for near vision; however, with multifocal lenses, both eyes have good distance vision, with variations of the near focal depth.

Accommodative lenses are different; in order to allow good distance and near vision, a compromise is necessary—one eye will be better for distance/intermediate vision and one eye will be better for intermediate/near vision (mini monovision).

It could be said that monovision is no longer as important as the comparable preoperative refractive situation that the patient wishes to preserve.

The use of monofocal lenses should be targeting a balance in the 2 eyes, with a symmetrical focal distance for near and distance vision, with the other focal distance corrected with spectacles.

The issues are more challenging with multifocal lenses; currently available lenses offer 2 focal points, for distance and near vision.

Every company has a different philosophy for near correction. Tecnis ZMB00, for example, has an add of +4 D at the lens plane, Zeiss AT LISA is +3.75 D, and finally Alcon ReSTOR is +3.00 D.

The near add is also determined by other factors, namely the portion of light intensity dedicated to near vision. The Tecnis lens has a 50:50 ratio of distance/near light distribution, the Zeiss lens is 65:35 ratio, and Alcon lenses have a variable amount depending on the pupil diameter (with a maximum of 50:50 with a small pupil under good lighting conditions).

In recent years, the market for multifocal IOLs has enjoyed significant growth, and this has led to a growing need to improve intermediate vision, to allow good vision for computer work or looking at the dashboard when driving. Currently available multifocal IOLs allow good distance and near vision, at the expense of intermediate vision. According to recent information, Alcon will soon launch a new model of the ReSTOR lens, with an even lower near add. A lens with a near add of +2.50 will no longer offer good near vision but better intermediate vision.

This will benefit people who spend a lot of time at the computer, with mild reduction of near vision. However, some surgeons suggest mixing the 2 lenses, providing a deeper focus value, resulting in one eye having good near vision and one eye for intermediate vision, and this alters the binocular summation.

In a recent publication, some authors evaluated the efficacy of asymmetrical implantation between 2 categories of lenses: an apodized diffractive refractive AcrySof ReSTOR D3 lens and a refractive M-flex 630F (Rayner) (the classical Mix and Match that has been widely discussed), examining the potential of a deeper focus for patients with a combination of the 2 lenses and less dependency on pupil diameter, compared to patients who receive the asymmetrical implant.[14] The Mix and Match approach that combines refractive and diffractive lenses is still used today as it exploits the advantages of the 2 types of the lenses. This optimizes the vision of the refractive IOLs, and offers an intermediate focus but has lower contrast sensitivity and greater development of glare and haloes, with diffractive IOLs that produce sharper distance/near vision and lower reduction in contrast sensitivity. The combination of the 2 lenses provides a greater focal depth, offset by worse contrast sensitivity (achievable with 2 diffractive lenses) and lower visual performance for reading.

Some surgeons have suggested hybrid monovision,[15] or rather, the combination of one monofocal and one multifocal lens, particularly in patients who complain about waxy vision with multifocal lenses implanted in both eyes.[15] According to the authors, distance vision is not compromised, and in 62.5% of patients, stereopsis is maintained; 18.8% of patients require spectacles for reading.

It is not easy to define guidelines for different combinations of multifocal lenses, even because the advantage of greater focal depth offered by the Mix and Match approach is countered by compromised stereopsis and visual performance when reading. Especially under these circumstances, it is essential to examine the patient carefully and determine his or her expectations, professional responsibilities, and hobbies—all factors that must be taken into consideration.

Total independence from spectacles is not necessarily always the main objective, if this is actually possible.

Visual Quality and Ocular Motility

When evaluating the patient and planning for surgery, measurements of ocular motility, ocular dominance, and binocular vision are essential. These provide important

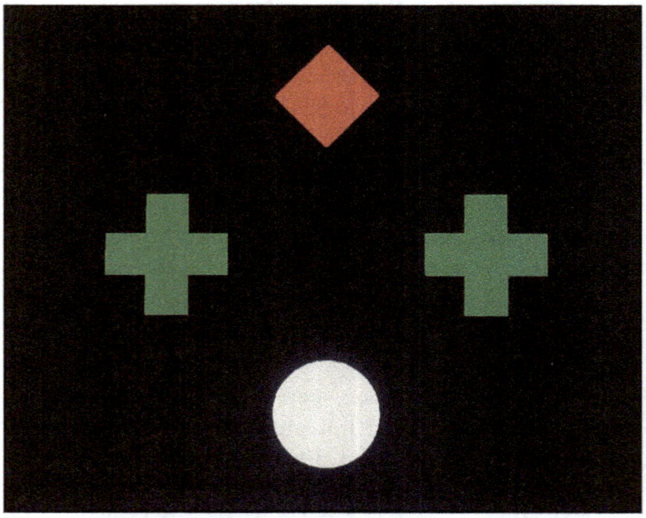

Figure 14-19. Worth's light test. Pattern of lights consisting of 2 green lights positioned at 3 o'clock and at 9 o'clock, a red light positioned at 12 o'clock, and a white light positioned at 6 o'clock.

information that can predict the postoperative visual result and the advisability of implantation of multifocal lenses.

Analysis of ocular motility will reveal the presence of strabismus and phorias, conditions that can compromise binocular vision and stereopsis. Refractive analysis of the patient and careful evaluation of his or her refractive history allow exclusion of amblyopia. A mature cataract may not always allow identification of the real "visual ability" of the eye in question, and some otherwise important information may be ignored. In these cases, analysis of near vision will provide invaluable information of macular function.

Strabismus, severe unilateral astigmatism, or significant anisometropia is the clinical sign that indicates abnormalities of the visual system that may compromise binocular function.

When the eye has an extremely mature cataract and there is decompensation of eye motility "ex non *uso*," it could suggest an incomplete recovery of visual function, or worse, postoperative diplopia.

In binocular function determination, a number of tests can be used to obtain a precise diagnosis.

Red-Green Test

The red-green test with moderate dissociation allows determination of binocular vision, the degree of dominance, and the extrinsic ocular motility. This test method involves placing a red glass filter over the right eye (by tradition) and a green glass filter over the left eye. The patient is asked to look at a light source and describe the numbers and color of the lights. If the patient sees a single light source of an indefinite color, somewhere between red and green (many patients observe white), it indicates good cooperation between the 2 eyes.

Vice versa, sight of just one color, either red or green, indicates a strong dominance of one eye and suppression of the other eye.

The third possible hypothesis is simultaneous vision of the 2 lights—one red and one green—with a variable distance between them. This third option indicates ocular codominance, with ocular misalignment, or diplopia.

It means that the mutual abnormal position of the 2 eyes is not associated with suppression of vision in one eye as opposed to another (eg, a child with one crossed eye) and the simultaneous presence of 2 images that are both valid though not coincident will produce uncomfortable double vision.

Worth's Light Test

This test closely resembles the previous test, and may be an improvement and complementary. Again using red and green glass filters, the patient is asked to look at a pattern of lights consisting of 2 green lights positioned at 3 and 9 o'clock, a red light at 12 o'clock, and a white light at 6 o'clock (Figure 14-19). The colors red and green are mutually exclusive, meaning that the red light is seen with the right eye only and the green light is seen with the left eye only (when the red glass filter has been placed over the right eye and the green glass filter has been placed over the left eye). The white light provides a parameter of superimposition between the 2 eyes. Consequently, the patient is asked to state how many lights he or she sees and their color.

Two red lights (one red and one white) indicate exclusion of the left eye (OS) (Figure 14-20).

Three green lights (2 green and 1 white) indicate exclusion of the right eye (OD) (Figure 14-21).

Four lights (1 red, 2 green, and a fourth of undefined color) indicate intact binocular vision.

Five lights (1 red, 2 green, and 2 white) indicate the presence of diplopia.

Even under these circumstances, the mutual position of the 2 white lights perceived as red and green indicate strabismus and diplopia.

Lang's Stereo Test

This test involves the patient looking at a card with simple 3-dimensional images that can be perceived only with binocular vision and stereopsis. There are 3 stereoptic images on the card, plus a third (a circle) that is also visible with monocular vision and by patients with compromised binocular vision. The 3 images illustrated are usually a cat, an elephant, and a star. The circle is included as a control system to reveal malingering patients (Figure 14-22).

The objective to achieve binocular vision is extremely important when planning a cataract procedure, particular when implantation of a multifocal lens is planned. As described previously, a diffractive or refractive multifocal lens will produce good visual performance when implanted in both eyes because of binocular summation. As described

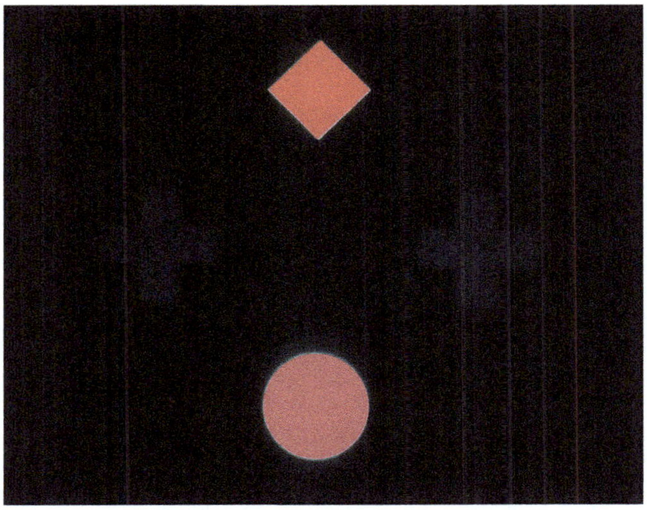

Figure 14-20. Exclusion of OS—left eye: 2 red lights (1 red and 1 white).

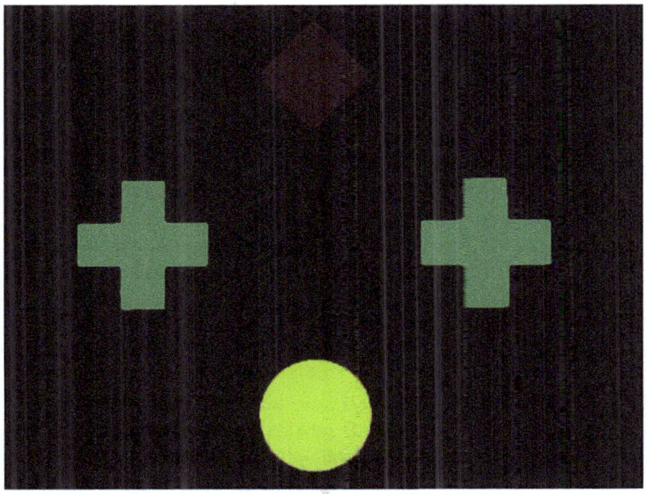

Figure 14-21. Exclusion of OD—right eye: 3 green lights (2 green and 1 white).

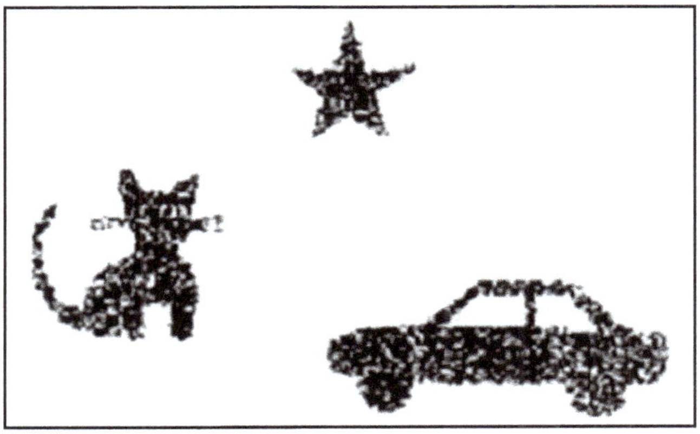

Figure 14-22. Lang's Stereo Test: 3-dimensional images that can be perceived only with binocular vision and stereopsis.

in the chapter on Mix and Match, binocular vision, particularly near vision, is greatly affected by symmetry between the 2 eyes. The perception of 2 identical and corresponding images translates into improved vision and better visual performance in patients with multifocal lenses, not just the ability to read smaller characters but also a faster reading speed. This is one of the reasons why the Mix and Match theory is not well accepted or promoted by all surgeons because the association of different IOLs with different focal distances, to improve intermediate vision, causes reduction of visual performance in reading.

Moreover, attempts to identify refractive abnormalities and associated amblyopia are extremely important in the planning and decision of lens power to be implanted. In a patient with anisometropic amblyopia in one eye, total correction of the post cataract surgical error may prove to be a satisfactory result. If the patient is used to suppressing the image from that eye, due to the uncorrected severe ametropia, total correction of the refractive error could lead to diplopia through image superimposition and abnormal retinal correspondence. The confusion induced by such a correction could create a considerable amount of discomfort,[16,17] and may sometimes require replacement of the IOL with one of a different power that will maintain a certain refractive difference between the 2 eyes.

Under these circumstances, a test with a contact lenses may be useful with an evaluation of the patient's acceptance of the final refractive result.[18]

References

1. Mainster MA, Turner PL. Multifocal IOL and maculopathy: how much is too much. In: Chang DF, ed. *Mastering Refractive IOLs: The Art and Science.* Thorofare, NJ: SLACK Incorporated; 2008:389-394.
2. Kirk KR, Werner L, Jaber R, Strenk S, Strenk L, Mamalis N. Pathologic assessment of complications with asymmetric or sulcus fixation of square-edged hydrophobic acrylic intraocular lenses. *Ophthalmology.* 2012 Mar 14. [Epub ahead of print] 2012 Mar 14.
3. LeBoyer RM, Werner L, Snyder ME, Mamalis N, Riemann CD, Augsberger JJ. Acute haptic-induced ciliary sulcus irritation associated with single-piece AcrySof intraocular lenses. *J Cataract Refract Surg.* 2005;31(7):1421-1427.
4. Gimbel HV, DeBroff BM. Intraocular lens optic capture. *J Cataract Refract Surg.* 2004;30(1):200-206. Review.
5. Suto C, Hori S, Fukuyama E, Akura JJ. Adjusting intraocular lens power for sulcus fixation. *J Cataract Refract Surg.* 2003;29(10):1913-1917.
6. Müller LJ, Marfurt CF, Kruse F, Tervo TM. Corneal nerves: structure, contents and function. *Exp Eye Res.* 2003;76(5):521-542.
7. Jaimes M, Xacur-García F, Alvarez-Melloni D, Graue-Hernández EO, Ramirez-Luquín T, Navas A. Refractive lens exchange with toric intraocular lenses in keratoconus. *J Refract Surg.* 2011;27(9):658-664. doi: 10.3928/1081597X-20110531-01. Epub 2011 Jun 10.
8. Bellucci R, Morselli S, Pucci V. Spherical aberration and coma with an aspherical and a spherical intraocular lens in normal age-matched eyes. *J Cataract Refract Surg.* 2007;33(2):203-209.

9. Guo H, Goncharov A, Dainty C. Intraocular lens implantation position sensitivity as a function of refractive error. *Ophthalmic Physiol Opt.* doi: 10.1111/j.1475-1313.2011.00888.x. Epub 2011 Dec 10.
10. Adamson I, Rubin GS, Taylor HR,Stark WJ. The effect of early cataracts on glare and contrast sensitivity: a pilot study. *Arch Ophthalmol.* 1992;110:1081-1086.
11. Elliot DB, Situ P. Visual Acuity versusletter contrast sensitivity in early cataract. *Vision Res.* 1998;38:2047-2052.
12. Holladay JT, Piers PA, Koranyi G, van der Mooren M, Norrby NE. A new intraocular lens design to reduce spherical aberration of pseudophakic eyes. *J Refract Surg.* 2002;18(6):683-691.
13. Piers PA, Norrby NE, Mester U. Eye models for the prediction of contrast vision in patients with new intraocular lens designs. *Opt Lett.* 2004;29(7):733-735.
14. Korkhov EA. Long-term results of binocular symmetric and asymmetric correction of aphakia using different multifocal intraocular lenses. *Vestn Oftalmol.* 2011;127(5):54-56.
15. Iida Y, Shimizu K, Ito M. Pseudophakic monovision using monofocal and multifocal intraocular lenses: hybrid monovision. *J Cataract Refract Surg.* 2011;37(11):2001-2005.
16. Krzizok T, Kaufmann H, Schwerdtfeger G. Binocular problems caused by aniseikonia and anisophoria after cataract operation. *Klin Monbl Augenheilkd.* 1996;208(6):477-480.
17. Gobin L, Rozema JJ, Tassignon MJ. Predicting refractive aniseikonia after cataract surgery in anisometropia. *J Cataract Refract Surg.* 2008;34(8):1353-1361.
18. Höh H. Management of unilateral refractive errors with contact lenses. *Fortschr Ophthalmol.* 1989;86(1):64-66.

Suggested Readings

Creuzot-Garcher C, Lafontaine PO, Gualino O, D'Athis P, Petit JM, Bron A. Study of ocular surface involvement in diabetic patients. *J Fr Ophtalmol.* 2005;28(6):583-588.

Donnefeld ED, Solomon K, Perry HD Doshi SJ, Ehrenhaus M, Solomon R, Biser S. The effect of hinge position on corneal sensation and dry eye after LASIK. *Ophtalmology.* 2003;110(5):1023-1029; discussion 1029-1030.

Hawkins AS, Szlyk JP, Ardickas Z, Alexander KR, Wilensky JT. Comparison of contrast sensitivity, visual acuity, and Humphrey visual field testing in patients with glaucoma. *J Glaucoma.* 2003;12(2):134-138.

Kamath GG, Prasad S, Danson A, Phillips RP. Visual outcome with the array multifocal intraocular lens in patients with concurrent eye disease. *J Cataract Refract Surg.* 2000;26(4):576-581.

Kohlhaas J. Corneal sensation after cataract and refractive surgery. *J Cataract Refract Surg.* 1998;24(10):1399-1409.

Kumar BV, Phillips RP, Prasad S. Multifocal intraocular lenses in the setting of glaucoma. *Curr Opin Ophthalmol.* 2007;18(1):62-66.

Petternel V, Menapace R, Findl O, et al. Effect of optic edge design and haptic angulation on postoperative intraocular lens position change. *J Cataract Refract Surg.* 2004;30(1):52-57.

Piers PA, Fernandez EJ, Manzanera S, Norrby S, Artal P. Adaptive optics simulation of intraocular lenses with modified spherical aberration. *Invest Ophthalmol Vis Sci.* 2004;45(12):4601-4610.

Ravalico G, Parentin F, Pastori G, Baccara F. Spatial resolution threshold in pseudophakic patients with monofocal and multifocal intraocular lenses. *J Cataract Refract Surg.* 1998;24(2):244-248.

Regan D, Neima D. Low-contrast letter charts in early diabetic retinopathy, ocular hypertension, glaucoma, and Parkinson's disease. *Br J Ophthalmol.* 1984;68(12):885-889.

Seiple WH. The clinical utility of spatial contrast sensitivity testing. In: Tasman W, Jaeger EW, eds. *Duane's Foundations of Clinical Ophthalmology.* Philadelphia, PA: Lippincott; 1991.

Stoffelns BM, Vetter J, Keicher A, Mirshahi A. Pars planavitrectomy for visually disturbing vitreous floaters in pseudophacic eyes. *Klin Monbl Augenheilkd.* 2011;228(4):293-297. Epub 2011 Apr 11.

Wood JM, Lovie-Kitchin JE. Evaluation of the efficacy of contrast sensitivity measures for the detection of early primary open-angle glaucoma. *Optom Vis Sci.* 1992;69(3):175-181.

15

Viscoelastic Substances

Lucio Buratto, MD; Stephen F. Brint, MD, FACS; and Domenico Boccuzzi, MD, PhD

When the surgeon selects the most suitable viscoelastic substance (VES) to use during cataract surgery, the most important characteristic is the substance's ability to coat and protect the corneal endothelium, in addition to creating space for intraocular lens (IOL) implantation.

The characteristics used to classify a VES are its viscoelasticity, viscosity, pseudoplasticity, cohesiveness, dispersiveness, and finally, surface tension.

Viscoelasticity is the term given to the ability of a fluid or solution to return to its original shape once it has been subjected to pressure. In practical terms, elasticity is the force that allows the anterior chamber to return to its original shape when the pressure that deformed it is released. A nonelastic solution such as balanced salt solution (BSS) will not return to its original shape when the compression is released.

Viscosity, on the other hand, is the measurement of a solution's resistance to flux and is a function of the substance's molecular weight. The molecular weight reflects the size of the molecules in the solution; the greater the molecular weight of a substance, the greater its resistance to flux.

The viscosity of the VES is measured in centipoise (cP) or in centistokes (cSt) that are the measurements of resistance to flux at a given cut rate (also known as *shear rate*).

The viscosity of water is 1.001 cP at 20°C; oily substances have a density of 1000 cP, and gelatinous substances (such as honey) have a density of approximately 10,000 cP.

Viscoat, for example, has a viscosity of approximately 40,000 cP; Vitrax has a viscosity of 50,000 cP. The viscosity of a substance is the degree of movement of a solution, also known as the shear rate, and its variation is inversely proportional to temperature.

The viscosity of a solution can be increased, by increasing the concentration or the molecular weight of the solution, and it can be changed by varying the temperature.

The density (more correctly referred to as the volumetric mass or the specific mass) of a body (often indicated with the symbol ρ or δ) is defined as the ratio between the mass and the volume of a body.

Pseudoplasticity, on the other hand, refers to the ability of a solution to be transformed when it is subjected to strong compression, with the transition from a gelatinous state into a more liquid state. This is a characteristic of non-Newtonian fluids that, in practical terms, is the ability of a substance to modify its resistance in response to stimuli.

Graphically, pseudoplasticity is represented as the logarithm of dynamic viscosity with respect to the logarithm of the shear rate (Figure 15-1). The ideal VES should have high pseudoplasticity or should maintain spaces and protect tissues (high viscosity with a low shear rate), allowing manipulation of surgical instruments inside the eye, and permit safe implantation of the IOL (moderate viscosity with a moderate shear rate); finally, it should have low resistance when injected into the eye through a cannula (low viscosity with a high shear rate).

Cohesiveness is the tendency of a material to adhere to itself and is an expression of the molecular weight and viscoelasticity. An extremely cohesive substance has an extremely high molecular weight and a very long molecular chain length.

Dispersiveness is the tendency of the VES to disperse when it is injected into the anterior chamber. This

Buratto L, Brint SF, Boccuzzi D.
Cataract Surgery and Intraocular Lenses (pp 119-124).

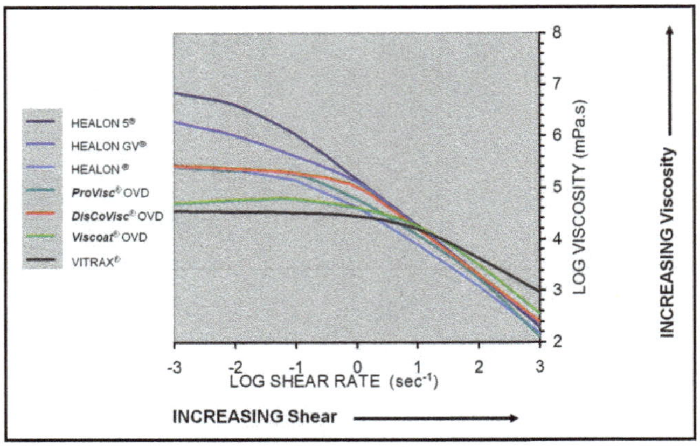

Figure 15-1. Pseudoplasticity: shear rate is shown on the x axis and viscosity is shown on the y axis.

Table 15-1

Chemical and Physical Characteristics of Ophthalmic Viscosurgical Device

PRODUCT	VOLUME (mL)	VISCOSITY*	PSEUDOPLASTICITY
Healon	0.55/0.95	40,000	++++
Healon GV	0.55/0.85	60,000	+++++
IAL	2.0/5.0	8000 to 10,000	++
ILA-F	1.1	20,000 to 22,000	+++
Provisc	0.4/0.55/0.85	25,000 to 28,000	+++
Viscoat	0.5	45,000	+++
Biolon	0.5/1	30,000	+++
Ophthalin	0.5	32,000 to 35,000	++++
Ocucoat	1	4000	+
Amovitrax	0.7	40,000	+++
Amvisc Plus	0.5/0.8	55,000	++++
*Expressed in cps and measured at 1 sec^{-1} (shear rate) and 20°C.			

parameter is also a function of the molecular weight and the viscoelasticity.

Generally speaking, highly dispersive molecules will have a low molecular weight and a short molecular chain.

Finally, the surface tension (coatability) measures the ability of a substance to coat fabrics, instruments, etc. Low surface tension is translated into a smaller contact angle.

Contact angle (α) is the angle created between the solid surface beneath the VES and the tangent of the VES bubble at the contact point. The smaller the contact angle, the lower the surface tension and the greater the wettability and coatability of the substance (Table 15-1).

A VES largely consists of hyaluronic acid (HA) at concentrations that vary between 1% and 3%. There are VES of hydroxypropyl methylcellulose (HPMC) (not popular at present) and others containing chondroitin sulfate (CDS). For example, the concentration of CDS in Viscoat and DisCoVisc is 4%; the concentration of HA in DisCoVisc is 1.65% and 3% in Viscoat (Table 15-2).

The advantage of CDS is based on the presence of 2 supplementary negative charges with respect to HA. This leads to better adhesion of the VES to the corneal endothelium.[1,2]

Moreover, CDS provides better protection against free radicals than sodium hyaluronate alone.[3]

Finally, the persistence of VES in the anterior chamber following removal of the lens was also evaluated. The use of in vivo confocal microscopy demonstrated that VES with CDS persists for a longer period of time in the anterior chamber following removal of the lens, and this translates into greater protection of the corneal endothelium[4] (Figure 15-2), lower inflammatory response of the tissues, and more rapid postoperative recovery times.

Table 15-2

Ophthalmic Viscosurgical Devices

PRODUCT	PRODUCTOR (PRODUCTOR, RAW MATERIAL)	COMPOSITION		MOLECULAR WEIGHT (MILLIONS OF DALTON)	ORIGIN	pH	OSMOLARITY
Healon	AMO (Biomatrix)	1%	HA	4.0	Natural	7.0 to 7.5	302
Healon G.V.	AMO (Biomatrix)	1.4%	HA	5.0	Natural	7.0 to 7.5	302
IAL	Bausch + Lomb (Fidia)	1.2%	HA	1.2	Natural	7.2 to 7.4	300
IAL-F	Bausch + Lomb (Fidia)	1.8%	HA	1.2	Natural	7.2 to 7.4	300
Provisc	Alcon (Genzyme)	1.0%	HA	0.5	Fermented	7.0 to 7.5	310
Viscoat	Alcon (Genzyme)	3% 4%	HA CDS	0.5 0.02	Fermented Natural	7.0 to 7.5	325
Biolin	SIFI (General Biotechnology)	1.0%	HA	2.8	Fermented	7.2 to 7.4	300
Ophthalin	Zeiss (Fermentech)	1%	HA	3.6	Fermented	7.0 to 7.5	305
Ocucoat	Bausch + Lomb	2%	HPMC	0.1	Natural	7	285
Amovitrax	AMO	3%	HA	0.5	Natural	7.2 to 7.4	310
Amvisc	Bausch + Lomb	1.6%	HA	1.5	Fermented	7.2 to 7.4	340

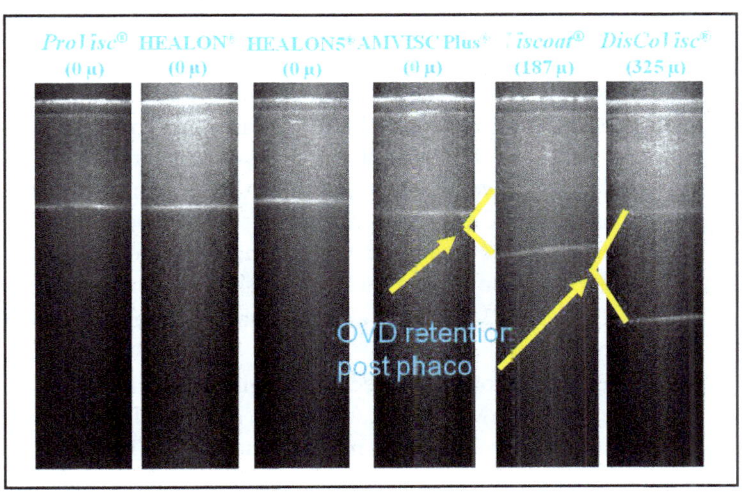

Figure 15-2. Quantitative evaluations of the VES that contain CDS compared to those that contain hyaluronate, using the confocal microscope in vivo. Viscodispersive VES guarantees greater residual thickness post phaco. The thickness of the VES adhered to the endothelium is an indication of its persistence post phaco. There will be less damage to the endothelial cells post phaco when the VES persists in the anterior chamber. (Reprinted from *J Cataract Refract Surg*, 31, Petroll WM, Jafari M, Lane SS, et al, Quantitative assessment of ophthalmic viscosurgical device retention using in vivo confocal microscopy, 2363-2368, Copyright 2005, with permission from Elsevier.)

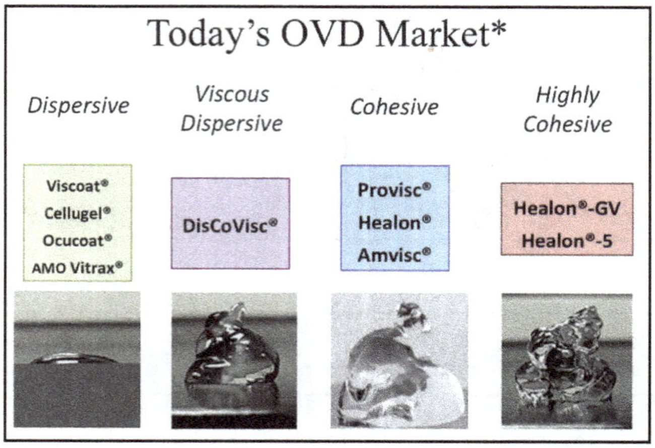

Figure 15-3. New classification of the VES. (Reprinted from *J Cataract Refract Surg*, 31, Arshinoff SA, Jafari M, New classification of ophthalmic viscosurgical devices—2005, 2167-2171, Copyright 2005, with permission from Elsevier.)

The molecular weight (expressed in Daltons) is another important characteristic of the VES; it expresses the length of the chain of HA, HPMC, or CDS. The molecular weight changes the characteristics of the VES and this leads to the expression of different rheological-chemical-physical properties.

High molecular weight is a typical feature of a cohesive VES, normally used to create space, for example, when the anterior chamber is shallow or the cataract is intumescent.

This VES can also be used when the surgeon requires a higher pressure in the anterior chamber compared to the pressure in the posterior chamber. This pressure increase is extremely useful during capsulorrhexis because it can flatten the convex surface of the lens capsule and prevent rhexis escape. Finally, cohesive VES can be used to dilate small pupils, dissect areas of adhesion, and may be useful during IOL implantation.

VES with high cohesive properties must be used with caution during the delicate phases of surgery because excessive maneuvers will lead to a rapid and sudden escape of the VES from the anterior chamber. Consequently, maneuvers must be extremely precise and the surgical technique must be performed with maximum attention. During aspiration, large molecules will be aspirated in a single mass, and this ensures that the removal is straightforward, rapid, and complete; consequently, the surgeon will not have to "search for" any residual VES in the anterior chamber or behind the IOL.

Due to its large structure, if left inside the anterior chamber, the VES will block the trabecular meshwork and can lead to large increases in intraocular pressure. Healon and Healon G.V. are high-molecular-weight cohesive VES with values of 4.0 and 5.0 million Dalton, respectively.

Low molecular weight is a characteristic of a dispersive VES. These substances resist aspiration and have the ability to split in the spaces (ie, to create areas with remaining VES and others that do not).

Their dispersive nature, the presence of negative electrical charges (2 more per molecule with CDS, eg, with Viscoat or DisCoVisc), and the presence of HA that binds to specific sites on the corneal endothelium increase retention of these substances in the anterior chamber during surgery. During rhexis, for example, they can inflate the chamber well and create good stability of the chamber during the movements, maneuvers, and compression that occur during this step, without provoking sudden shallowing (different from that of a cohesive VES).

Moreover, these substances can separate the anterior chamber into spaces occupied by the VES and surgical areas that are free from the VES; consequently, irrigation/aspiration can continue, without the 2 areas mixing. This phenomenon is called *surgical compartmentalization.*

These VES are particularly indicated in eyes in which surgeons suspect pathology of the endothelium because of their high ability for protecting the endothelium.

Dispersive VES are used to move or isolate intraocular structures, for example, as a tamponade with a posterior capsule dialysis, or vitreous that has prolapsed because of zonular detachment or to move the iris.

Dispersive VES are more difficult to remove than cohesive VES, and smaller molecules are usually not completely removed during irrigation/aspiration.

During cataract surgery, dispersive VES is used in the initial part of the procedure, during rhexis and phacoemulsification, particularly during ultrasound; this step of surgery brings larger nuclear pieces into the anterior chamber with fairly high fluid dynamics. At this point, the amount of residual VES is minimal (only the VES that contains CDS remains in the anterior chamber until the lens is removed).

In the final step of cortical aspiration with a coaxial handpiece, or with separate irrigation/aspiration cannulas, surgeons may have to perform complete removal of dispersive VES from the anterior chamber. The surgeon must check that all residual VES has been removed by moving the aspiration cannula into all areas of the anterior chamber, without waiting for the VES to be drawn toward the opening of the aspiration cannula (as is the case with cohesive VES). This is caused by the chemical-physical composition of these substances, formed by short-chain molecules.

Dispersive VES in the anterior chamber does not lead to a pressure spike.

Examples of low-molecular-weight dispersive VES are Viscoat and AMO Vitrax, which are composed of HA with a molecular weight of 0.6 million Dalton (Figure 15-3).[5]

Under some circumstances, combination of a cohesive and a dispersive VES can improve stability of the anterior chamber, particularly when the nucleus of the cataract is extremely hard or when the surgeon has to manage complications.

This technique, based on using 2 different types of VES, is called the *soft shell technique* (Figures 15-4 and 15-5). The procedure involves first an injection of a dispersive VES

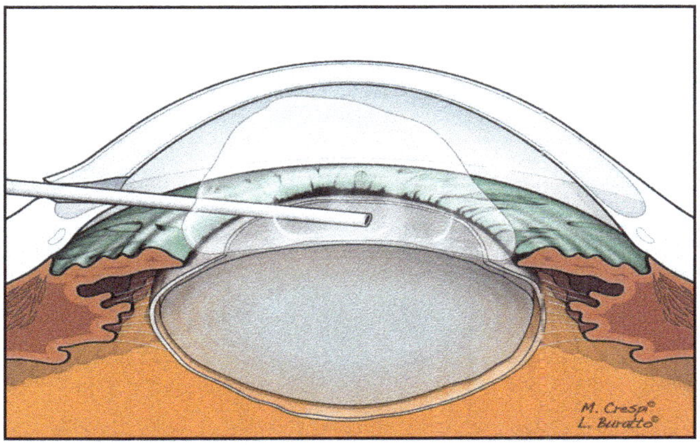

Figure 15-4. Soft shell technique. Injection of dispersive VES that will spread over the endothelial surface.

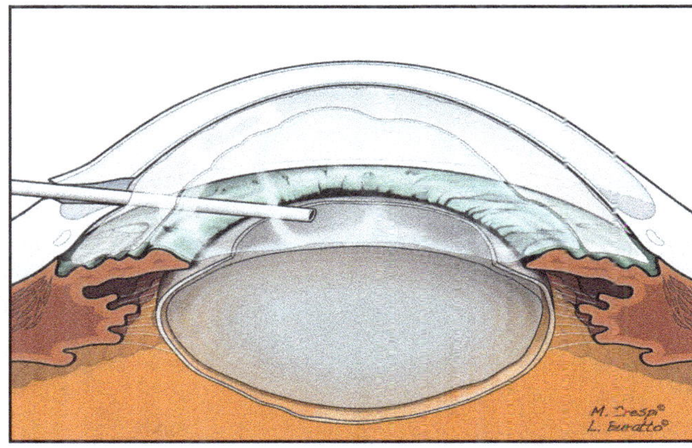

Figure 15-5. The surgeon injects a cohesive VES in the portion that is in contact with the anterior capsule of the crystalline to deepen the chamber, flatten the anterior capsule, and push the dispersive VES underneath the corneal endothelium.

that coats the endothelial surface and then a second injection of a cohesive VES in contact with the anterior capsule of the lens to distend and deepen the chamber, flatten the anterior capsule, and push the dispersive VES against the corneal endothelium. This will increase endothelial protection particularly in patients with Fuchs' endothelial dystrophy, and will result in more rapid postoperative recovery.[6]

Viscoelastic substances have a pH that varies between 7.0 and 7.5 with an osmolarity that ranges between 285 and 325 mOsm/L, the limit to prevent inflammation and toxic phenomena that may damage the corneal endothelium specifically, and more generally, all of the ocular structures. In addition to dispersive and cohesive VES, there is an additional category of VES called *viscodispersive* VES. One example of a viscodispersive VES is DisCoVisc.

It is a monophasic VES that can be used both in the early part of surgery (eg, during the rhexis and phaco) and in the final phases of IOL implantation. Like Viscoat, this VES contains HA and CDS (HA 1.65%, CDS 4%). Similar to the other VES containing CDS, the presence of the dual negative charge, in addition to the HA content, makes a contribution to increasing adhesion to corneal endothelium, improving protective qualities during phacoemulsification.

Finally, there is a fourth category of VES called the *adaptive VES*. The adaptive VES consist of long-chain molecules; thus, they are very dense and highly cohesive and can be split by a water flow. They have the same properties as a dispersive VES under certain situations such as a high cut rate, for example, when movements in the anterior chamber are at a high frequency (eg, during phaco); they demonstrate the properties of a cohesive VES in phases using low cut rates (eg, during insertion of the IOL). If these substances are not removed completely at the end of surgery, they can lead to significant increases in IOP.

Healon 5 is one example of an adaptive VES.[7]

The Role of Viscoelastic Substance During Cataract Surgery

During cataract surgery, VES has the following roles:

- Inflating and maintaining anterior chamber depth, particularly during rhexis.
- Flattening the anterior surface of the lens, particularly when the lens is intumescent, to reduce expulsion, that may lead to extension or escape of the rhexis.
- Covering the corneal endothelium and protecting it from the turbulence created by the irrigation fluids or floating lens fragments.
- Pushing the iris back from the entrance of the ultrasound probe; stabilizing the iris so that its movements are minimized during the turbulence.
- Buffering the friction caused when surgical instruments are introduced through small incisions.
- Temporarily tamponading a posterior capsular rupture until phacoemulsification has been completed or until the surgeon converts to a manual extracapsular technique.
- Creating space inside the anterior chamber and inside the capsular bag for IOL implantation (Tables 15-3 and 15-4).

References

1. Poyer JF, Chan KY, Arshinoff SA. New method to measure the retention of viscoelastic agents on a rabbit corneal endothelial cell line after irrigation and aspiration. *J Cataract Refract Surg.* 1998;24:84-90.

Table 15-3

Role of the Viscoelastic Substance in the Various Phases of Cataract Surgery

Maintain the spaces	During the rhexis	Dispersive
	Insertion of the IOL	Cohesive
Create space	Creates the groove Moves the crystalline lens material	Cohesive
Isolate	Closes the capsular ruptures Keeps the iris at a safe distance	Dispersive
Coating and protection	Protects the endothelium during phaco	Dispersive

Table 15-4

Behavior of the Viscoelastic Substance in the Various Phases of Cataract Surgery

STEP	COHESIVE	DISPERSIVE
Capsulotomy	Fills the anterior chamber easily but also escapes readily during the capsulotomy procedure	Fills the chamber and provides excellent stability during the rhexis procedure
Phaco	Escapes with initial vacuum	Adheres to the endothelium Protects the endothelium from impact from vagrant fragments
IOL insertion	Ideal for filling and maintaining the bag Easily removed	Difficult to remove

2. Craig MT, Olson RJ, Mamalis N, Olson RJ. Air bubble endothelial damage during phacoemulsification in human eye bank eyes: the protective effects of Healon and Viscoat. *J Cataract Refract Surg.* 1990;16:597-602.
3. Vasavada A, Ong M, Cordova D, Hartzer M. *Protective Effect of Ophthalmic Viscosurgical Devices (OVDs) Against Hydrogen Peroxide-Induced Oxidative Damage to Corneal Endothelial Cells: an In-Vitro Model.* Accepted for presentation: San Francisco, CA: American Society of Cataract and Refractive Surgeons; 2009.
4. Petroll WM, Jafari M, Lane SS, et al. Quantitative assessment of ophthalmic viscosurgical device retention using in vivo confocal microscopy. *J Cataract Refract Surg.* 2005;31(12):2363-2368.
5. Arshinoff SA, Jafari M. New classification of ophthalmic viscosurgical devices—2005. *J Cataract Refract Surg.* 2005;31(11):2167-2171.
6. Tarnawska D, Wylegala E. Effectiveness of the soft-shell technique in patients with Fuchs' endothelial dystrophy. *J Cataract Refract Surg.* 2007;33:1907–1912.
7. Dick HB, Krummenauer F, Augustin AJ, Pakula T, Pfeiffer N. Healon 5 viscoadaptive formulation: comparison to Healon and Healon GV. *J Cataract Refract Surg.* 2001;27(2):320-326.

16

Instruments Used for Intraocular Lens Insertion

Lucio Buratto, MD; Stephen F. Brint, MD, FACS; and Domenico Boccuzzi, MD, PhD

The intraocular lens (IOL) is a fragile, delicate product that must be handled and inserted with care and attention; surgical instruments have been developed for intraoperative management of the IOL and to facilitate insertion of the IOL, allowing the lens to be manipulated and positioned without damage. We are referring to forceps that can be used to handle and introduce rigid IOLs, the "holder and folder," and the more modern injection systems (screw-controlled or piston) that allow foldable IOLs to be injected directly into the anterior chamber, through mini- or micro-incisions created for implantation.

Folders and Holders for Rigid Intraocular Lenses

Before the advent of foldable IOLs, in order to implant rigid polymethylmethacrylate (PMMA) IOLs, the surgeon had to enlarge the incision to allow the entrance of the IOL. Irrespective of whether the surgery was a phaco or an extracapsular procedure, for insertion of the IOL, the size of the corneal incision needed to be similar to the diameter of the optic of the IOL.

The implantation of a rigid PMMA IOL required special care and attention because this type of rigid lens, particularly the 1-piece lens, could damage the endothelium or the posterior capsule during insertion.

To complete implantation, the surgeon could use forceps, such as McPherson forceps; however, this was not ideal because of the angulation of the arms; alternately, the surgeon could opt for specially designed forceps, such as Buratto forceps, consisting of 2 atraumatic tips that hold the optic and introduce it into the capsular bag. Once the first haptic and the optic have been inserted, the second haptic is introduced using McPherson forceps or by rotating the lens using a Sinskey Buratto hook (or similar) positioned at the junction between the optic and the haptic.

Holder and Folder for Soft Intraocular Lenses

The development of foldable IOLs was a major improvement and allowed surgeons to use the size of the initial phaco incision without enlarging it. This led to a reduction in surgical time (multiple sutures were not required), a reduction in postoperative recovery times, and avoidance of induced astigmatism. There are 2 distinct methods for insertion of foldable lenses: the first involves the use of a surgical instrument called "holder and folder"; the second involves use of injectors and cartridges.

The holder and folder require enlargement of the incision from 3.6 to 3.8 mm to facilitate introduction of the IOL into the capsular bag.

The recent introduction of injectors, on the other hand, has improved and simplified the procedure used to insert the IOL, through the phaco incision with no incision size enlargement necessary.

Generally speaking, foldable IOLs that are implanted using forceps are made of hydrophobic acrylic.

Buratto L, Brint SF, Boccuzzi D.
Cataract Surgery and Intraocular Lenses (pp 125-133).

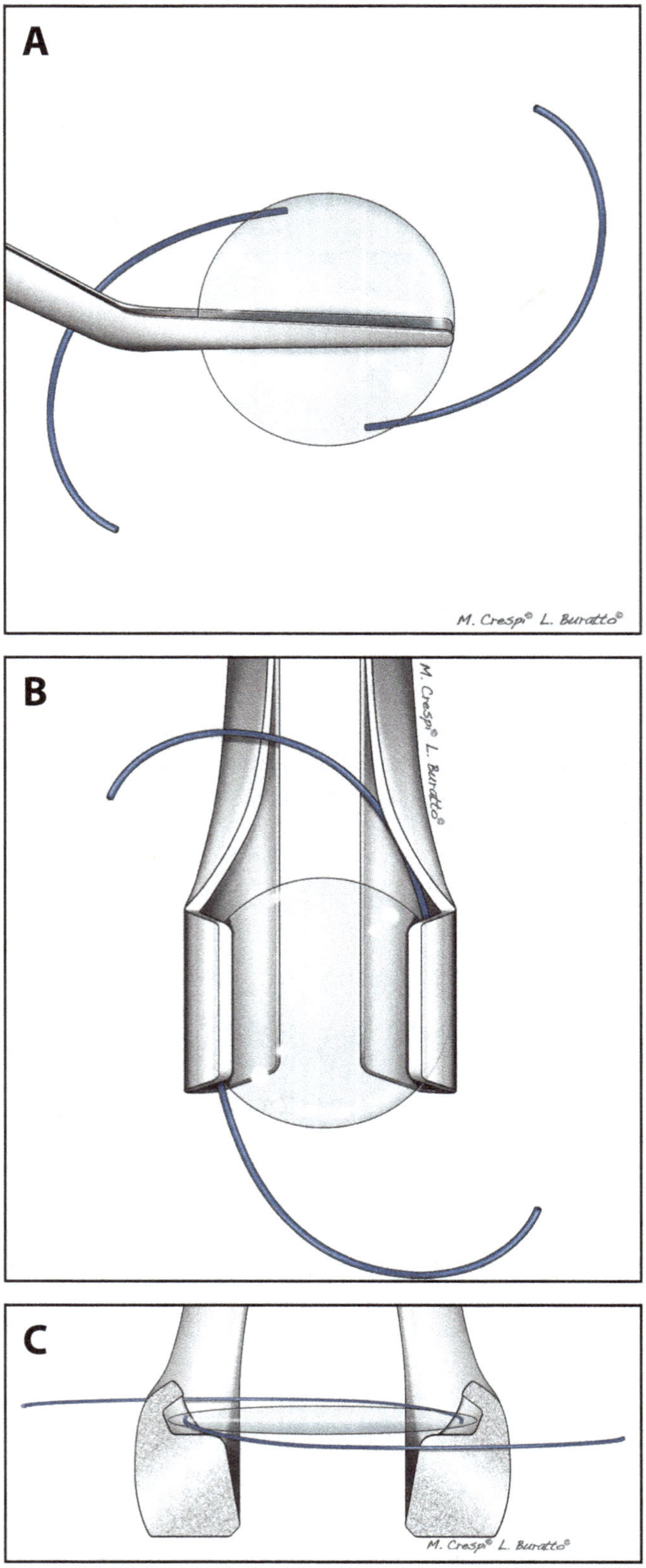

Figure 16-1. (A) The lens is removed from its container. If the tips of the forceps touch the lens surface, the optic may be scratched. (B) The lens is placed horizontally on the plate of the folder. (C) The edge of the optic must correspond to the internal angle of the folder plate.

Because of the structure of acrylic IOLs, some surgeons suggest warming the lens to soften it, as this facilitates the folding and unfolding processes.

Numerous instruments have been designed for this procedure, all of them developed to fold the IOL and facilitate its insertion in the eye.

We will give a brief description of the some of these instruments, illustrating appropriate insertion techniques and possible complications, with special reference to a specific folder (F-300 Micra or Janach's); the procedures are similar for all of the other instruments.

The surgeon must ensure that the instruments that come into contact with the IOLs are clean and free from debris deposited during sterilization. The lenses must be handled very carefully, to avoid scratching the extremely delicate surface of the lens.

The folder has 2 arms where the tips are slightly tilted inward; at the bottom, there are 2 feet that rest on the lens, and finally, along the valve a full depth groove, to catch the 2 arms of the holder to lift the lens and insert it into the eye.

Folding of the Intraocular Lens

Once the IOL has been removed carefully from its container, it is positioned on the 2 feet at the base of the folder, with the upper surface facing upward (the surgeon can orient it by observing the position of the haptics); the surgeon must ensure that the edge of the optic rests on the internal angle of the plate (Figure 16-1). The folder has been specifically designed to hold the lens firmly and not slip out of the folder's grasp; it also ensures that the lens is folded in the correct direction (meaning that the surfaces of the 2 halves face each other when the lens has been folded).

Correct positioning of the lens at the base of the folder ensures that the lens has been folded symmetrically (Figure 16-2). Any abnormal or incorrect position of the lens on the folder will result in the lens being folded asymmetrically and the 2 halves will have different dimensions (Figure 16-3); thus, a larger incision will be required to insert the lens into the eye.

When the lens has been folded correctly, the holder is used to insert the lens inside the eye (Figure 16-4). This is also an extremely delicate step; the position of the forceps' arms on the lens will determine the outcome of the entire procedure. If the forceps' tips are too close to the edge of the lens, problems may arise when the lens is released inside the eye. Occasionally, a second instrument may be necessary to disengage the lens from the forceps.

When the IOL is being inserted, it is not necessary to fold the distal haptic. With the forceps held in the right hand, the surgeon simply rotates his or her hand in a counterclockwise direction (moving his or her wrist toward a prone position) and insert the haptic inside the tunnel to place it in the anterior chamber (Figure 16-5).

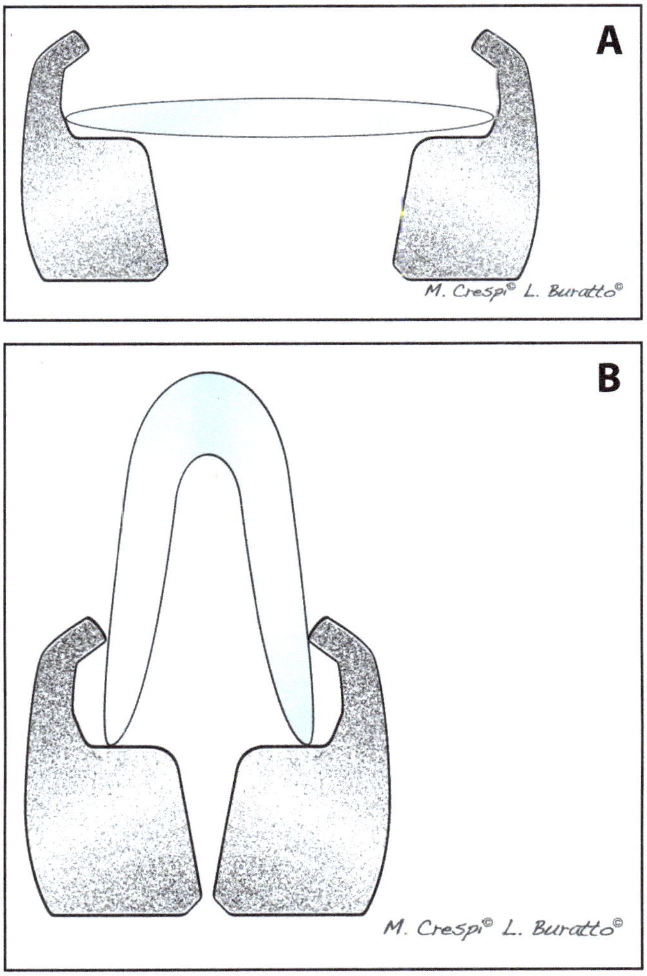

Figure 16-2. The lens is folded symmetrically.

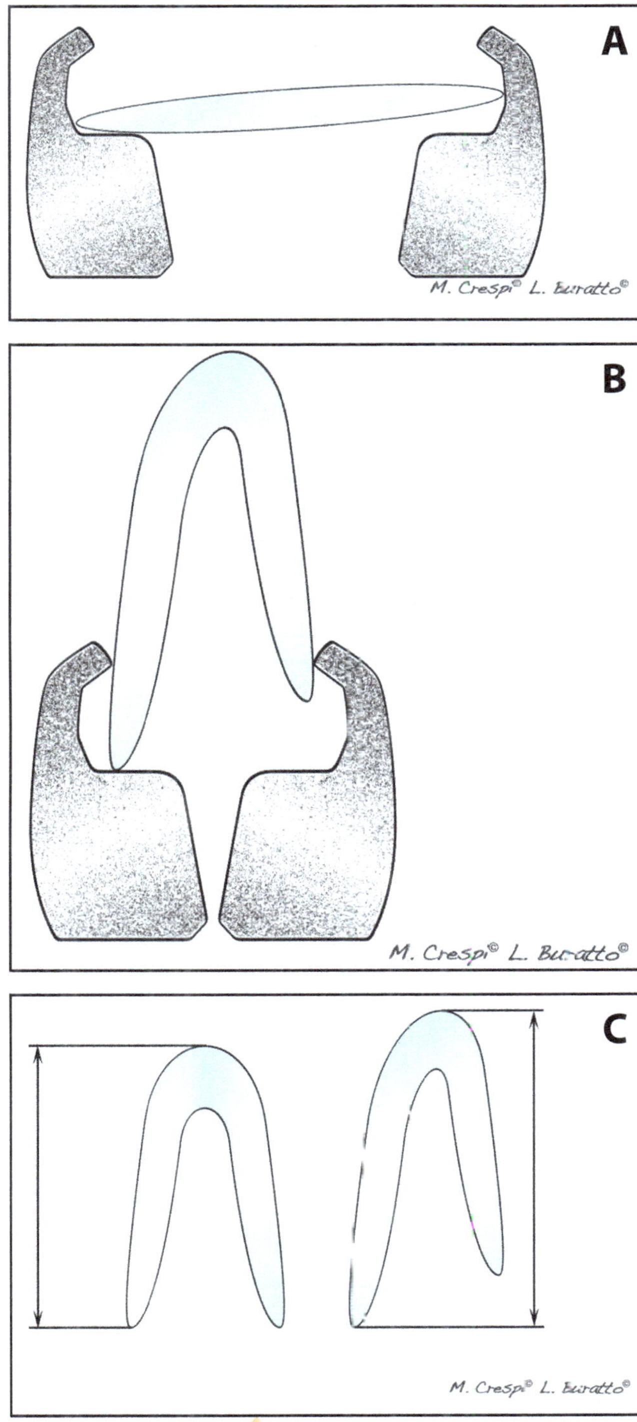

Figure 16-3. (A) The edge of the optic is not positioned correctly on the internal angle of the folder. (B, C) This incorrect position will result in the lens being folded asymmetrically.

At this point, the closed portion of the optic will be on the left side. Once the optic has been positioned inside the tunnel, the forceps should be withdrawn slightly to facilitate the positioning of the distal haptic below the rhexis. The longer the tunnel length, the greater the distance the forceps must be withdrawn. It is essential to direct the distal haptic into the capsular bag before the optic of the lens has been inserted in the anterior chamber and unfolds.

Once the distal haptic has been inserted below the edge of the capsulorrhexis, the forceps is rotated in a clockwise direction (with the surgeon's wrist moving to a supine position) (Figure 16-6). The surgeon gently releases the arms of the forceps; the lens will unfold and disengage from the forceps (Figure 16-7).

Using small movements of compression and rotation of the lens, the optic enters the capsular bag followed by the second haptic (Figure 16-8). A hook can assist this maneuver; the surgeon must ensure that the hook's tip engages the junction between the optic and the proximal haptic. The lens should be rotated gently clockwise, under gentle pressure. Another option is to use atraumatic forceps (McPherson) to grasp the proximal haptic and place it below the capsulorrhexis (Figures 16-9 and 16-10).

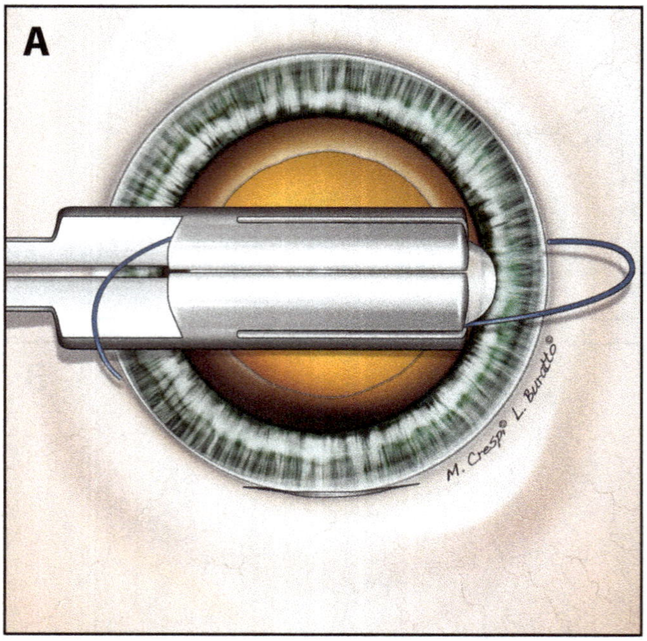

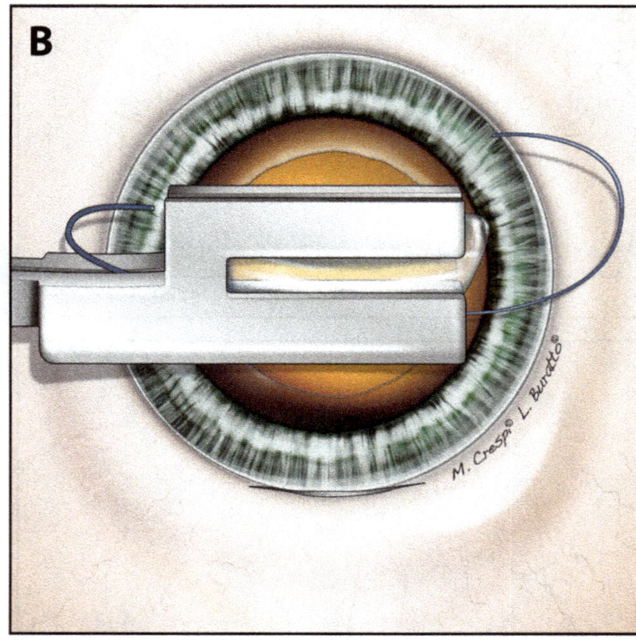

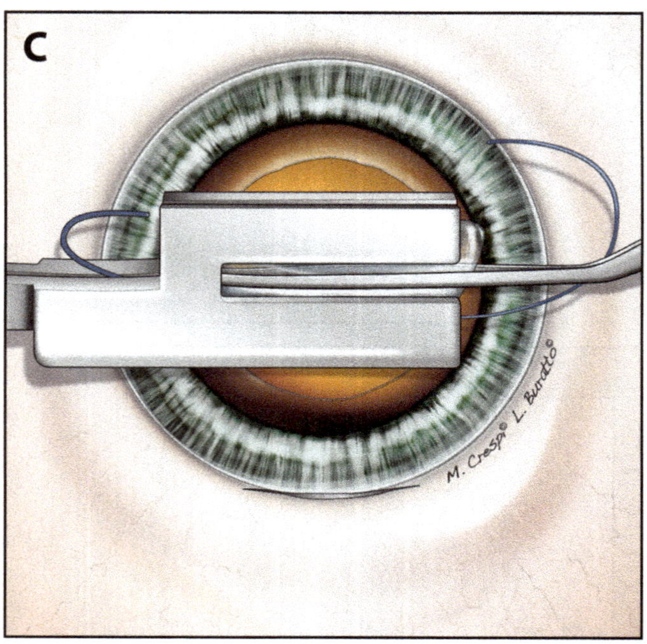

Figure 16-4. (A) The folder is closed and the lens has been folded correctly. (B) A side view of the closed folder. (C) The lens is grasped by the forceps for implantation, using a folder.

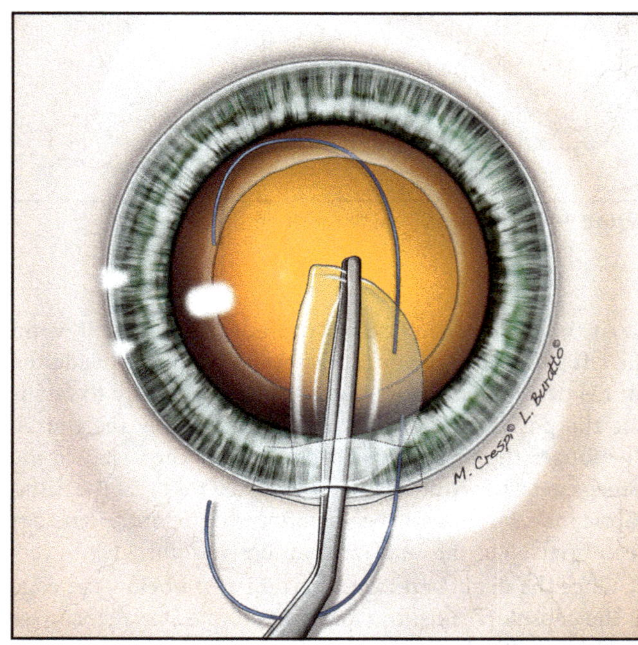

Figure 16-5. The forceps are rotated in a counterclockwise direction for the implantation; the distal loop is positioned inside the tunnel and implanted in the anterior chamber. The closed portion of the optic is positioned on the left.

Useful Suggestions

The position of the arms of the holder on the surface of the optic is also an important step of correct lens implantation (Figure 16-11). If the arms of the forceps grasp the lens in a position that is too peripheral with respect to the optic (in comparison to the folded portion) (Figures 16-12 and 16-13), the lens may remain trapped and the surgeon will have to use a second instrument to disengage it (Figure 16-14).

If the lens is grasped in a position that is too central, too close to the point where the lens has been folded (Figures 16-15 and 16-16), the surgeon will have to apply a greater amount of pressure to keep the lens folded, and runs the risk of tearing or damaging the lens.

Regarding the horizontal position of the forceps with respect to the lens, it is essential that the arms of the forceps exactly cover the entire length of the optic (Figure 16-17).

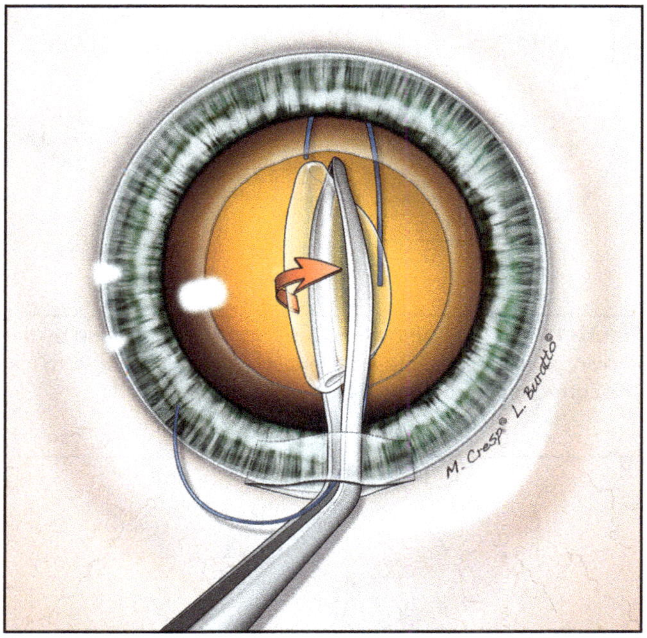

Figure 16-6. As the optic progresses into the tunnel, the forceps for the implantation are repositioned posteriorly to ensure that the distal loop is positioned underneath the opposite edge of the anterior capsule. The longer the tunnel, the more posterior the position of the forceps. The distal loop must be positioned in the capsular bag before the optic is introduced and has unfolded inside the anterior chamber.

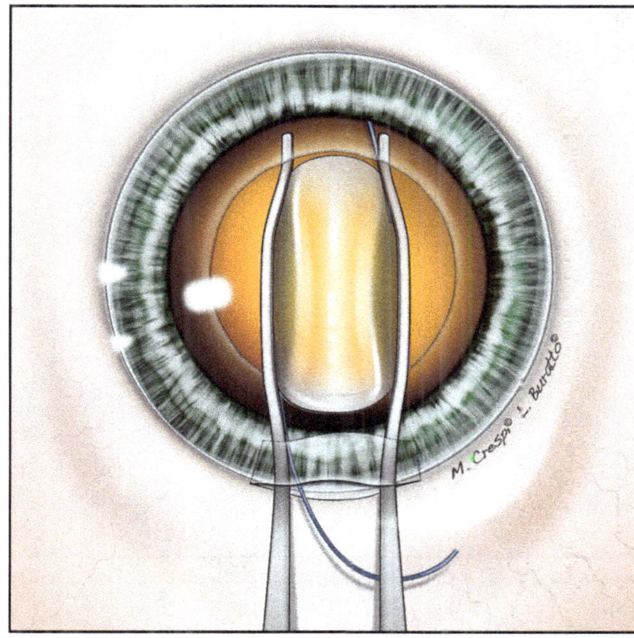

Figure 16-7. When the distal haptic has been positioned below the edge of the anterior capsulorrhexis, the forceps must be rotated in a clockwise direction.

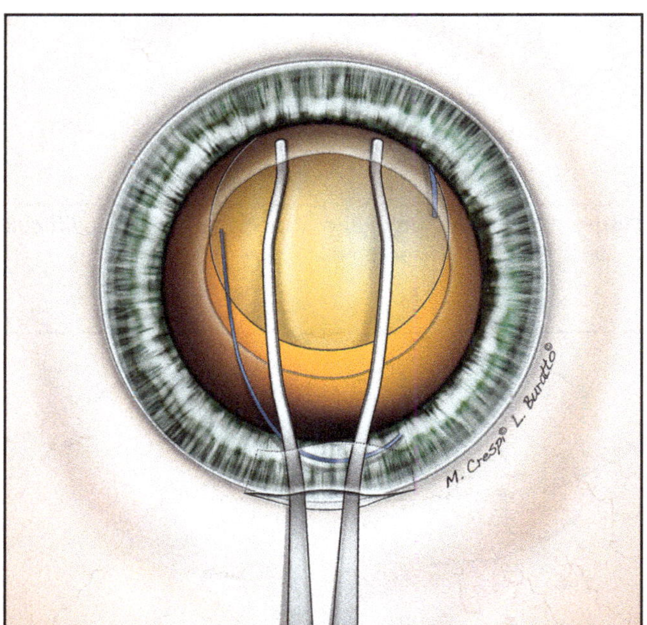

Figure 16-8. Opening the forceps allows the optic plate to open slowly and disengage from the forceps.

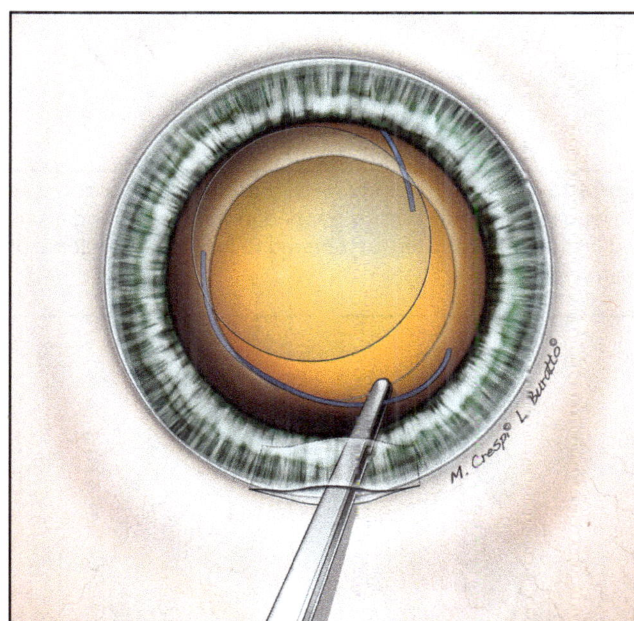

Figure 16-9. The optic is pushed downward and rotated in a clockwise direction using the implantation forceps.

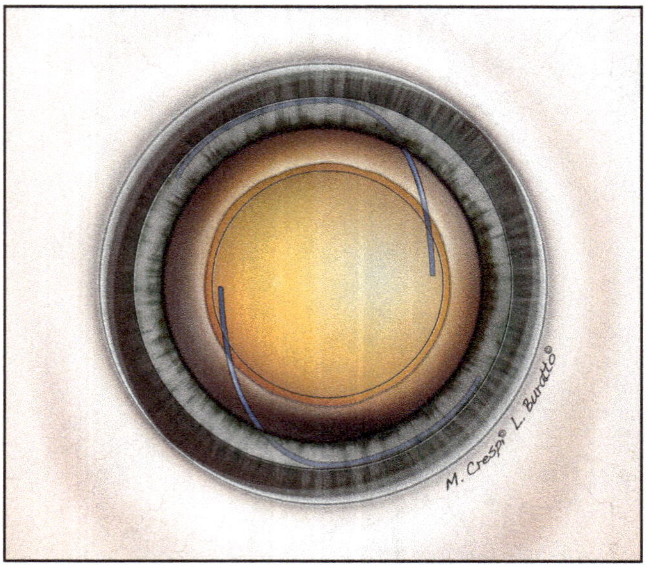

Figure 16-10. The proximal loop is introduced into the capsular bag.

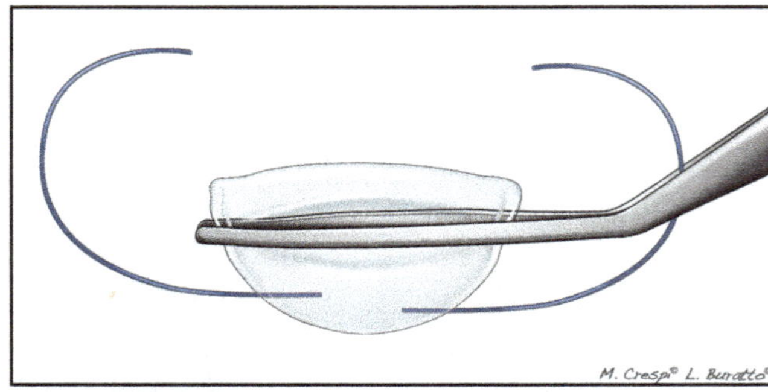

Figure 16-11. The point where the lens optic is grasped by the implantation forceps (grasping phase) is of crucial importance. The correct point to grasp the lens is in the center.

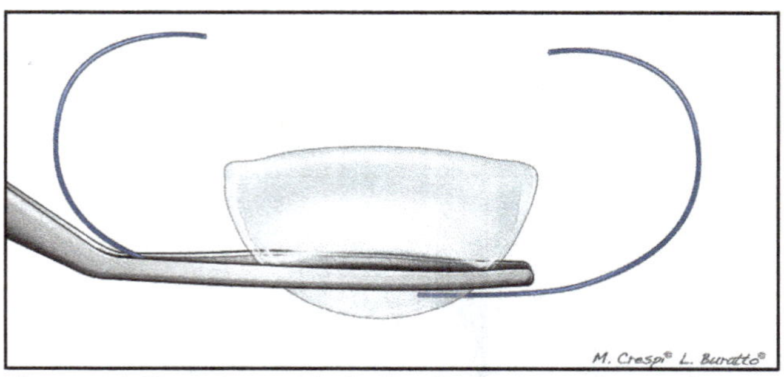

Figure 16-12. An excessively distal grasping point. In this way the lens will probably remain trapped in the forceps and a second instrument will often be required to facilitate the release of the forceps.

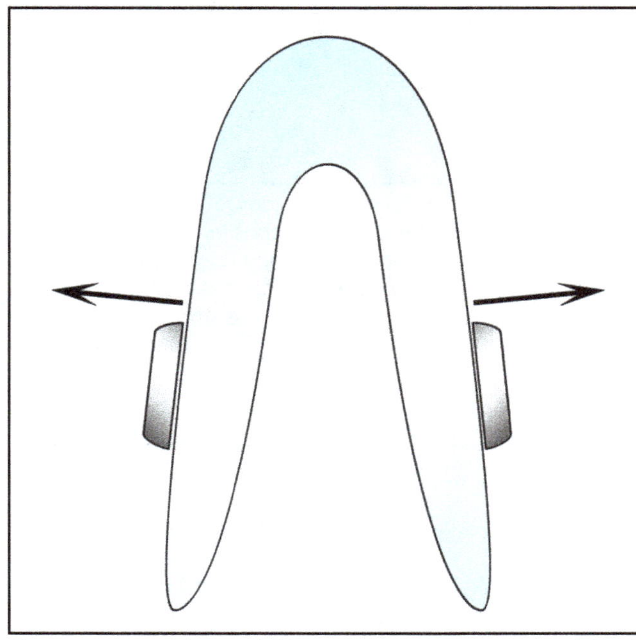

Figure 16-13. The unfolding process is proving difficult because the optic was grasped at the wrong point.

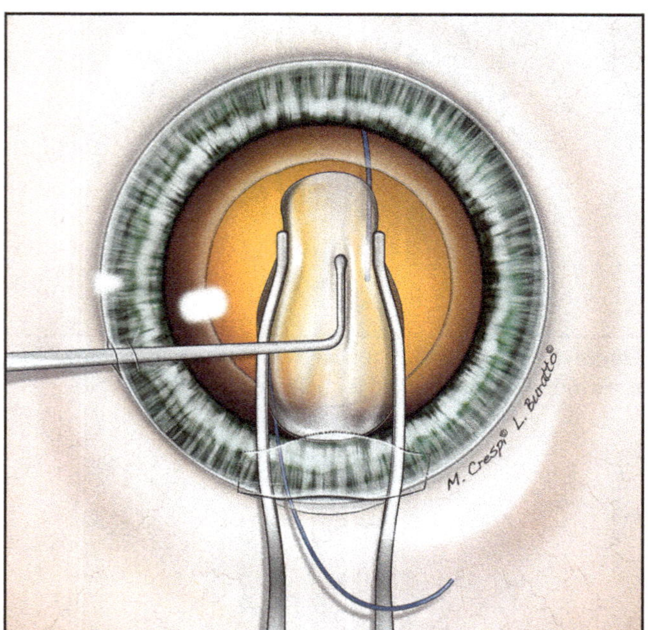

Figure 16-14. A second instrument is required to release the lens that has become stuck between the arms of the forceps.

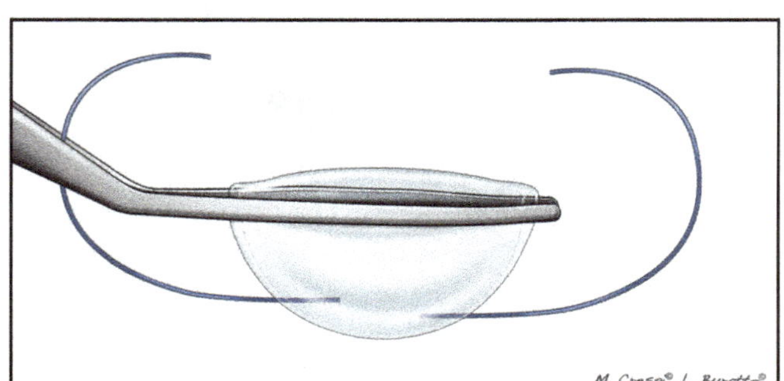

Figure 16-15. An excessively proximal grasping point in relation to the fold. Under these circumstances, greater pressure is required to keep the lens folded and this may result in tears of or cracks in the optic plate.

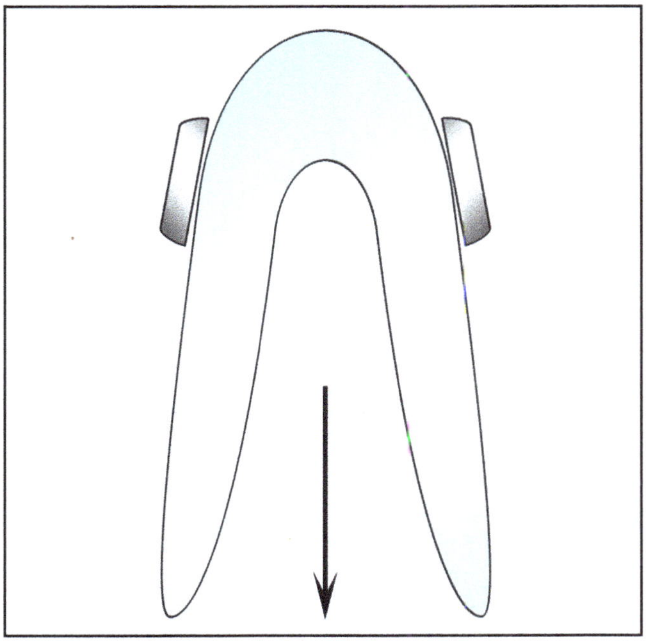

Figure 16-16. The correct lens unfolding process.

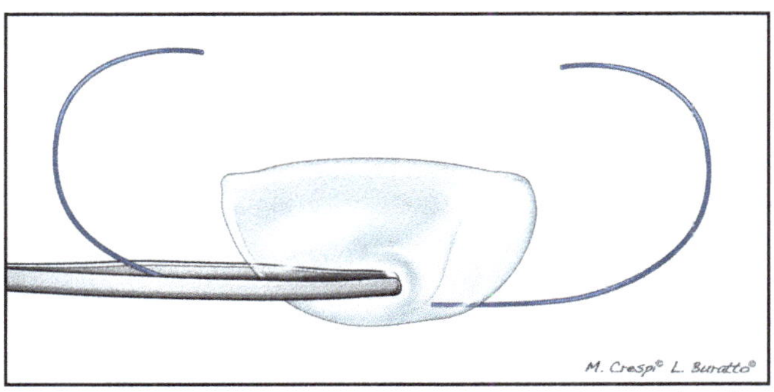

Figure 16-18. If the grasp point is excessively peripheral, a "fishmouth" may develop and this will complicate the implantation procedure as shown.

Partial engagement of the optic will create a "fishmouth" because of the lens' elastic properties. This situation will complicate the insertion of the lens through the tunnel (Figure 16-18).

On the other hand, when the arms of the forceps are positioned too far across the optic (Figure 16-19), the "protruding" portion of the forceps may become trapped in the tissue of the scleral tunnel.

A number of instruments have been designed to fold lenses. For example, there is a paddle-type folder that was developed exclusively to grasp the optic and facilitate the folding. This folder lacks the groove for holding the lens with the insertion forceps (Figure 16-20).

The lenses can also be folded without special instruments being required, by simply using 2 forceps as shown (Figures 16-21 and 16-22).

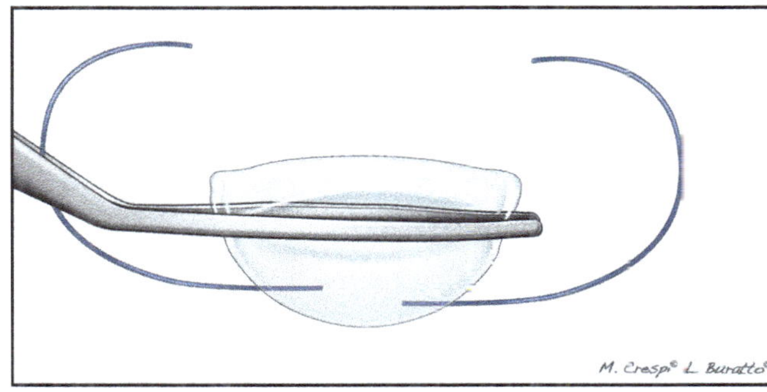

Figure 16-17. The implantation forceps must grasp the surface of the lens as shown.

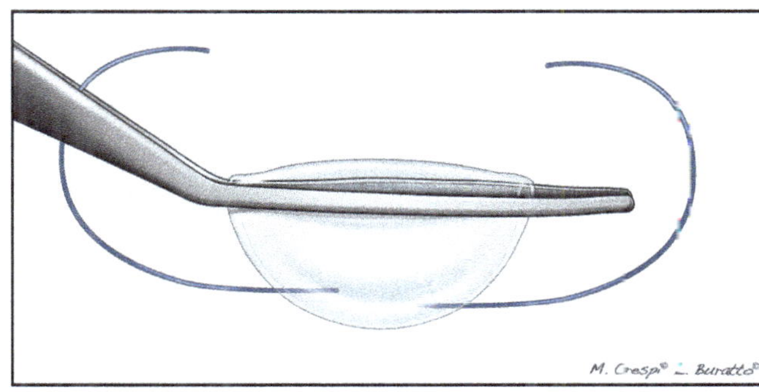

Figure 16-19. If the tips of the forceps extend beyond the far edge of the lens, it is likely that the lens will remain trapped in the corneal tissue or in the tunnel and this will complicate the implantation procedure.

The insertion forceps also have a variety of different shapes. In addition to forceps with straight arms, there are forceps with curved arms. These facilitate the release of the lens inside the eye because the shape of the arms creates more space for the maneuvers; however, the incision must be larger. Compared to forceps with straight tips, forceps with a curved tip do not have the same degree of agility inside the anterior chamber.

Suggested Reading

Oshika T. Acrylic foldable IOL: implantation tecnique, complication, management and clinical results. In: Fine IH, Agarwal A, et al. *Phacoemulsification, Laser Cataract Surgery and Foldable IOLs.* New Delhi, India: Jaypee; 1998: Chapter 32.

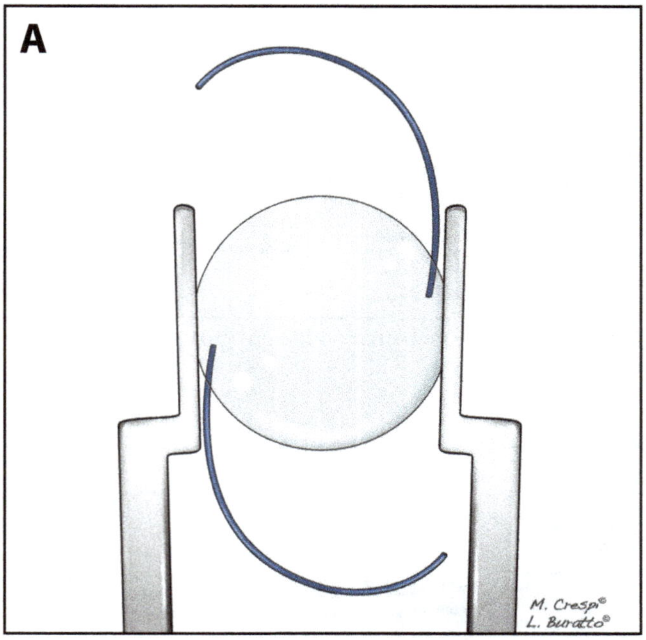

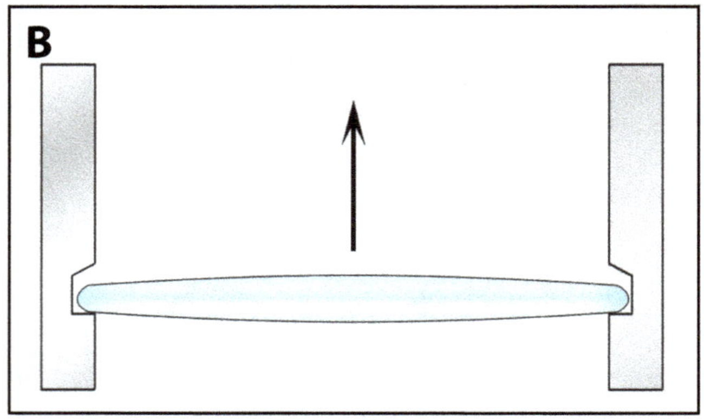

Figure 16-20. (A) Paddle-type folder. (B) Both edges of the optic have been perfectly engaged in channel created inside the folder.

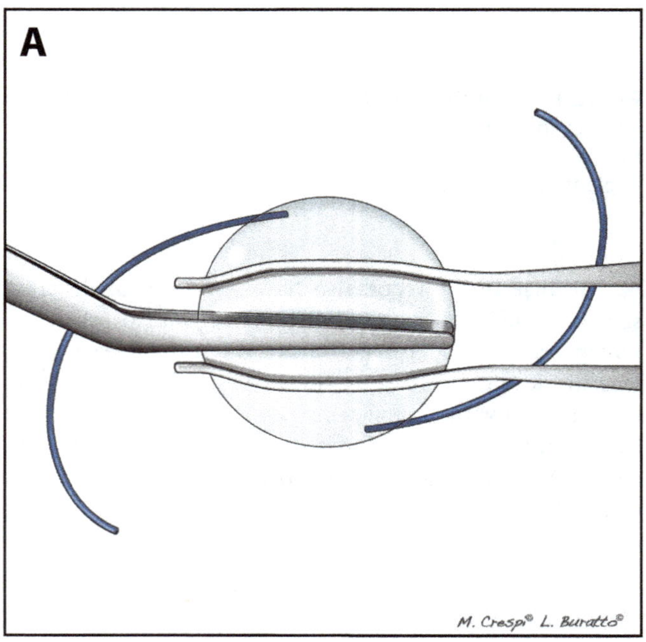

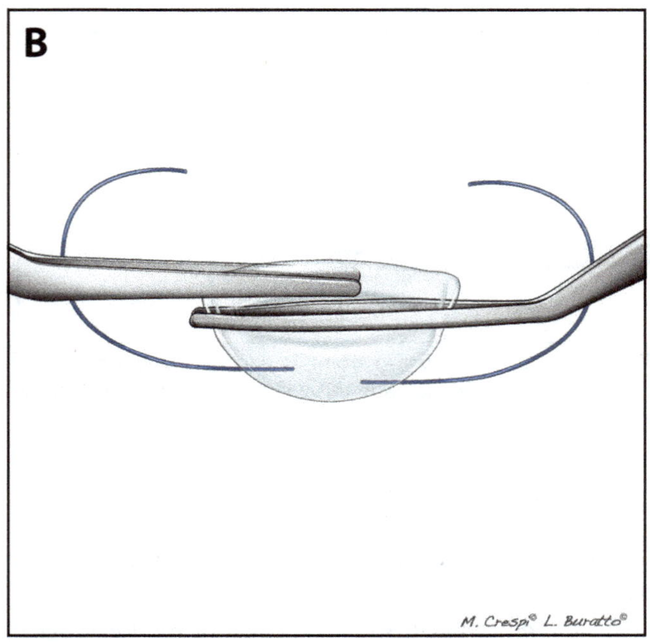

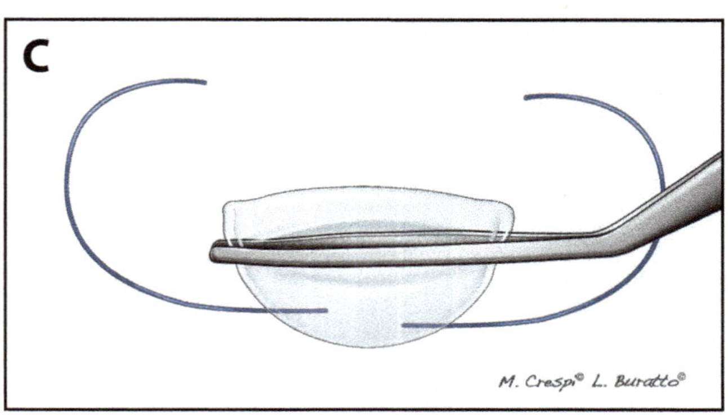

Figure 16-21. The horizontal or longitudinal method for the 2-step implantation method.

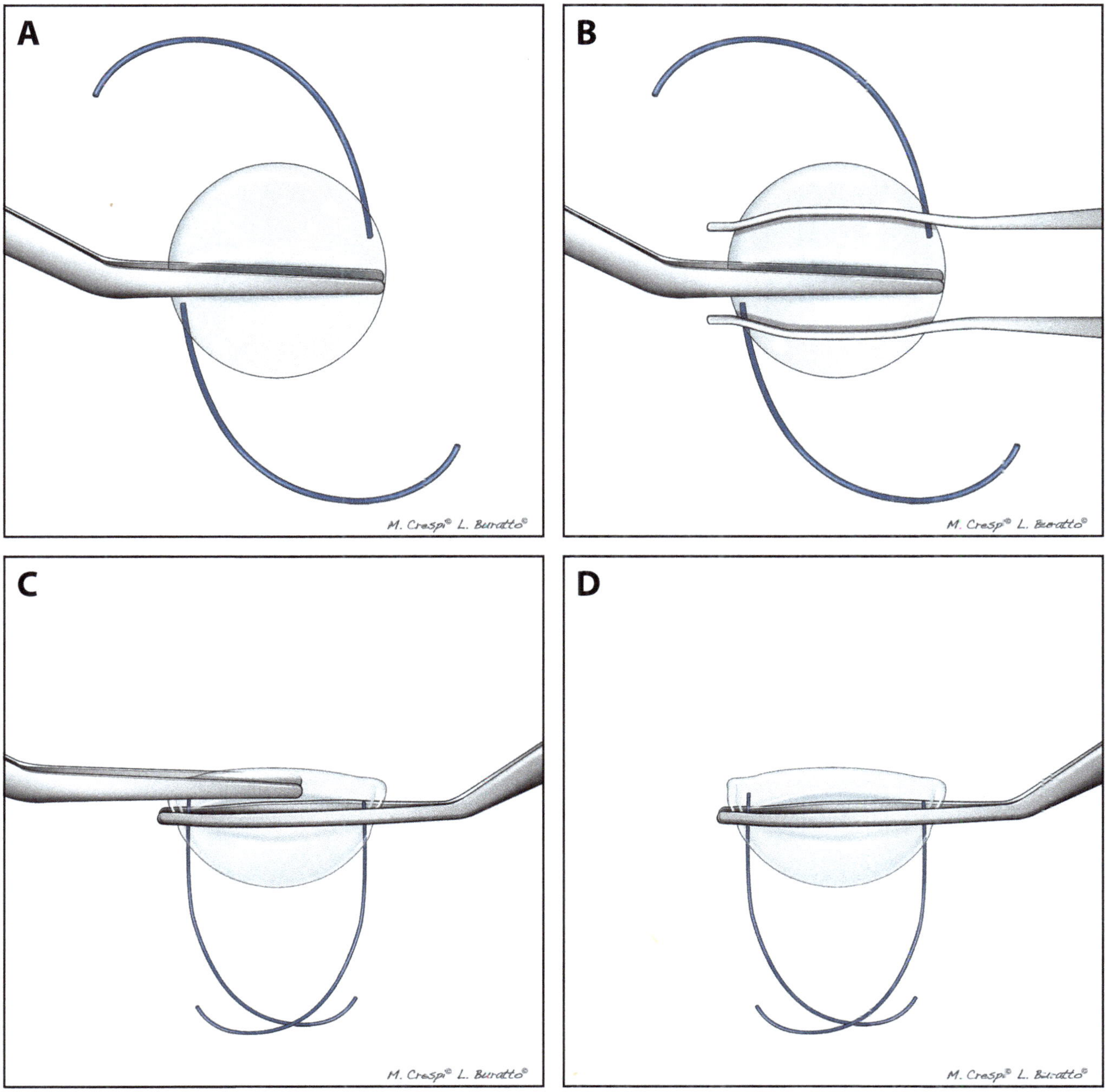

Figure 16-22. The vertical or transversal method for the 1-step implantation method.

17

Injectors and Implantation of Foldable Intraocular Lenses

Lucio Buratto, MD; Stephen F. Brint, MD, FACS; and Domenico Boccuzzi, MD, PhD

The need to insert intraocular lenses (IOLs) through increasingly smaller incisions and the requirement of safer methods led to the development of injectors. There are many variations available and they all allow foldable IOLs to be inserted through very small incisions without damaging the lens.

There are several injector models: screw controlled, piston injectors, preloaded, disposable, automated, etc. The mechanism of action of the injector is dependent on the cartridge for loading and folding the lens. The cartridge has a small chamber that receives the lens from the injector and allows the rolled-up IOL to be injected through very small incisions.

Each injector and each cartridge has been designed and developed for a specific type of lens, on the basis of the material and the design features of the lens itself. The piston, the propulsion mechanism that expels the lens from the injector, the shape of the cartridge, the procedure for loading the IOL, and the dimensions of the injector tip are specific for every type of lens. The injectors allow a straightforward and safe insertion of the lens, and there is little risk of damaging the eye or the IOL even with small incisions.

The first injectors were screw controlled. By turning the screw, the surgeon inserts the IOL slowly and progressively with no sudden change in advancement speed; however, the surgeon has to use both hands for this procedure: one holds the injector and the other activates the mechanism for injecting the lens. When used correctly, this injector is safe and allows the IOL to be introduced into the eye with a controlled gradual progression.

The second type of injector uses a piston- or a syringe-like mechanism; the advantage of this injector is that it can be operated with one hand, leaving one of the surgeon's hands free to hold another instrument. For example, in bimanual microincision surgery, which uses very small incisions to insert the IOL (even as small as 1.8 mm) the use of a piston-operated injector is almost mandatory, as the surgeon's fellow hand often holds a second instrument to keep the eye steady. This is because the lens is not inserted by pushing the injector's cannula inside the corneal tunnel, but by simply positioning the open tip of the injector against the tunnel incision (wound-assisted method). Compared to the success of the screw-controlled version, the first models of the piston or syringe injector did not always produce controlled constant progression of the lens. The injection was often quite sudden, sometimes explosive expulsion of the lens into the anterior chamber, and this can result in unexpected and undesired events.

Development of the cartridges has progressed as cataract surgery techniques have evolved, with smaller incisions and evolution of the IOLs themselves; the surgeon now has a number of safe effective options available.

As mentioned, each cartridge is designed for a specific type of lens and its corresponding injector. The cartridge consists of 3 fundamental parts: a part for loading and folding the IOL, a nozzle, and a system to attach to the injector.

The IOL loading method is specific for every lens type and normally has a portion with a groove used to engage the optic of the IOL.

The open cartridges have a semicircular groove that forms a circle when the 2 arms of the cartridge face each

Buratto L, Brint SF, Boccuzzi D.
Cataract Surgery and Intraocular Lenses (pp 135-153).

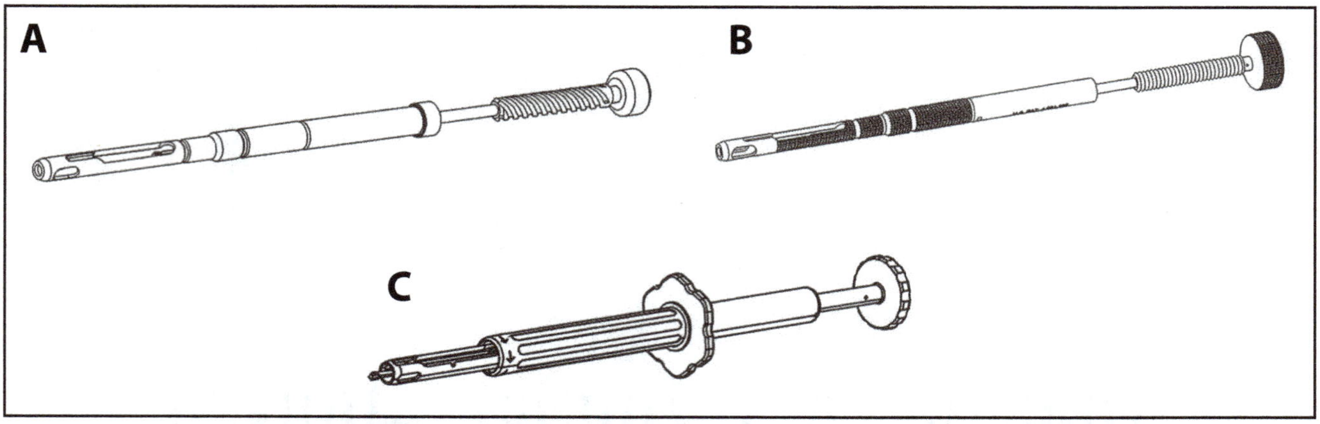

Figure 17-1. Models of the Emerald Unfolder produced by AMO. (A) Model Emerald T with a screw mechanism. (B) Model Emerald XL with a screw mechanism, a large progression wheel, and a narrow screw thread. (C) Model Emerald Ease with a piston mechanism.

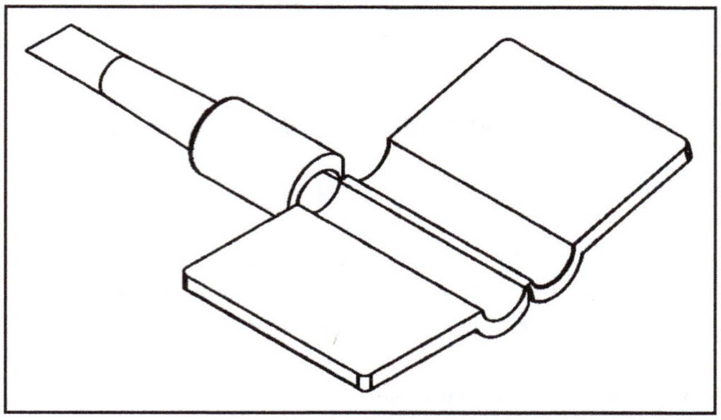

Figure 17-2. Unfolder cartridge, Emerald series, a device that can be used with 3-piece lenses with OptiEdge (in relation to the edge of the optic), the ReZoom lens, and the Sensar lens through an incision measuring 2.8 mm.

other and are folded together. This portion is suitable for loading the "open" optic of the lens; the lens is folded when the 2 arms are closed and it allows the plunger to progress and insert the IOL. One of this type of cartridges is the Emerald produced by Abbott Medical Optics (AMO); it can be loaded with a 3-piece IOL (hydrophobic acrylic) such as Sensar AR40 models and the ReZoom multifocal lens (also a hydrophobic acrylic).

A second type of cartridge (closed) consists of a single unit with a large posterior opening, designed to allow an "open" IOL. This type of cartridge folds the IOL as the lens progresses into the nozzle when the plunger is depressed.

The nozzle is shaped like a funnel, allowing the IOL to be introduced through the reduced diameter of the corneal incision. This cartridge is designed with a system that allows it to engage the injector, creating a single unit that allows the plunger to push the lens first into the nozzle and subsequently into the eye. This type of cartridge can be loaded with 1-piece hydrophobic acrylic IOLs and 3-piece hydrophobic IOLs.

The preloaded IOL injection systems deserve special mention. The advantage of this type of device is that the surgeon does not handle the lens, and this minimizes the risk of damaging and/or contaminating the lens.

Moreover, the disposable systems provide a higher standard of sterility and reduce surgical times. This group includes the SofPort Easy-Load Lens Delivery System that will be described in detail later in this chapter.

The Emerald Injector Produced by Abbott Medical Optics

The Emerald Injector was one of the first injectors produced and it is still being used today. It is extremely effective and currently has 3 different models: the Emerald T with a screw-controlled mechanism (Figure 17-1A); the Emerald XL with a screw-controlled mechanism, a large progression wheel, and a narrow screw thread (Figure 17-1B); and the Emerald Ease with a piston mechanism (Figure 17-1C). These are joined by a fourth, recently developed model, the Emerald AR, with a different system for progression of the plunger. It avoids having to rotate the injector for insertion of the IOL.

These injectors use different types of cartridges that depend on the type of lens to be implanted and the type of incision. There is a cartridge in the Emerald series called the Unfolder and this can be used with 3-piece lenses with OptiEdge (in reference to the shape of the optic), ReZoom, and the Sensar through an incision measuring 2.8 mm (Figure 17-2).

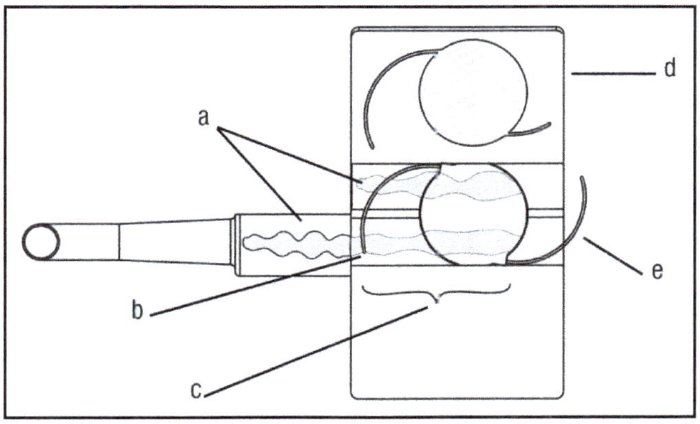

Figure 17-3. After filling the cartridge with VES, the lens is positioned, as illustrated, on the internal surface of the cartridge. The surgeon must carefully position the optic of the lens below the 2 grooves on the edges of the cartridge. The cartridge must be closed slowly to allow the lens to fold with the convex shape facing the base of the cartridge. The loops of the IOL must therefore be positioned correctly and not folded over on themselves. The distal loop must enter the launch chamber without forming a loop. The proximal loop must follow the lens plate without being trapped in the injector's piston.

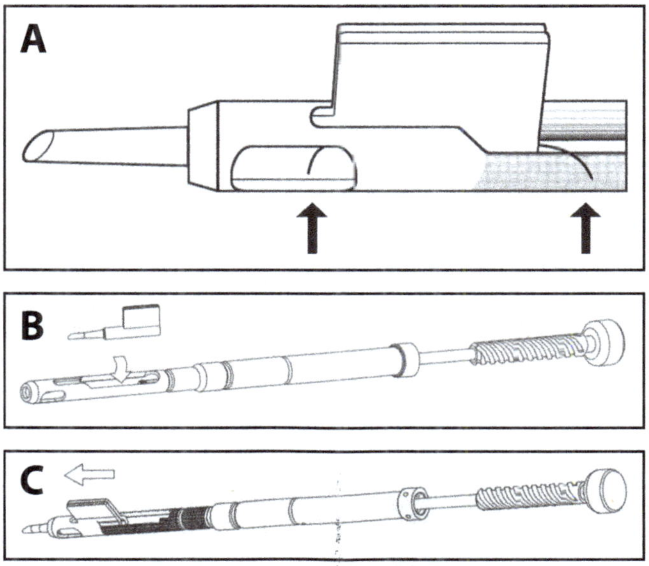

Figure 17-4. (A) The IOL positioned correctly inside the cartridge. The haptics in the correct position. (B) Insertion of the cartridge in the injector. (C) Once the cartridge has been loaded in the injector, it is pushed forward to engage.

Intraocular Lens Loading Technique (for a Three-Piece Acrylic Lens) and Insertion in the Eye

When the cartridge is still in its cassette, inject viscoelastic substance (VES) into the cartridge channel and along the lower part of both of the channels. The lens is positioned on the upward facing the anterior portion on the central hinge of the cartridge with the haptics of the lens positioned according to the drawing on the wing of the cartridge. Carefully place the lens at the center of the loading area. Position the anterior loop inside the cartridge loading channel and position the posterior loop external to the wing tips. Slide the edge of the lens underneath the portion of the cartridge in relief, pushing it from the edge inward (Figure 17-3).

Using round-tipped forceps, push the edges of the lens along the tubular portion of the wings and the central inferior portion while the wings are closing; avoid nipping the edge or haptics of the IOL with the wings as they close. The surgeon should also ensure that the anterior haptic folds reverse. The anterior haptic should be visible with the relative tip facing the tubular portion of the cartridge, and the haptic must be placed in a straight position inside the canal. The posterior haptic should extend beyond the back of the cartridge. If either of the haptics is trapped between the arms of the forceps when they close, the haptic in question may tear from the IOL as it progresses along the cartridge (Figure 17-4A). (Alternately, the IOL can be loaded into the cartridge from the posterior section using a similar procedure.)

When the wings have been closed, they must be kept closed; the cartridge is placed in the handpiece, paying maximum attention to avoid damage to the tip. The cartridge is delicately pushed forward along the slit in the handpiece until it stops. The surgeon must check that the tip of the cartridge has not been damaged during the progression to its final position inside the handpiece (Figures 17-4B and C). The plunger should not advance.

Check that the trailing haptic is on the left side of the plunger and has not been blocked. The tip of the posterior haptic must face to the outside of the handpiece (Figure 17-5A).

If the surgeon uses the Emerald T or the Emerald XL injector, he or she must push the plunger forward without turning the screw-controlled mechanism until the plunger reaches the end of the run (when it can no longer slide forward) inside the handpiece. At this point, the screw mechanism is turned to move the IOL forward until the anterior tip of the loop is positioned 1.0 to 2.0 mm from the blunt tip of the cartridge. The direction of progression of the plunger should not be reversed until the body of the lens has not been completely released (Figure 17-5B).

The anterior haptic should be positioned 1.0 to 2.0 mm from the blunt exit portion of the cartridge.

The implant must be completed immediately after having pushed forward the plunger of the handpiece. The lens is therefore loaded into the cartridge, only when the eye is ready to receive the IOL. The lens and the cartridge must be replaced if the lens remains in the advanced position for

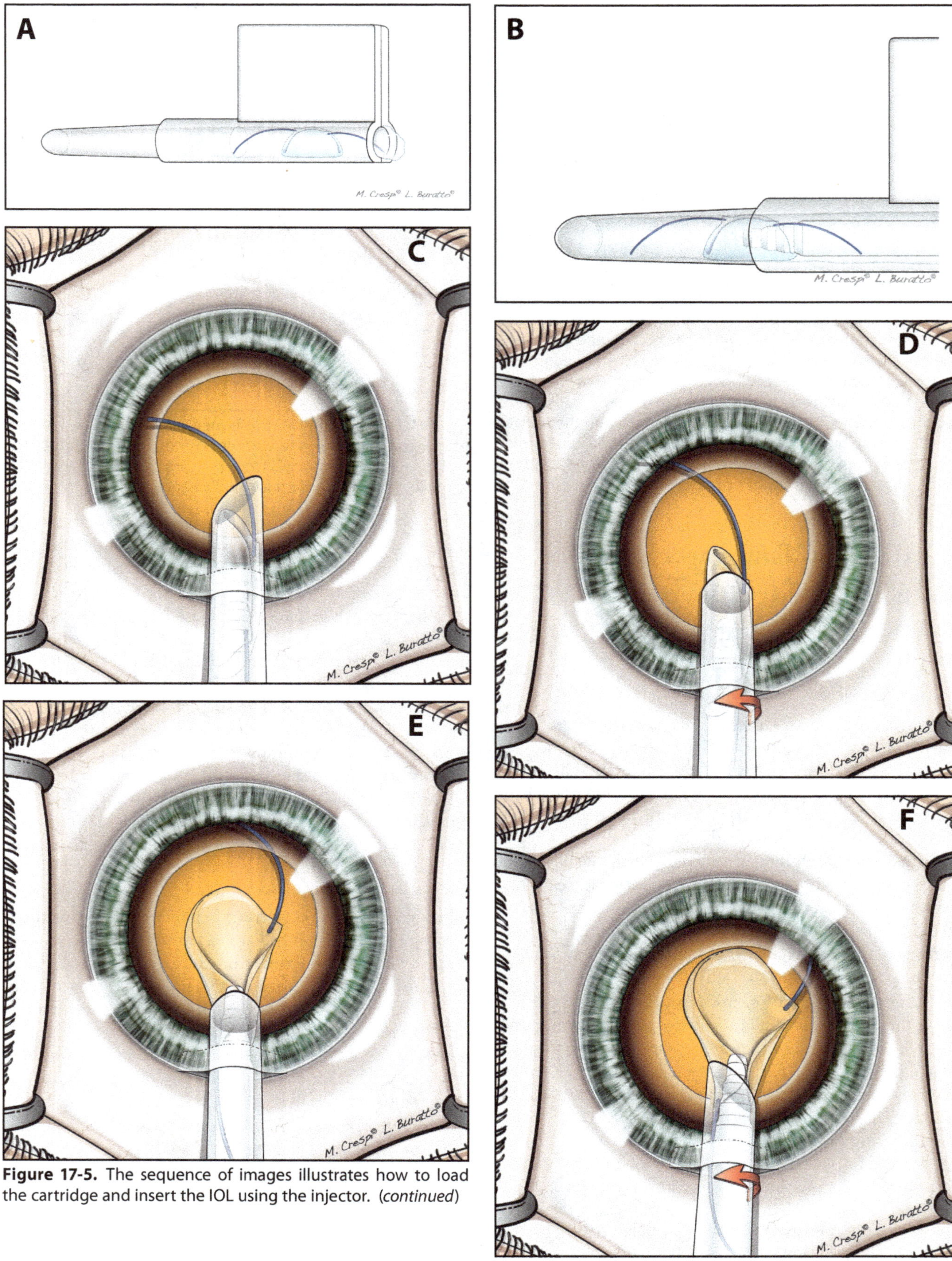

Figure 17-5. The sequence of images illustrates how to load the cartridge and insert the IOL using the injector. (*continued*)

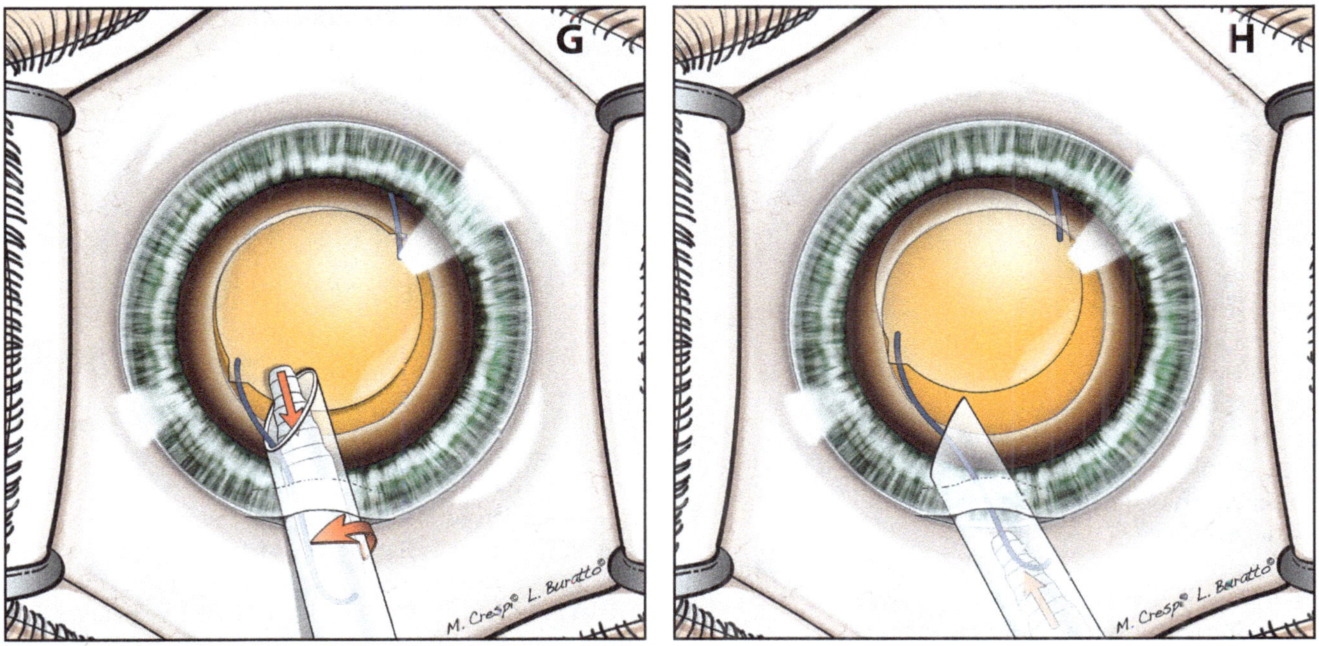

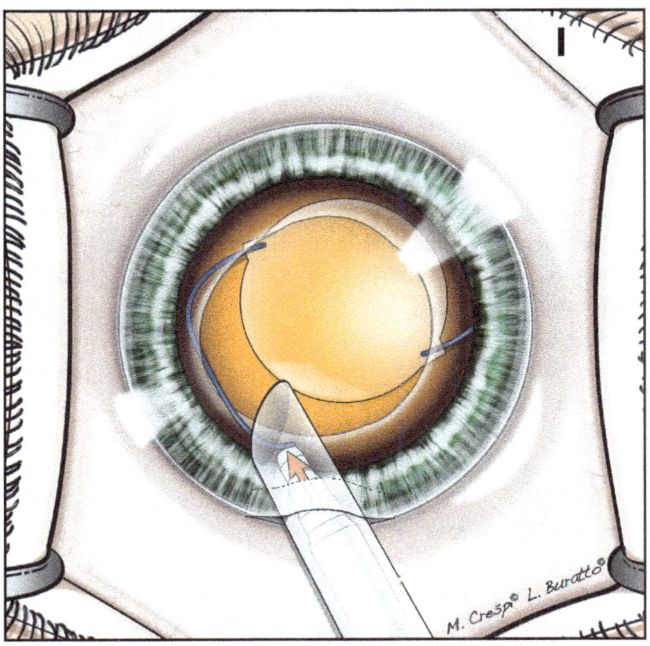

Figure 17-5. (continued) The sequence of images illustrates how to load the cartridge and insert the IOL using the injector.

more than 30 seconds or if the lens has remained folded in any position inside the cartridge for more than 5 minutes.

Insert the tip of the cartridge into the incision with the oblique angle facing downward (bevel-down) (Figure 17-5C).

Rotate the cartridge and position the blunt part and the anterior haptic to the left of the surgeon. If the surgeon opts to use the Emerald T or Emerald XL injector, he or she should push the optic of the lens forward using the screw-controlled mechanism until the tip of the anterior optic reaches the blunt portion of the cartridge. When the anterior tip of the optic reaches the point of the cartridge, the surgeon turns the screw and injector to the right as required, to ensure that the tip of the anterior haptic is always to the left of the surgeon and that it has not been damaged (Figures 17-5D through F). If the IOL is completely released with the oblique angle facing downward (bevel down), the lens could flip over when it is released. Moreover, if the tip of the anterior haptic is not facing to the left after the rotation, the IOL could flip over after it has been released inside the cartridge tube. If the tip of the haptic is directed toward the posterior capsule, it could tear it.

When using the Emerald T and Emerald XL injectors, if the haptic does not face to the left on exiting the cartridge, the surgeon should remove his or her hand from the screw-controlled mechanism and rotate the handpiece containing

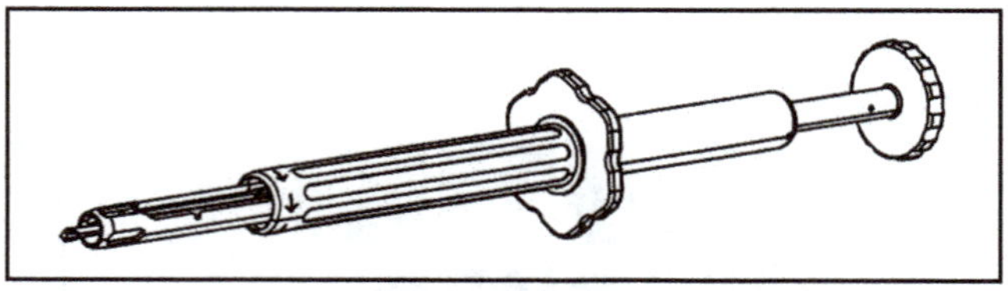

Figure 17-6. The AMO injector with the screw-progression mechanism.

the cartridge until the haptic faces to the left. At this point, the surgeon should rotate the screw mechanism and the handpiece as required until the IOL has been released completely into the capsular bag.

Due to the large thread on the handpiece of the Emerald T, the IOL may move backward if the screw mechanism is released before the lens reaches the oblique angle of the cartridge.

Continue pushing the plunger forward until the lens is free from the cartridge with the plunger protruding approximately 1 mm beyond the tip of the tube.

The plunger should never move backward until the body of the lens has been totally released; if this occurs, the haptic could be damaged.

The surgeon should watch the position of the leading haptic inside the cartridge. The tip of the cartridge can be used to maintain the lens in position when the plunger is being withdrawn (Figure 17-5G).

The end of the plunger should not be withdrawn beyond the posterior haptic. The cartridge should be rotated in a clockwise direction until the oblique angle faces downward (bevel down). The trailing haptic should be captured with the plunger and positioned inside the capsular bag (Figures 17-5H and I). Alternately, the instrument should be withdrawn from the eye and the trailing haptic placed using a McPherson forceps or a hook to catch the junction between the IOL optic and the haptic; a clockwise rotation movement and mild downward pressure introduces the second haptic into the capsular bag.

The Emerald Ease Injector

The Emerald Ease injector differs from the previous models that use screw-controlled progression of the plunger. It operates with a syringe- or piston-type mechanism.

The plunger system is equipped with a stop mechanism that is used in the preloading step of the IOL, prior to its injection into the eye (Figure 17-6).

Pushing the plunger will advance the IOL in the nozzle with injection of the IOL into the capsular bag. With this type of injector, when the lens is being injected, the surgeon should ensure that the leading haptic is oriented in an inferior left position, to ensure that during insertion in the capsular bag, it is positioned beneath the rhexis.

Again with this type of handpiece, the surgeon must adjust as the opening movement of the IOL occurs and rotate his or her wrist in a clockwise direction during the expulsion of the optic to avoid the IOL flipping; this maneuver facilitates correct insertion of the lens into the bag.

The Easy-Load One Series Produced by Abbott Medical Optics

The 1-piece Tecnis lens (model ZCB00 produced by AMO) deserves mention. This type of lens is injected using a cartridge and injector that is different from those required for 3-piece lenses. The cartridge is the model Easy-Load One, Ultra series, which is closed with a posterior loading opening (Figure 17-7A). The injector is the One Series model produced by AMO with a syringe-like plunger progression system (Figure 17-7B). A screw-controlled system may also be used (Figure 17-7C). The technological innovations of the cartridge and the injector optimize the properties of the 1-piece Tecnis lenses.

The cartridge has a closed 1-piece structure with an ergonomic shape to improve the surgeon's grip. This 1-piece cartridge has been designed with a posterior opening for loading the IOL and a micro tip for insertion of the lens in small microincisions with a coaxial method. The inside of the cartridge is coated with a special smooth substance that facilitates the progression of the lens.

The name "easy load" of the cartridge comes from the presence of 2 small technological innovations that improve and simplify the loading process of the IOL: the posterior opening for loading the lens is designed with a small indentation that assists correct folding of the distal haptic of the lens over the optic (Figure 17-8A, detail "a"); there is also a small superior and inferior groove in a position perpendicular to the opening of the cartridge and this allows easy entrance of the 2 arms of the forceps (eg, McPherson forceps) that hold the IOL steady during the loading procedure. This simple yet important structural variation prevents the lens becoming trapped between the arms of the forceps; the forceps are unable to open and do not release the IOL optic that has been placed into the cartridge (see Figure 17-8A). During the insertion procedure of the lens optic into the cartridge, the surgeon should push the optic gently downward to initiate folding.

Once the cartridge has been filled with VES (Figure 17-8B) and the optic of the IOL has been loaded, with care taken to fold the distal haptic over the lens optic (Figures 17-8C and D), the surgeon folds the proximal loop over the superior face of the lens (Figure 17-8E). The initial progression of the lens is accompanied and assisted by forceps, and with advancement, the folding of the lens begins (Figure 17-8F).

This procedure allows complete insertion of the lens into the bag with a single movement, with no need to withdraw the piston or push the distal loop forward again.

When the cartridge has been loaded with the lens, it is connected to the injector by a simple ergonomic handle (Figures 17-8G and H).

This latest generation of injector is made of titanium; it is ergonomic with a monomanual syringe-like progression, typical of the systems designed to be used with microincisions (Figure 17-9). The part that attaches to the cartridge is on the upper surface of the injector and the unit allows straightforward insertion. The blue plunger does not reflect light emitted from the operating microscope; there is a small notch at the tip (fishmouth) that is used to engage the optic of the IOL and allows progression with no risk of trapping or damaging the lens.

Monarch III Injector Produced by Alcon

Alcon uses a screw-controlled injector for its IOLs, of reusable sterilizable titanium attached to a disposable polypropylene cartridge.

The Monarch III injector evolved from the previous Monarch II model, and operates with a screw-controlled mechanism for advancing the lens, allowing both 1- and 3-piece IOLs to be loaded.

The cartridge of the Monarch D model consists of a single polypropylene unit with a fenestration positioned in the portion that is diametrically opposite the injection aperture; this is useful for loading IOLs; 2 small lateral wings lock in the cartridge to the injector (Figures 17-10A and B).

The process for loading the IOL into the cartridge varies depending on the lens.

Three-piece lenses (MA60AT): The lens is carefully removed from its container with atraumatic forceps (with no ridging or teeth); through the opening it is gently inserted into the cartridge that had been previously filled with VES. When the lens is inserted, the surgeon must push gently downward to commence the folding process; the lens advances under the effects of this pressure exerted on the injector plunger. Once the lens has been inserted in the cartridge, the cartridge is firmly attached to the injector using the 2 side wings.

For correct positioning of the 3-piece lens, the surgeon should ensure that the distal haptic is fully extended and not folded on itself. The surgeon can check its position by pushing the lens with the plunger and turning the screw control to advance the lens. If the haptic appears to have been folded on itself, the surgeon must unfold it to avoid compressing the narrow distal portion of the cartridge and possibly deforming it. In this (rare) situation, the surgeon can introduce a chopper or a Sinskey hook through the distal portion and gently pull the haptic toward the outside (before it becomes firmly trapped inside the exit tunnel).

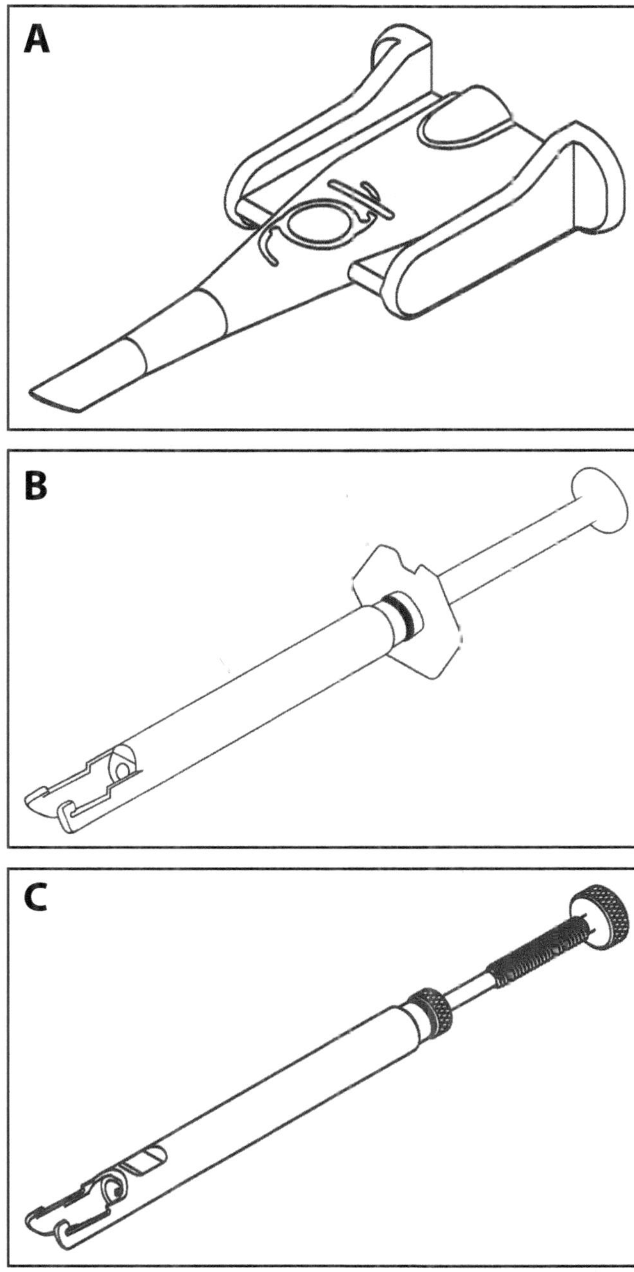

Figure 17-7. (A) The cartridge produced by AMO, Model Easy-Load One Series. (B) The injector produced by AMO with piston-controlled progression. (C) An injector with screw-controlled progression.

The proximal loop slides into the outer lower left portion of the cartridge, to prevent it obstructing the progression of the plunger and becoming trapped. Prior to lens insertion, it should be advanced until the distal loop is positioned 1.0 to 2.0 mm from the exit point. The cartridge is then introduced into the eye and the plunger advances.

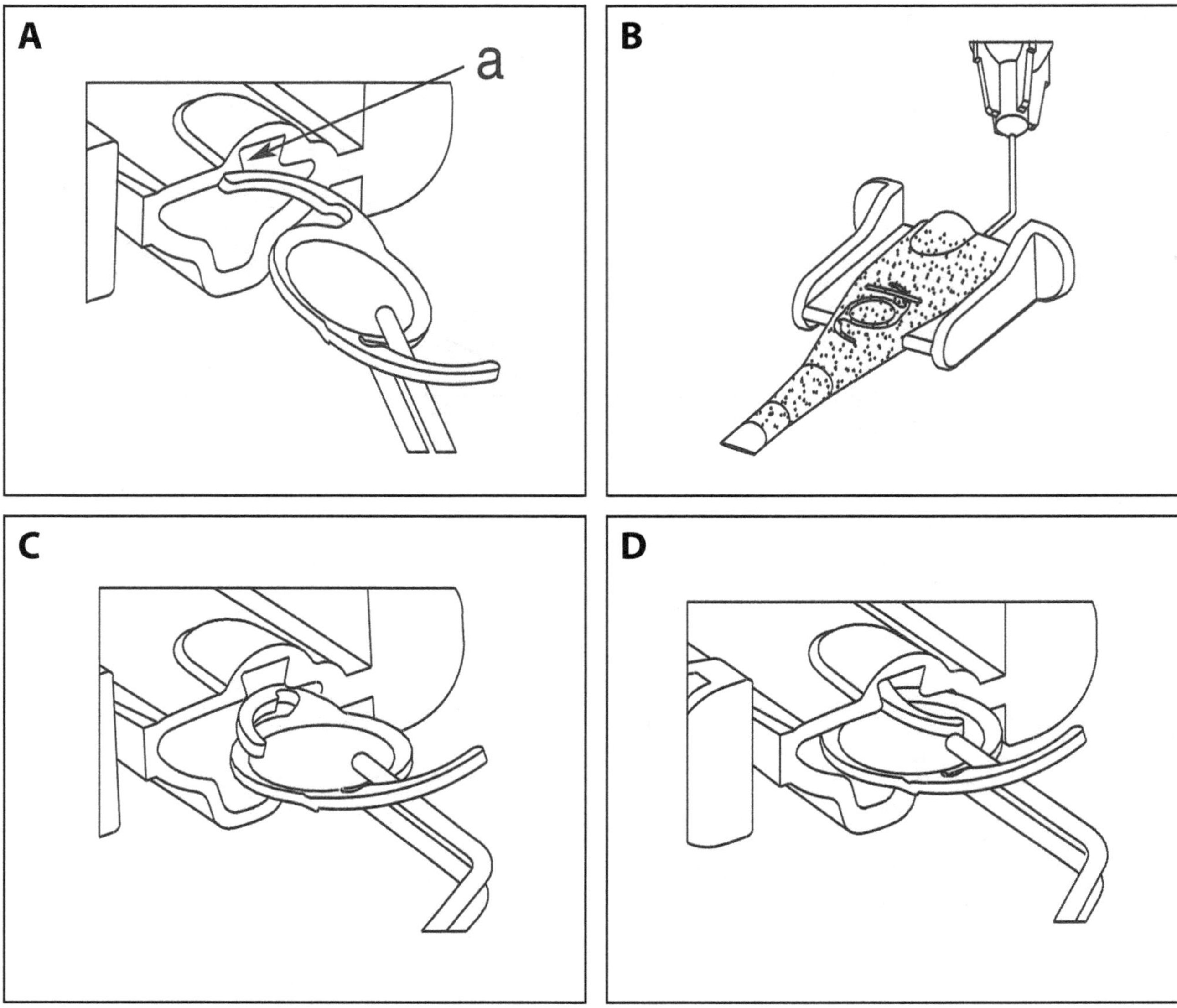

Figure 17-8. The sequence of images shows the procedure for loading the lens in the cartridge and the attachment of the cartridge to the injector (A). Once the cartridge has been filled with VES (B), the lens is grasped by blunt forceps and gently positioned inside the cartridge through the posterior fenestration (C). A small upper groove assists the folding of the distal loop over the anterior face of the lens (D). (*continued*)

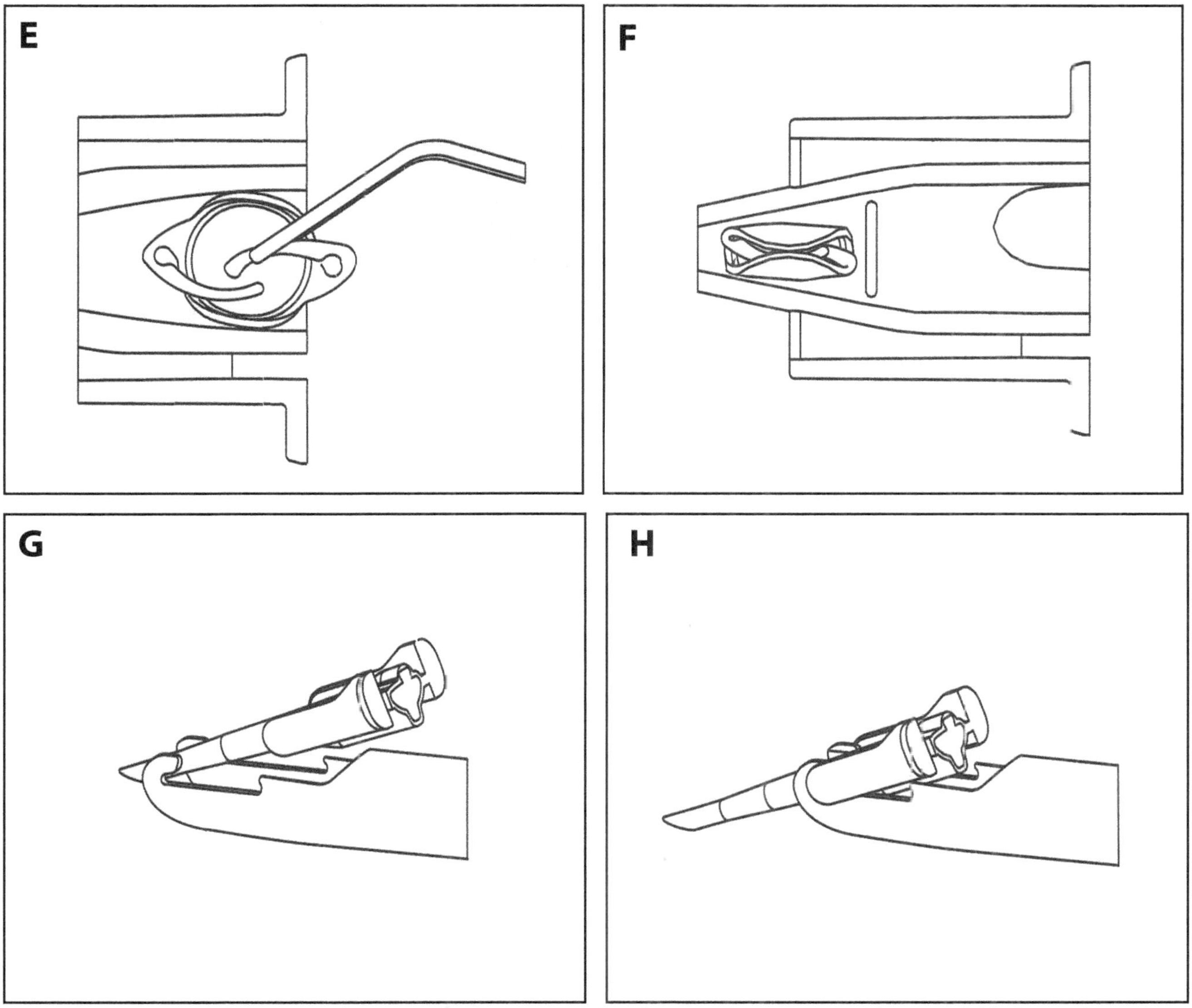

Figure 17-8. (continued) Once the lens optic has been inserted in the cartridge, the second haptic is folded over the anterior face of the optic (E), using the groove on the upper edge of the cartridge to assist opening the forceps that were used to insert the IOL in the cartridge. The surgeon proceeds with the insertion by pushing the IOL toward the launch chamber (F). The cartridge is attached to the injector as shown (G, H); the lens is engaged with the tip of the piston. The lens is pushed to a distance of 1 to 2 mm from the mouth of the launch chamber. The lens is now ready to be injected into the eye.

This lens insertion technique does not require forward or backward rotation movements of the handpiece, and the advancement of the plunger allows insertion of the lens into the capsular bag. Once the optic has been inserted, it is possible to withdraw the plunger, fold the second haptic, and insert it into the bag. If this maneuver proves difficult, the cartridge can be removed from the eye and the insertion of the IOL in the capsular bag completed using a Buratto or a Sinskey hook, carefully positioned at the junction between the optic and the haptic. Once the optic has been inserted inside the capsular bag, through rotation it is easy to slip the second haptic inside the bag.

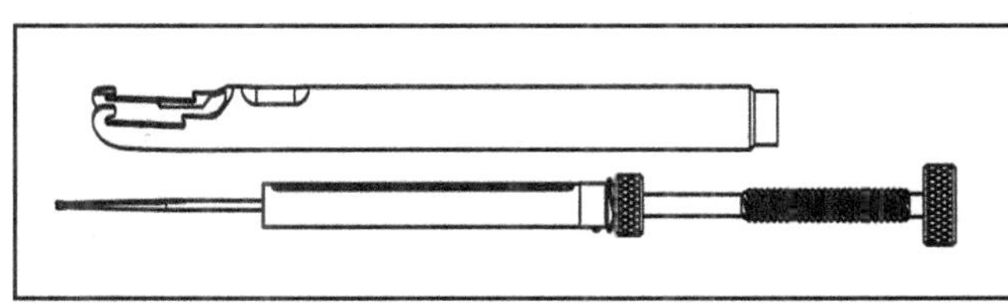

Figure 17-9. The AMO injector for the Easy-Load One Series cartridge in titanium with a 1-handed piston-controlled progression system.

For the 1-piece IOL (SA60AT, SN60, or SN6A), the process for loading the lens and insertion of the IOL is completely different.

The lens is carefully removed from its container using atraumatic forceps (Figure 17-10C); it is inserted through

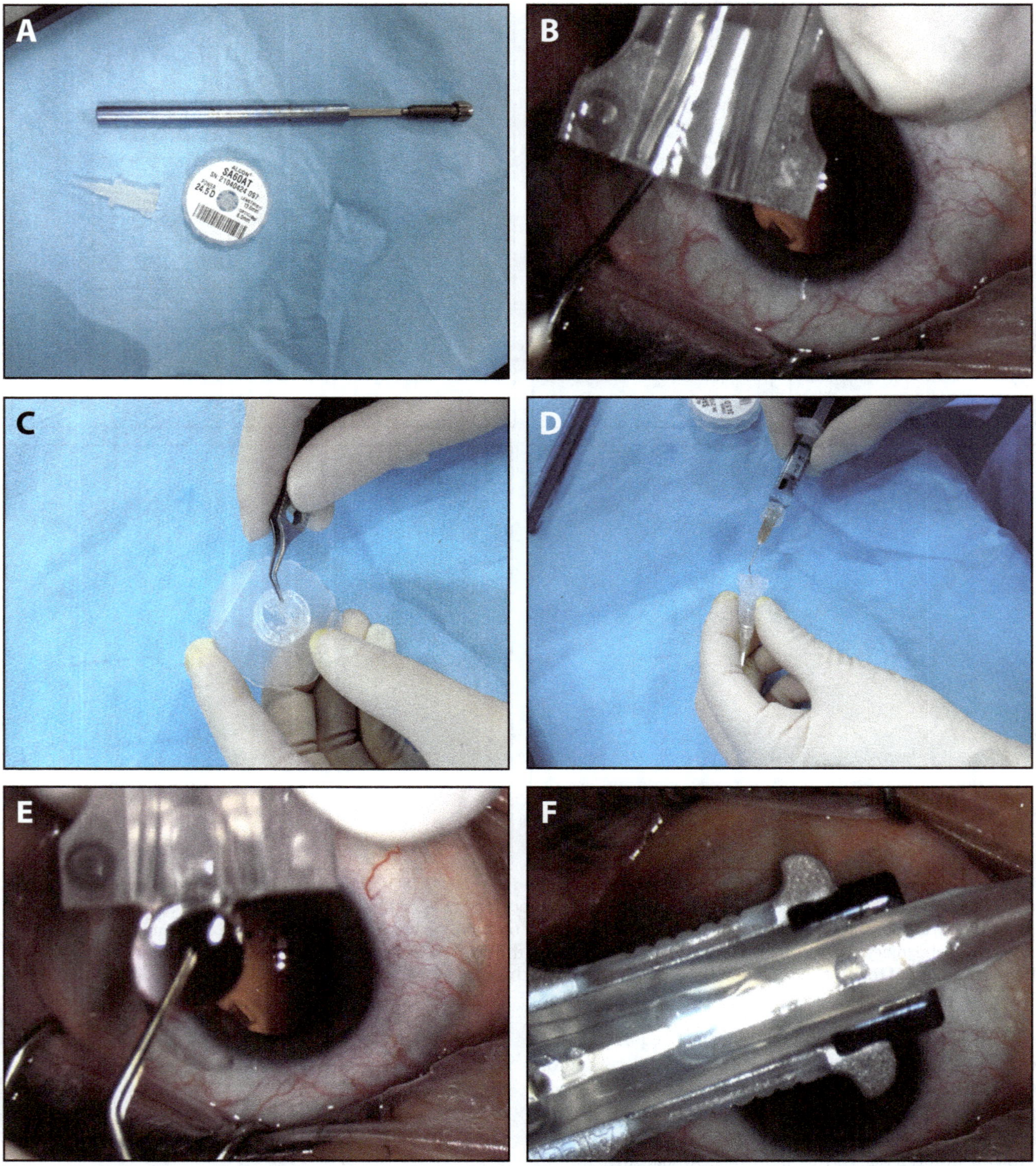

Figure 17-10. The figures illustrate the procedure for loading the Alcon IOL in the cartridge and the insertion of the IOL into the eye using an injector. (*continued*)

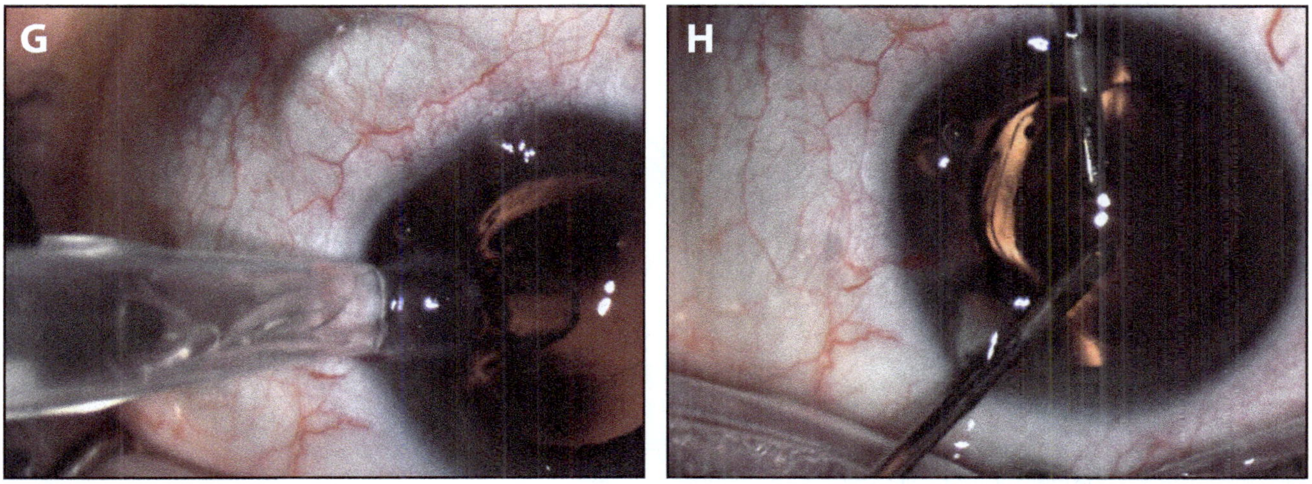

Figure 17-10. (continued) The figures illustrate the procedure for loading the Alcon IOL in the cartridge and the insertion of the IOL into the eye using an injector.

the posterior opening and positioned in the cartridge that has been previously filled with VES (Figure 17-10D); the surgeon should ensure that the distal haptic is folded on the superior face of the IOL (Figure 17-10E). During insertion of these IOLs, mild downward pressure is exerted on the optic to facilitate the folding of the lens. The proximal loop must also be positioned on the upper face of the IOL; the lens is then delicately pushed inside the cartridge. The 2 haptics are thus folded over the upper face of the lens and will tend to wrap around this surface. This procedure allows insertion of the lens into the bag with a single movement, without withdrawing and advancing the plunger.

When the IOL has been loaded into the cartridge, the cartridge is attached to the injector and anchored using the 2 lateral wings (Figure 17-10F). The surgeon advances the plunger to touch the lens and creates smooth progression of the IOL, while slowly rotating the screw-controlled device. Prior to inserting the lens inside the eye, it is necessary to advance it to a distance of 1.0 to 2.0 mm from the exit point. The cartridge is introduced into the eye and the plunger is pushed farther (Figure 17-10G). When the lens is injected into the capsular bag, if it has been loaded correctly, it will be rolled up with the 2 haptics folded inside. The lens and the haptics will unfold slowly. At this point, the surgeon can use a blunt instrument to assist the movement of the haptics and the unfolding of the optic and ensure the correct position of the lens inside the capsular bag.

Aspiration of VES will facilitate the complete unfolding of the haptics (Figure 17-10H).

The Akreos Insertion Device Produced by Bausch + Lomb

The Akreos single-use insertion device is a disposable injector that folds and inserts the 1-piece IOL Akreos AO lens. The lens insertion system consists of a syringe injector (operated with direct pressure), with a plunger and a groove for positioning the IOL, and a cartridge that connects to the injector and folds the lens (Figure 17-11).

The correct procedure for loading the IOL in the injector is described below.

1. Open the box on the injector designed for loading the lens; add a drop of VES (Figure 17-12).
2. Open the blister containing the lens and remove it using the lens holder. Orient the lens holder with the arms facing downward (Figure 17-13A).
3. Using atraumatic forceps, transfer the lens from the lens holder to the box on the injector, taking care to not reverse the lens. There are 2 markers on the haptics that are useful for checking that the IOL has been positioned correctly; the marks must be seen on the upper left and the lower right portions (Figure 17-13B).
4. When the lens has been positioned, add a drop of VES to the surface of the IOL and check once again that it is well positioned in its groove prior to closing the box (Figure 17-14).
5. When the box has been closed, align the cartridge and connect it to the injector, once the anterior opening has been filled with VES (Figure 17-15).
6. To connect the 2 pieces correctly, push the cartridge into the injector until the safety spring is released. Check that the 2 pieces are firmly connected by exerting mild pressure on the unit. Fill the cartridge once again with VES to eliminate any air bubbles present (Figure 17-16).
7. At this point, the injector is ready and loaded for insertion of the IOL. Introduce the tip of the injector in the bevel-down position, and with a constant and progressive movement, inject the lens into the eye. Movements of withdrawal and advancing can damage the lens. The

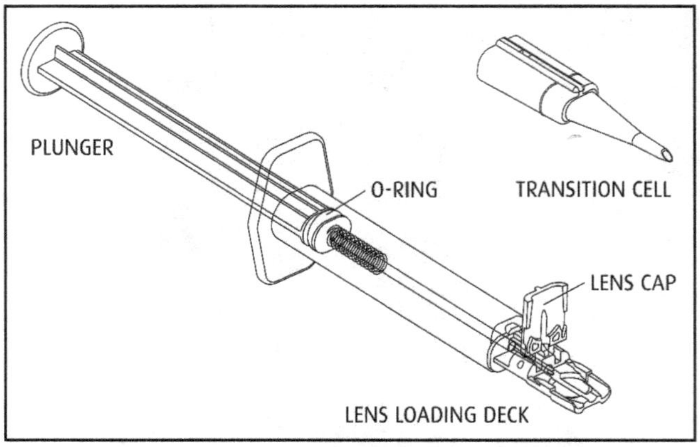

Figure 17-11. The figure illustrates the disposable piston-controlled injector. The portion for containing the IOL is located on the distal portion of the injector. Moreover, the launch chamber is visible; this attaches to the injector to create a single device.

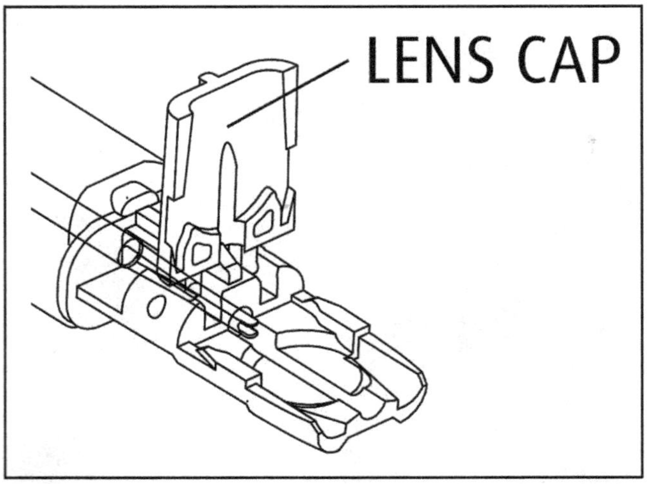

Figure 17-12. Open the box on the injector that will receive the lens and add one drop of VES.

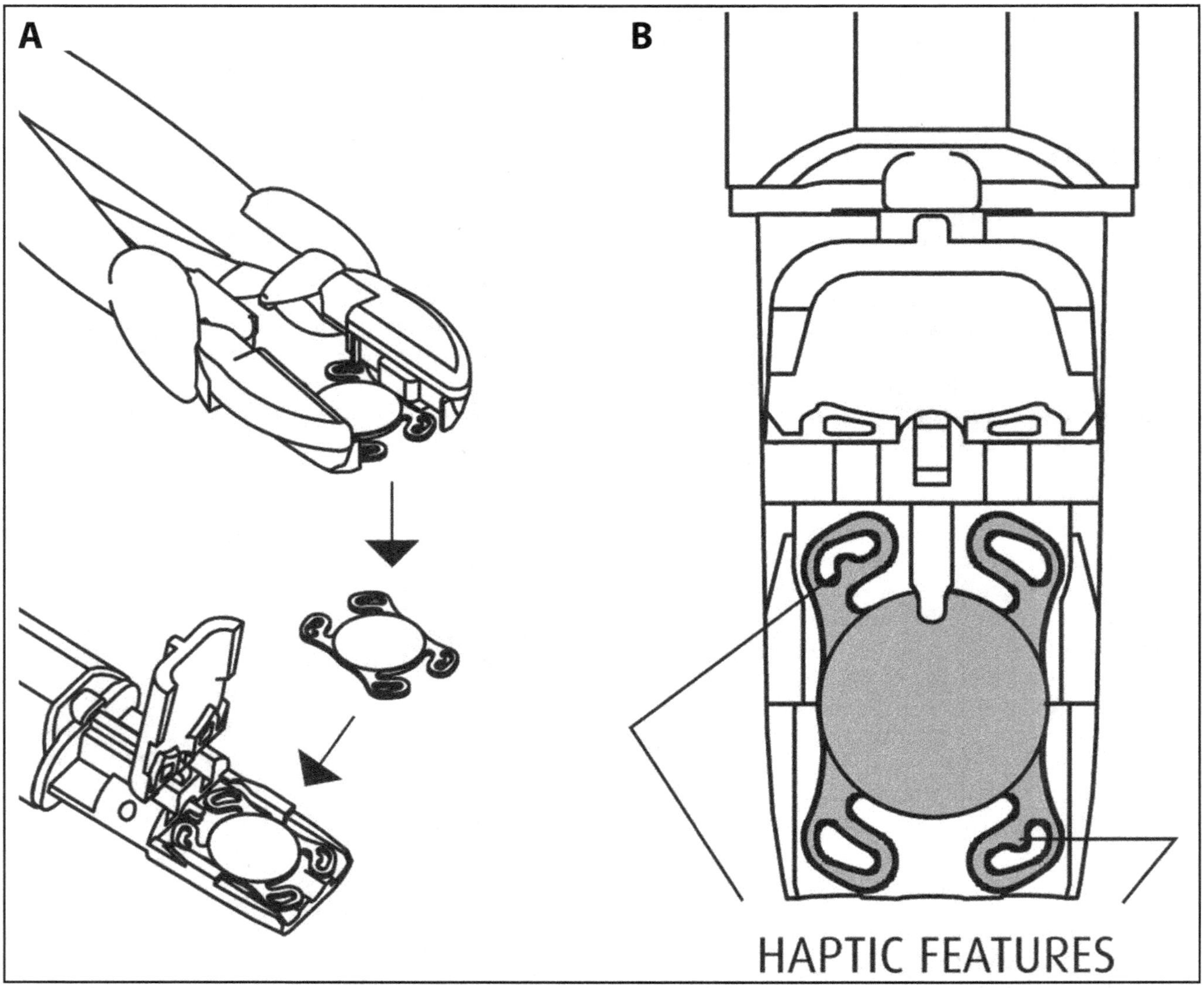

Figure 17-13. (A) Open the vial that contains the lens and extract the lens holder. Position the lens holder with the valves facing downward. (B) Using atraumatic forceps, transfer the lens from the lens holder to the container in the injector, taking care to avoid overturning the lens.

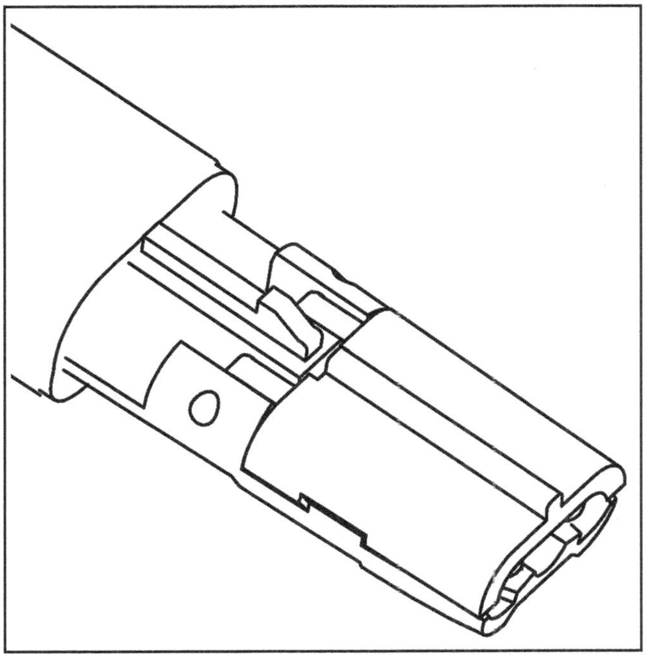

Figure 17-14. Check the correct position of the lens and add a drop of VES onto the IOL before closing the launch chamber.

surgeon should continue exerting pressure until the distal haptic and the optic have exited the cartridge into the capsular bag.

8. At this point, the pressure in the plunger is released and it is withdrawn to catch the proximal haptic. Once again the surgeon exerts gentle pressure on the plunger to facilitate the insertion of the distal haptic into the capsular bag.

The SofPort Easy-Load Lens Delivery System for Bausch + Lomb SofPort Lenses

The IOL is preloaded in a device that is attached to the injector, and this avoids manipulating the lens; the resulting operative benefits can be summarized as increased simplicity of use, increase in sterility and less risk of lens damage.

The Easy-Load Lens Delivery System consists of several components: an injector with a syringe-like mechanism, a small tip inserted close to the injector for straightening the haptic of the IOL after this has been loaded; and finally, a device for housing the lens with a sliding box that folds the lens as it advances (Figure 17-17A).

The injector is sterile and single use or disposable, and the device allows problem-free loading of the lens without the surgeon handling it. A monomanual syringe-like movement inserts the IOL. The IOL loading process requires the loading chamber to be filled with VES (Figure 17-17B).

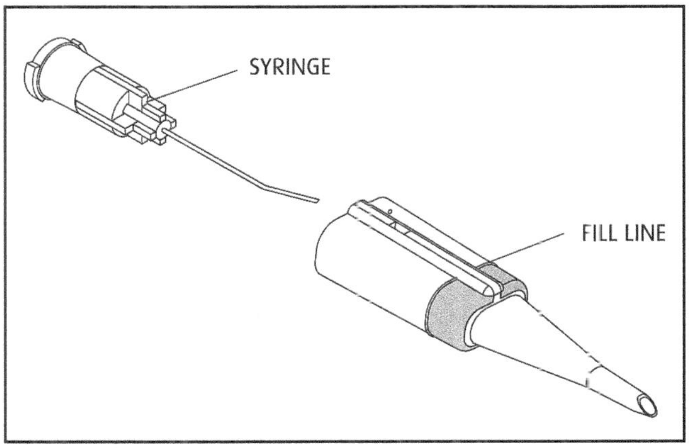

Figure 17-15. Fill the launch chamber with VES as far as the reference line.

The lens holder is inserted into the loading chamber of the injector (Figures 17-17C and D).

The box is then pushed gently forward until the lens holder stops its movement. At this point, the lens holder can be removed and detached from the injector (Figure 17-17E). The lens holder is then raised slightly from the box lid, which is raised vertically and discarded (Figure 17-17F).

Immediately prior to insertion of the IOL, the box is closed completely to compress the lens (Figure 17-17G). As the plunger is pushed forward, the loop extractor begins to remove itself from the tip of the injector. At approximately halfway, the plunger inserted in the injector tip is removed manually, the distal haptic is distended and positioned correctly for insertion into the eye. The piston is discarded (Figure 17-17H).

The surgeon now fills the distal portion of the injector with VES (or with BSS) to reduce the risk of injecting air bubbles into the eye. The surgeon places the tip of the injector inside the corneal tunnel (Figure 17-17I). The forward pressure on the plunger facilitates the injection of the lens into the capsular bag, with correct orientation. By releasing the pressure on the plunger, the rod is withdrawn to capture the proximal axis. The forward progression of the plunger will then insert the proximal haptic into the capsular bag.

The Crystalens Insertion Device

The insertion system for the accommodative lens, Crystalens, produced by Bausch + Lomb, is characterized by a syringe-type single-use injector cartridge device (Figure 17-18). The loading procedure for the IOL involves loading the IOL in the opening that has been coated with VES (Figures 17-19A and B). The correct orientation of the lens is essential here so that when the lens is inserted in the eye, it can move forward and allow accommodation. Consequently, it is important to inspect the positioning of the loops with the button-tip loop in the upper right and lower left positions (Figures 17-19C and D).

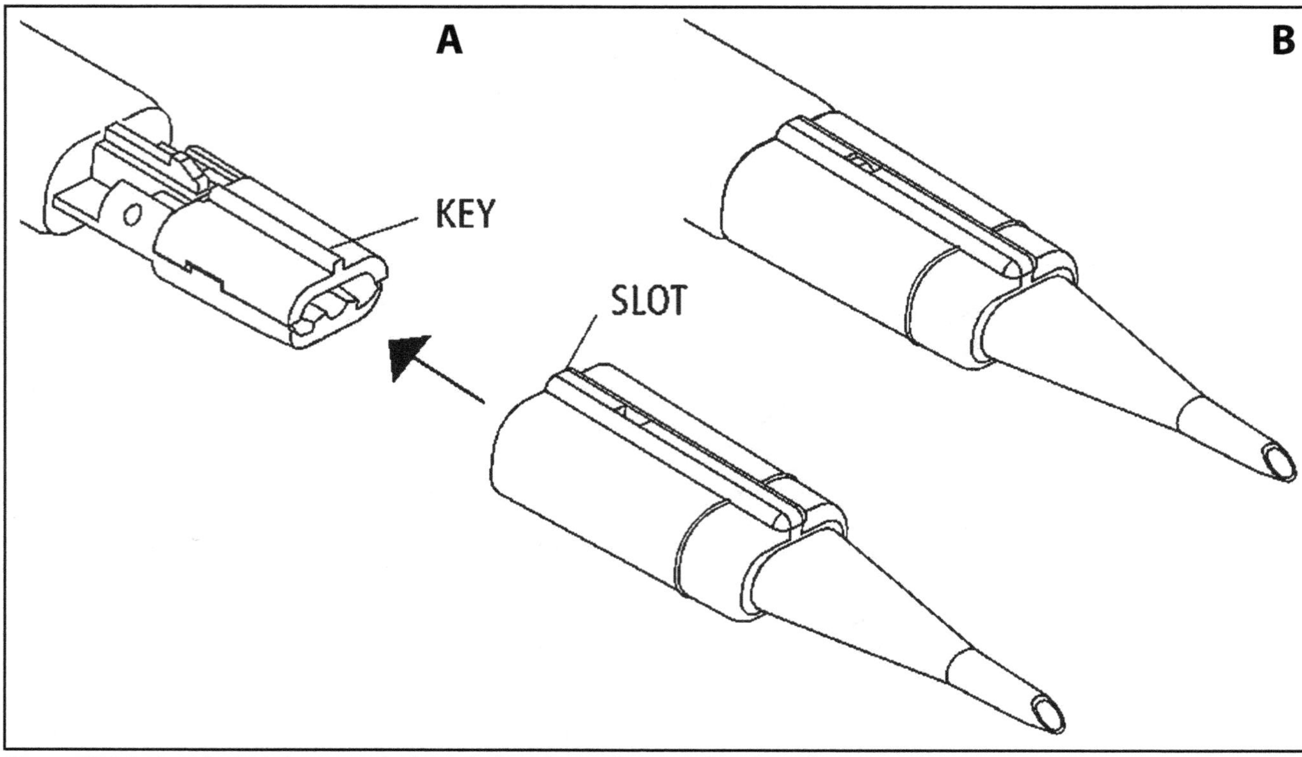

Figure 17-16. Attach the injector to the launch chamber and ensure that the safety device is engaged.

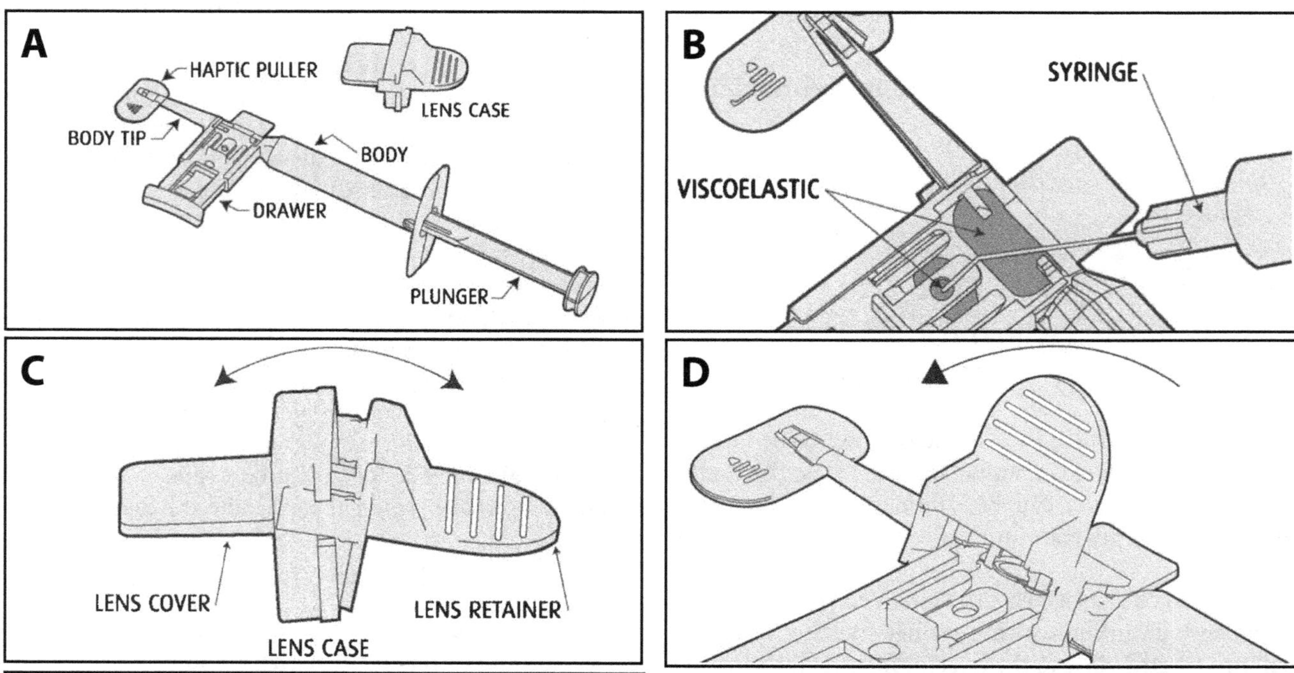

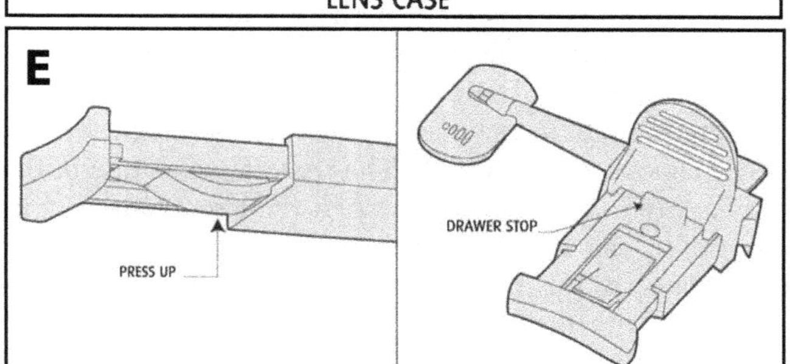

Figure 17-17. (A) Disposable injector with a preloaded lens. The distal portion of the syringe-type injector grasps the lens. (B) Fill the lens chamber with VES. (C) Open the IOL container and prepare it for attachment to the injector. (D) Attach the lens holder to the loading bay. (E) The figure illustrates how the lens is loaded in the injector. Release the box and push it gently to engage the lens. This pressure will load the lens and the surgeon then removes the lensholder. *(continued)*

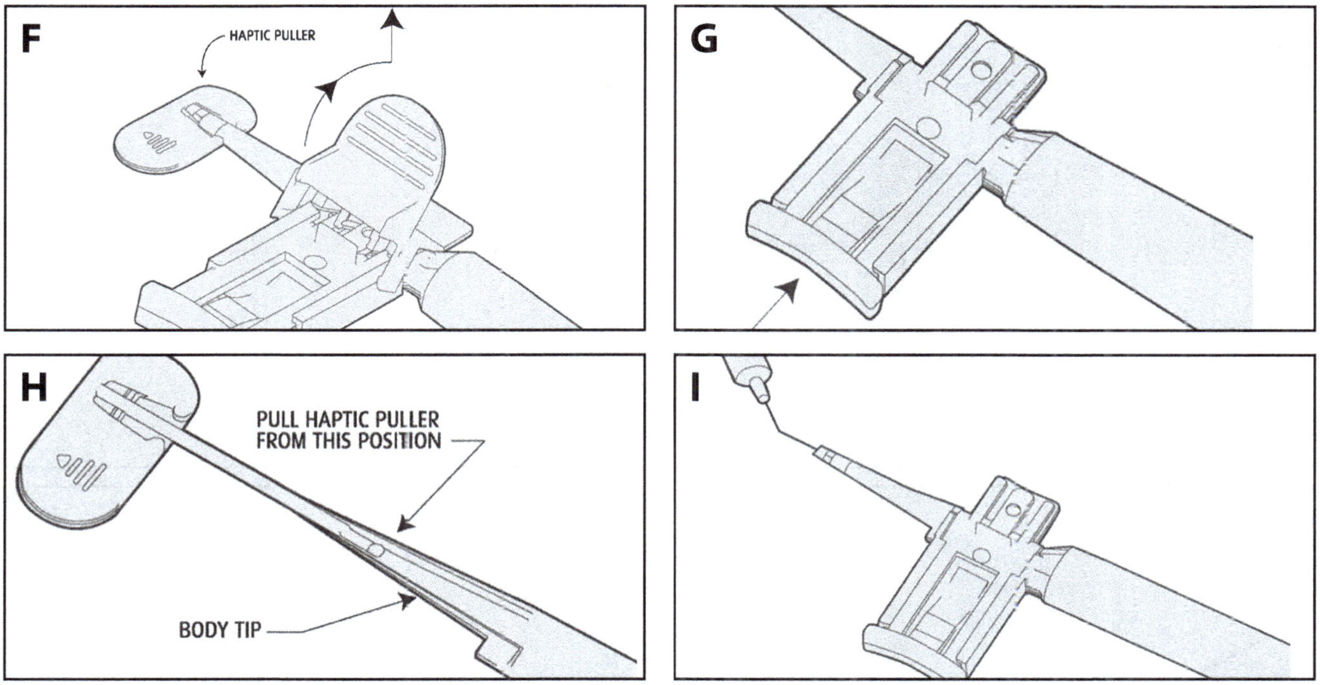

Figure 17-17. (continued) (F) The figure illustrates how the lensholder is removed once the IOL has been loaded in the injector. (G) Gently close the box completely until the docking mechanism has engaged. (H) As the piston is pushed forward, the loop extractor begins to distance itself from the tip of the injector. Halfway along, the piston inserted in the tip of the injector is removed manually; the distal loop is straightened and positioned for the correct insertion in the eye. The piston is discarded. (I) After filling the distal portion of the injector with VES (or with BSS) to reduce the possibility of introducing air bubbles into the eye, the surgeon can position the tip of the injector in the corneal tunnel.

When the IOL has been positioned correctly, the surgeon proceeds with the folding procedure; this occurs by sliding the box fitted to the side of the injector (Figure 17-19E); this will compress the optic and also fold the haptics. The surgeon must pay attention during this step and ensure that both haptics are folded forward when they enter the cartridge and are not in an oblique position (Figure 17-19F). Filling the cartridge with VES will help the plunger to slide and engage the optic of the IOL. The IOL is injected when the opening of the cartridge is positioned in the eye (Figure 17-19G). It is essential that the surgeon performs smooth continuous movements, taking care to orient the distal haptics correctly in the bag (Figure 17-19H).

These will be followed by the optic and the proximal haptics (Figures 17-19I through K). It should be remembered that the optic of this lens is silicone and will consequently unfold very rapidly.

If the movement is continuous and progressive, the lens will be injected into the capsular bag with one shot. However, if the movement is interrupted, the final step of the procedure to position the lens will involve the use of a blunt instrument to engage the proximal portion of the haptic and the optic pushing them gently into the capsular bag (Figure 17-19L).

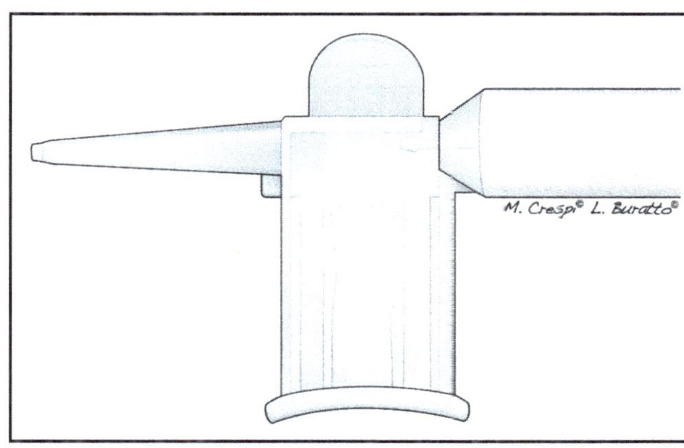

Figure 17-18. Crystalsert Crystalens delivery system.

The Zeiss Injector AT Shooter

The Zeiss injector for implanting lenses through a micro or mini-incision is called the AT Shooter A2-2000; it requires the ACM2 cartridge for the microincision that can inject the IOL through an incision of just 1.5 mm (Figure 17-20). Combined with the ACM2 cartridge, this type of injector can be used to implant all of the Zeiss IOLs characterized by "MICS design," or rather, all of the one-piece lenses with flat haptics. The standard cartridge is used

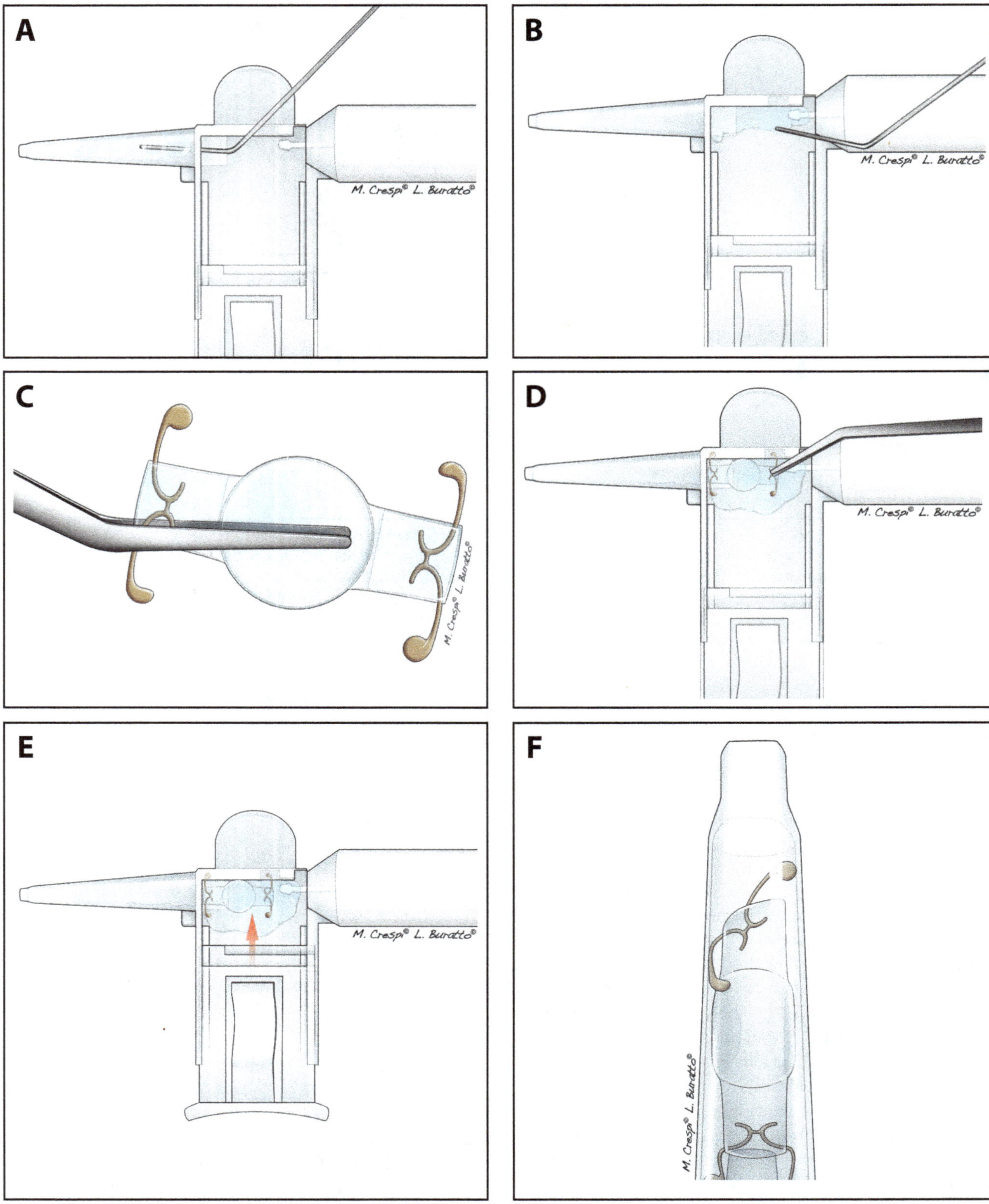

Figure 17-19. (A) Preparation of the Crystalens cartridge with addition of VES in the launch chamber. (B) Preparation of the Crystalens cartridge with addition of VES in the area that receives the lens. (C) The lens is removed from its container. The surgeon can control the orientation of the lens by positioning the button tips in the top right and bottom left positions. (D) The lens is positioned in the cartridge that has been filled with VES, respecting the orientation of the lens. This is possible by positioning the button tips at the top right and bottom left. (E) The lens is folded across the center of the optic when the box is closed. In this phase, the surgeon must ensure the haptics so that the 2 distal tips are both folded forward. (F) Bad positioning of the haptics in the launch chamber. *(continued)*

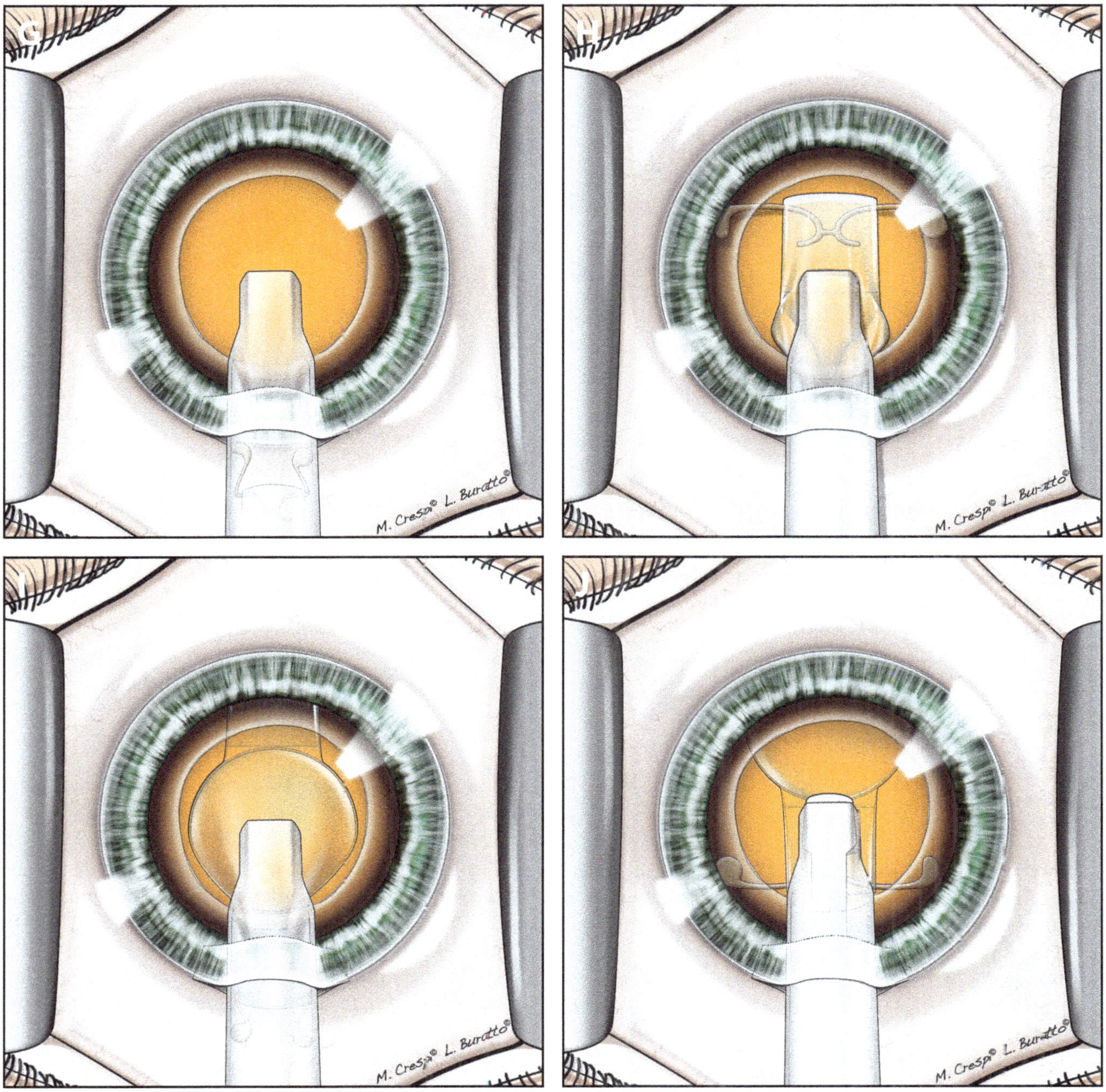

Figure 17-19. (continued) (G) Insertion of the injector in the eye with the smooth controlled progression of the haptics (both folded forward). (H) The progression of the piston encourages the opening of the distal haptics in the anterior chamber. In this phase, it is important to position the 2 haptics in the bag below the anterior rhexis. (I) The lens optic unfolds in the anterior chamber. It should be remembered that this lens is silicone and consequently will open very rapidly. The surgeon must control the procedure by exerting smooth gradual pressure on the piston. (J) The progression of the piston encourages the progression of the lens into the anterior chamber, until the proximal loops are inserted. By exploiting the elasticity of the lens, it is possible to insert the proximal loops in the bag with a "1-shot" maneuver. (*continued*)

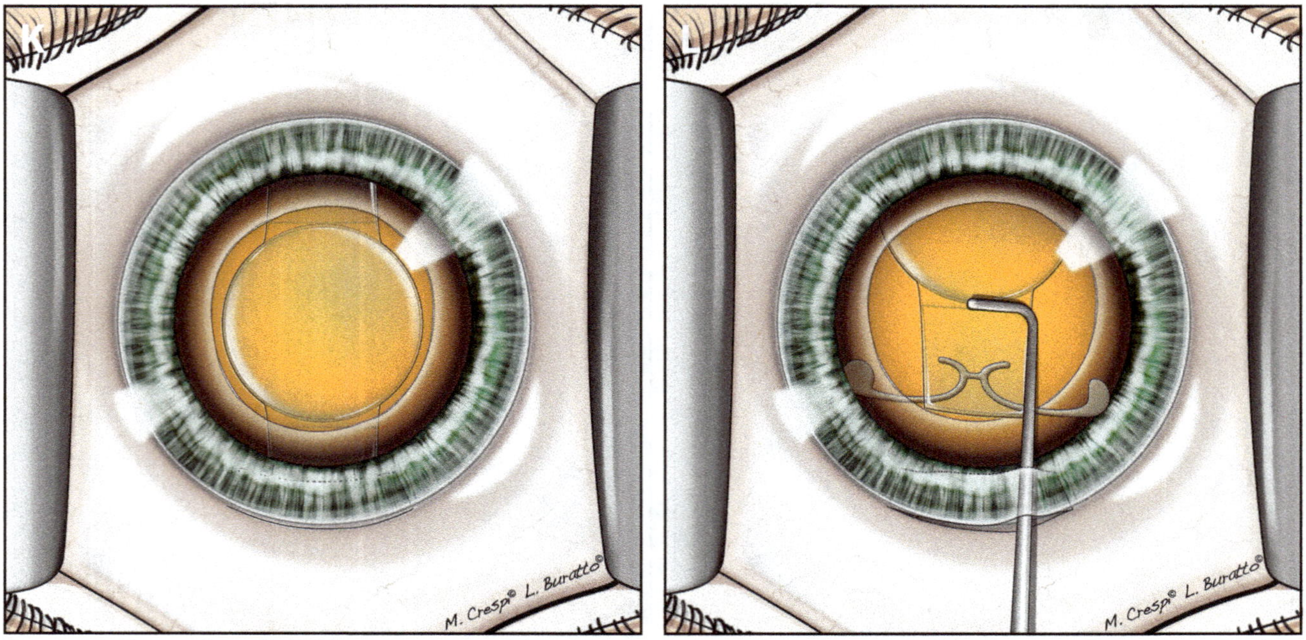

Figure 17-19. (continued) (K) The progression of the piston encourages the progression of the lens into the anterior chamber, until the proximal loops are inserted. By exploiting the elasticity of the lens, it is possible to insert the proximal loops in the bag with a "1-shot" maneuver. (L) In the event the insertion of the distal loops in the capsular bag is not completed with a "1-shot" of the piston, the surgeon can use a forked probe or a specific instrument that will facilitate the insertion of the distal loops in the bag.

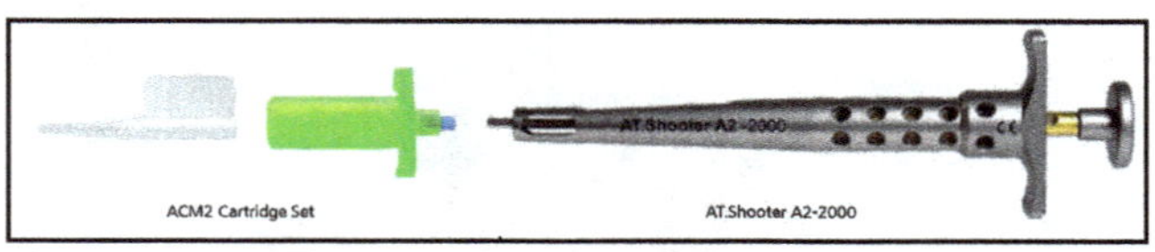

Figure 17-20. The complete kit of the injector AT Shooter A2-2000 and the ACM2.

for powers of between +16.0 and +24.0 D and for cylinder values of between +1.0 and +3.5 D; outside of these power levels, the appropriate cartridge is supplied with the IOL of different powers.

The injector is titanium and designed with a syringe mechanism, with a metal tip protected by a silicone sleeve supplied with the cartridge; this will protect the lens from damage as it is being inserted into the eye.

The cartridge has the classic "butterfly wing" design with 2 halves that open to receive the IOL. The "4 haptic design" models use the AT Shooter A1-2000 injector with the Viscojet 2.2-mm cartridge. The preloaded "4 haptic model" is an injector called Skyinvent.

Finally, the 2 "2-haptic design" models use the 2.8-mm Skyjet injection system for diopters of +27 to +30 D; the cartridge has a diameter of 3.2 mm.

Lens Loading and Implantation Technique

Remove the IOL from its container using atraumatic forceps (Figure 17-21A) and place it at the center of the cartridge that has been filled with VES (Figures 17-21B and C).

1. The 2 wings are closed; with closed atraumatic forceps the surgeon applies gentle pressure to the optic of the IOL to facilitate the folding of the lens (Figure 17-21D). Closing the 2 wings will activate the safety mechanism and this will prevent the 2 arms opening and scratching the lens during the injection process (Figure 17-21E).
2. Insert the cartridge into the injector and engage the lens with the tip of the plunger covered by the silicone sleeve; the surgeon should provide smooth gradual progression of the lens in the cartridge (Figures 17-21F through I).
3. The monomanual insertion procedure for the IOL is very straightforward and must be completed with a single smooth push, taking care to direct the IOL into the capsular bag.

The movement must be rapid and complete and must allow straightforward injection of the IOL into the capsular bag. Any hesitation in the movements may result in incomplete positioning of the IOL in the bag and the surgeon will have to maneuver the IOL with a blunt probe or with the VES cannula to push the 2 proximal loops into the bag. If

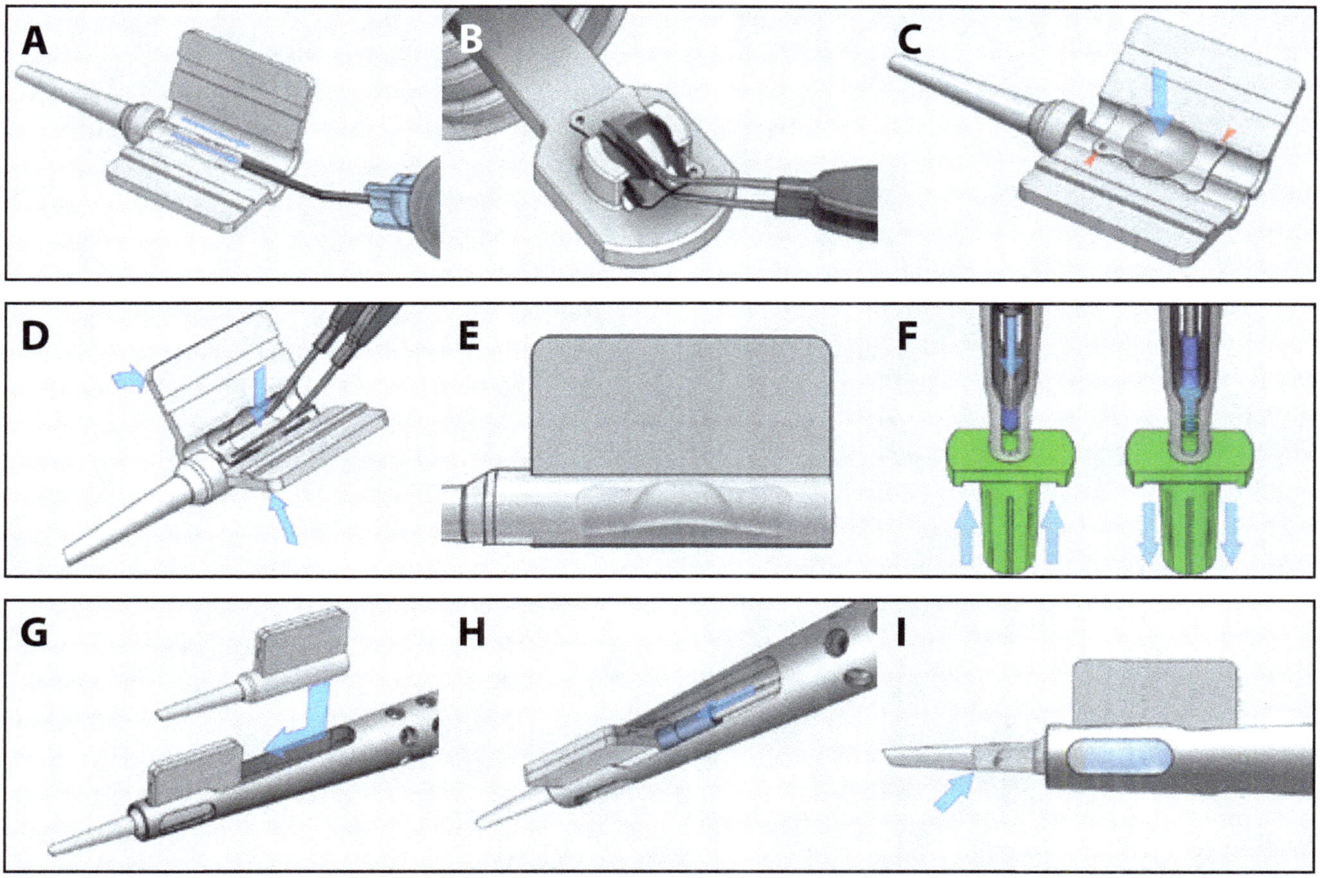

Figure 17-21. (A) The lens is supplied on a plastic support, allowing it to be removed from its package using atraumatic forceps. (B) Image of the butterfly-shaped cartridge, with the 2 valves that open to provide the structure for receiving the IOL. The lens must be inserted in the cartridge, respecting the orientation of the insertion with the 2 landmarks in the top left and bottom right positions. (C) The lens must be covered in VES before positioning it in the cartridge. (D) When the lens is positioned inside the cartridge, it must be pushed downward with the open arms of atraumatic forceps, to facilitate correct positioning. (E) The lens has been positioned correctly in the cartridge and folded on itself. (F) Attach a nontraumatic silicone tip to the end of the injector to allow the lens to be pushed into the launch chamber. (G) Attach the cartridge securely to the injector. (H) Engage the lens with the injector tip that has been covered with a silicone sleeve. (I) The correct position of the IOL in the cartridge. The distal portion of the haptics can be observed in the launch chamber.

the surgeon applies excessive pressure on the plunger, the silicone sleeve may protrude from the injector tip.

The silicone tip will tend to expand because it has a greater diameter compared to the injector and it may become trapped in the corneal tunnel; in this case, the surgeon will have to intervene and manually disengage it.

The insertion technique for the Zeiss IOL is straightforward and easy to learn, and the maneuver is safe and can be performed monomanually.

Suggested Readings

Picardo V, Vincenti P. Lenti precaricate. IOL ad avanzata tecnologia. Lenti Premium. Speciale La Voce AICCER. Fabiano; 2012.

Sachdev MS, Venkatesh P. In: Fine IH, Agarwal A, eds. *Phaco Intraocular Lenses; Phacoemulsification, Laser Cataract Surgery and Foldable IOLs*. New Delhi, India: Jaypee; 1998: Chapter 31.

18

Implantation of an Intraocular Lens With Capsular Rupture

Lucio Buratto, MD; Stephen F. Brint, MD, FACS; and Domenico Boccuzzi, MD, PhD

When the surgeon has capsular rupture with more or less obvious loss of vitreous, he or she will always be reluctant to abort the surgery before the procedure has been completed with the lens safely implanted. He or she may consider the option of aborting surgery as a failure; however, in many situations, it is the most sensible decision.

However, under some situations, the surgeon may continue the surgery after evaluating the risks and managing the vitreous; he or she may decide to implant the intraocular lens (IOL) in the sulcus and successfully finish the surgery. The first thing he or she has to consider when deciding to implant an IOL in the sulcus is the presence of a continuous circular anterior capsulorrhexis that is of a diameter sufficient to support the IOL.

When the anterior rhexis is intact and of an appropriate diameter, has been created just slightly below the IOL optic, and is well centered with respect to the pupil, the surgeon should attempt capsular capture of the IOL, where the haptics are positioned in the sulcus and the optic slides beneath the anterior rhexis.

This condition is ideal for anchoring the IOL that will remain centered irrespective of the position of the loops and the diameter of the optic of the IOL.

When this is not feasible because of a decentered rhexis, the simultaneous rupture of the anterior capsule, or rhexis escape, the IOL must be implanted in the sulcus.

In order to implant the IOL in the sulcus, the anterior or posterior capsule must provide sufficient support for the lens and the zonules must be intact to ensure that the IOL is stable and depends only on the sulcus for fixation.

Alternatively, the surgeon should postpone the operation by approximately 1 month and opt for scleral, iris, or angle fixation of a polymethylmethacrylate (PMMA) IOL.

There are 2 essential factors for the implantation of an IOL in the sulcus: correct centration of the IOL and uveal biocompatibility.

One-piece acrylic IOLs are not suitable for implantation in the capsular sulcus because they have a reduced total diameter and the haptics are excessively thick and excessively "soft"; these characteristics lack good support in the sulcus and consequently lack of good centration.

It stands to reason that IOLs with plate (biscuit-like) haptics are also contraindicated.

The circumstances are similar for capsular capture, and the surgeon should use a 3-piece IOL. Three-piece IOLs for implantation in the bag (Figure 18-1), with an optic diameter of 6.0 mm and a diameter of the haptics of 13.0 mm, are also ideal for implantation in the sulcus (even though a 1-piece PMMA IOL would be preferable). Only under some circumstances (eg, when the eye is large or severely myopic), should the IOL have an optic of 6.5 mm and a diameter between the haptics of 13.5 or 14.0 mm.

- Foldable IOLs should be acrylic and not silicone. There are 2 reasons for this: the first is immediately obvious because the silicone IOLs will open with an "explosive" movement and this could further compromise the already delicate situation the surgeon faces with capsule rupture.
- The second reason is that, in case of retinal detachment, the implantation of a silicone IOL and the absence of the posterior capsule would compromise the final surgical outcome if a silicone oil tamponade has

Buratto L, Brint SF, Boccuzzi D.
Cataract Surgery and Intraocular Lenses (pp 155-159).

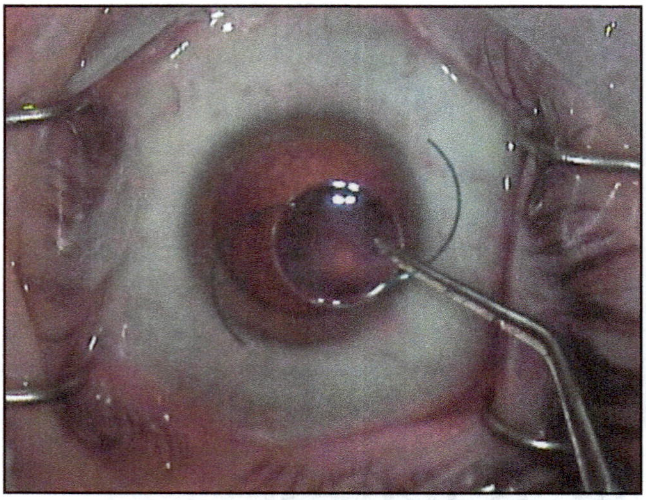

Figure 18-1. Three-piece IOLs for implantation in the capsular bag. (Reprinted with permission from Dr. V. Orfeo and Dr. D. Boccuzzi.)

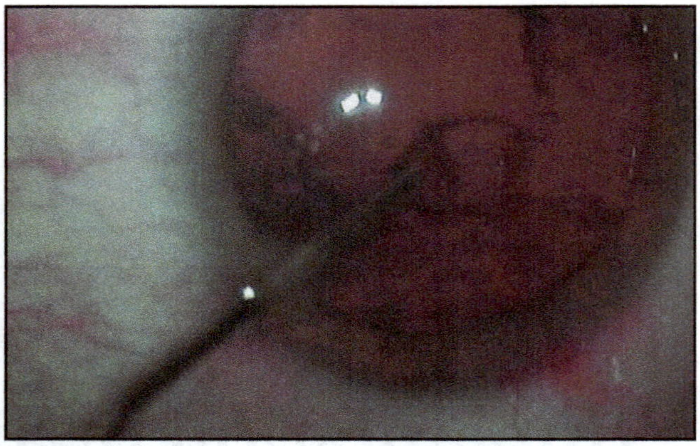

Figure 18-2. Aspiration of the capsular fragments with a fine cannula, taking care to avoid capturing vitreous fragments. (Reprinted with permission from Dr. V. Orfeo and Dr. D. Boccuzzi.)

been used. This is because contact between the silicone oil and the silicone IOL would lead to formation of a permanent interface between the 2 surfaces with a consequent reduction in visual quality.

Choosing Intraocular Lens Power

When the IOL is implanted in the sulcus with capsular capture, the effective lens position (ELP) will not change. The ELP is the ideal position of the IOL calculated by systems such as the IOL Master, Ocuscan, etc, and consequently, it is not necessary to vary the "A" constant.

If the surgeon implants the IOL in the capsular sulcus, he or she must remember that the lens will be anterior to its intended ELP. In this case, the surgeon should reduce the power of the IOL, as its more anterior position will lead to a myopic shift.

The degree of correction varies as a function of the dimensions of the eye and the power of the lens to be implanted.

For powers of between +15.0 and +23.0 D, it is necessary to reduce the power of the IOL in the bag by 1.0 D. For IOLs of less than +15.0 D, it is sufficient to reduce the power by 0.5 D. For powers greater than +23.0 D, the power of the lens must be reduced by 1.5 D. These reductions are based on the different impact the various powers of the lenses have on the optic system created, due to their anterior shift. In other words, if we compare the impact of a lens of high power with the impact of a lens of low power, with an equivalent anterior shift (for implantation in the sulcus), the lens with the higher power will cause a greater dioptric change than the lens with the lower power.

Surgical Technique

The implantation of an IOL in a nonintact capsular bag is contraindicated if there is a rupture of the posterior capsule, with the exception of a posterior rupture that can be converted into a continuous circular posterior capsulorrhexis, without a significant loss of vitreous; if possible, the lens can be implanted in the capsular bag.

Prior to implantation of the IOL, the surgeon must ensure that the capsular bag has been cleaned of all of the cortical remnants. If these remnants are left in situ, they may become hydrated and, among other things, affect the vision if they present in the pupillary field.

The capsular bag can be cleaned using the manual irrigation/aspiration of Simcoe or by coaxial irrigation/aspiration of McIntyre (Figure 18-2). During aspiration, the surgeon should avoid aspirating vitreous that may pull on the retina and cause serious complications. If there is a significant amount of vitreous, the surgeon must perform an anterior vitrectomy (Figure 18-3).

Once the surgeon has removed the vitreous that has prolapsed in the anterior chamber, he or she should inject viscoelastic substance (VES) into the anterior chamber and into the ciliary sulcus, prior to implanting the IOL.

The VES has a dual function. First, it tamponades the vitreous and avoids any escape through the capsular rupture into the anterior chamber; second, when injected in the ciliary sulcus, it creates space for implantation of the IOL.

When an IOL is implanted in the ciliary sulcus, the surgeon must do everything to ensure that both the loops are positioned in the sulcus. If one loop is in the sulcus and the other in the capsular bag, there is a risk of decentration of the IOL.

The IOL can be implanted with 1 of 2 procedures. The first involves injection of the IOL (a 3-piece acrylic lens) into the anterior chamber above the iris plane (Figure 18-4). Once the distal haptic and the optic have been

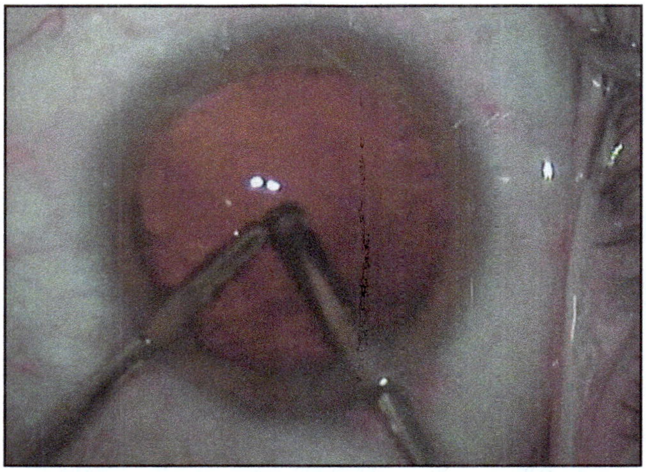

Figure 18-3. In the event there is a large amount of vitreous, the surgeon must perform a central anterior vitrectomy to eliminate the vitreous fragments from the anterior chamber. (Reprinted with permission from Dr. V. Orfeo and Dr. D. Boccuzzi.)

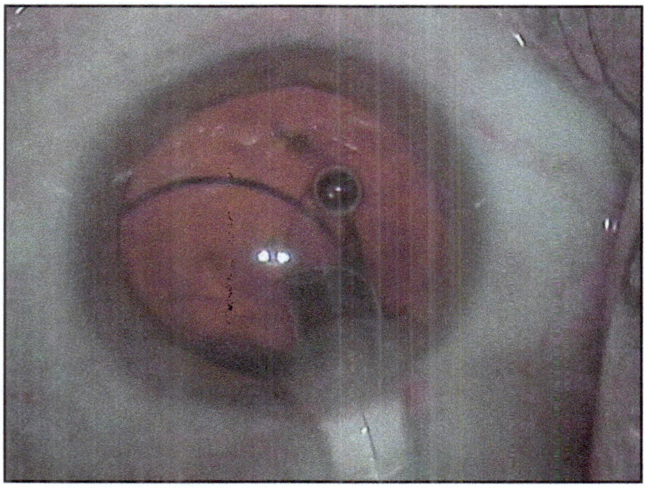

Figure 18-4. Insertion of the 3-piece IOL in the anterior chamber. The distal loop must be inserted above the anterior rhexis. (Reprinted with permission from Dr. V. Orfeo and Dr D. Boccuzzi.)

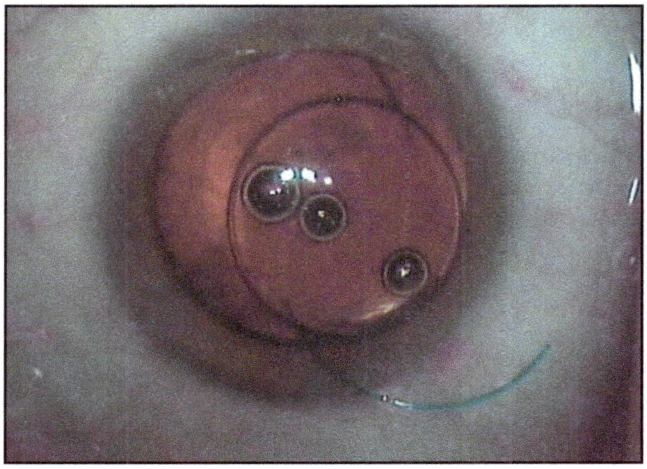

Figure 18-5. The lens should not be wholly inserted in the anterior chamber. It is recommended to position the distal loop and the IOL optic on the rhexis, leaving the proximal loop outside of the tunnel. (Reprinted with permission from Dr. V. Orfeo and Dr. D. Boccuzzi.)

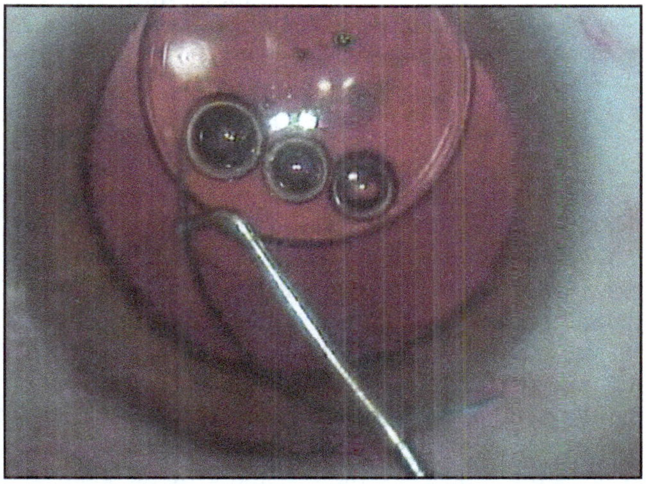

Figure 18-6. A Sinskey hook was used to facilitate the insertion of the IOL. The IOL can be grasped at the junction between the optic and the haptic. By rotating the lens in a clockwise direction, it can slide in the capsular sulcus between the anterior rhexis and the iris. (Reprinted with permission from Dr. V. Orfeo and Dr. D. Boccuzzi.)

introduced, the proximal haptic is positioned above the iris plane. At this point, using a long Sinskey hook, the surgeon captures the distal haptic and bends it until it slides below the iris. The haptic is allowed to unfold gently under the iris and above the anterior capsule. Using McPherson forceps, the surgeon repeats the maneuver for the proximal haptic, bending it until it slides underneath the edge of the iris and positions it above the anterior rhexis.

If there is good visualization of the anterior capsule and there is good mydriasis, the distal haptic and the optic of the IOL can be injected below the iris and directly above the anterior capsule (Figure 18-5), positioning the second haptic by rotating it with a Sinskey hook using the junction between the optic and the haptic (Figure 18-6)

When possible, the second option is preferable and a more straightforward technique.

If the capsulorrhexis is well centered and the diameter slightly smaller than the diameter of the optic of the IOL, the surgeon can capture the optic. Once the IOL has been completely positioned in the sulcus, the surgeon slides the optic underneath the rhexis by exerting moderate pressure at a distance of approximately 90 degrees from the optic–haptic junction (Figure 18-7). On completion of this movement, the rhexis will be deformed, from circular to oval, with the poles positioned related to the junctions between the optic of the IOL and the haptics (Figure 18-8). This maneuver will allow positioning of the IOL with no risk of decentration, and without worrying about the diameter

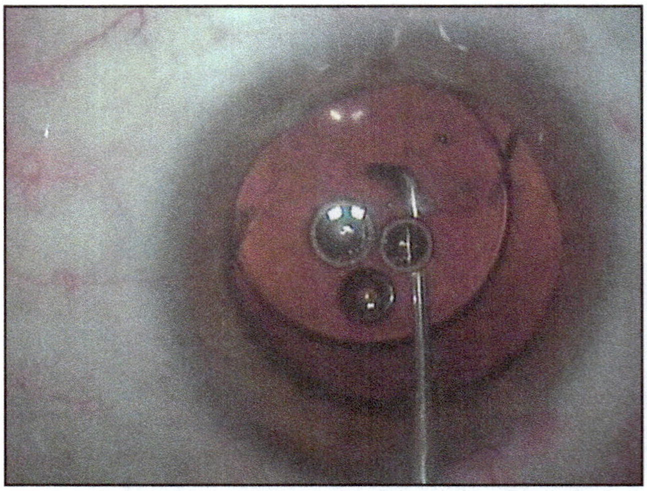

Figure 18-7. Capsular capture. It is possible to capture the capsule when a central rhexis of appropriate diameter has been created. The lens optic slides underneath the anterior rhexis, with the haptics positioned above the rhexis. When this procedure is performed correctly, the anterior capsule will assume a diamond shape. (Reprinted with permission from Dr. V. Orfeo and Dr. D. Boccuzzi.)

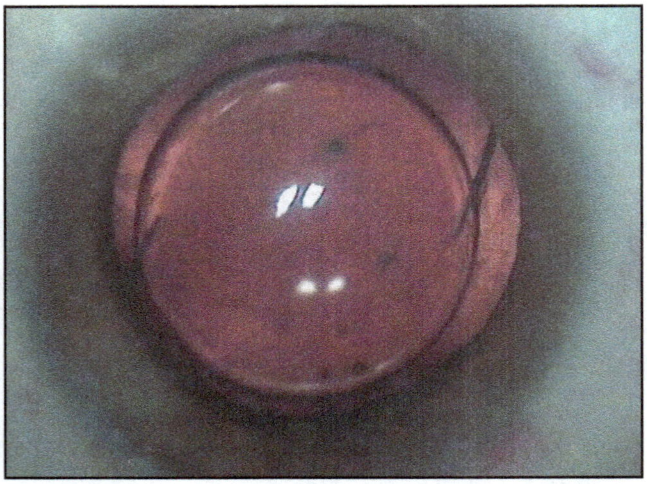

Figure 18-8. The lens has been captured. The correct completion of this maneuver will position the lens on a plane of the rhexis lower than the anterior chamber. This will allow correct centration of the IOL and the correct positioning of the lens on the anteroposterior axis. (Reprinted with permission from Dr. V. Orfeo and Dr. D. Boccuzzi.)

of the haptics with respect to the diameter of the sulcus, because the capsular opening will allow the correct position of the lens. Moreover, with this maneuver, the surgeon will avoid adhesion between the anterior and posterior capsules that would encourage and facilitate fibrosis formation. If the surgeon has any doubts that the lens implanted in the sulcus is sufficiently stable or centered, he or she may opt for mono or bilateral iris fixation, with 10/0 Prolene sutures positioned around the loops. For iris fixation of the haptic, the surgeon must create an appropriate degree of miosis, position the optic above the iris, and leave the loops well defined below the iris to allow the safe pass of a long needle with 10/0 Prolene suture. It should be pointed out that when the maneuvers prove to be long and laborious, the surgeon should postpone the implantation until a later date because these maneuvers can increase the risk of complications.

Loops in the Bag and Capsular Capture of the Optic in the Anterior Rhexis

This inverted capture of the optic can be performed if the posterior capsule ruptures after the surgeon has implanted the IOL in the bag. If the posterior capsule ruptures unexpectedly during the implantation of the IOL in the capsular bag (eg, when the surgeon is aspirating the VES from behind the IOL), and this may destabilize the lens in the bag, the surgeon can slide the optic of the lens in front of the anterior rhexis. This minimal stress procedure ensures that the lens is well attached to the anterior capsule and avoids dislocation of the lens into the vitreous and the associated complications.

Conclusion

- When there is capsular rupture with vitreous loss, the surgeon may postpone the implantation procedure until a later date.
- When simultaneous implantation process is feasible, the surgeon should perform an anterior vitrectomy in the retro iris zone, to avoid leaving vitreous strands in the anterior chamber, or worse still, wrapped around the IOL or in the corneal openings.
- Good support is essential, meaning that the anterior rhexis must be intact or almost intact.
- A 3-piece IOL must be implanted and the surgeon should capture the optic with the haptics in the sulcus and the optic below the anterior rhexis.
- Miosis should be induced with acetylcholine.
- The surgeon should remove as much of the VES as possible without excessive deepening of the anterior chamber.
- The main incision should be sutured with 10/0 nylon (Figure 18-9).

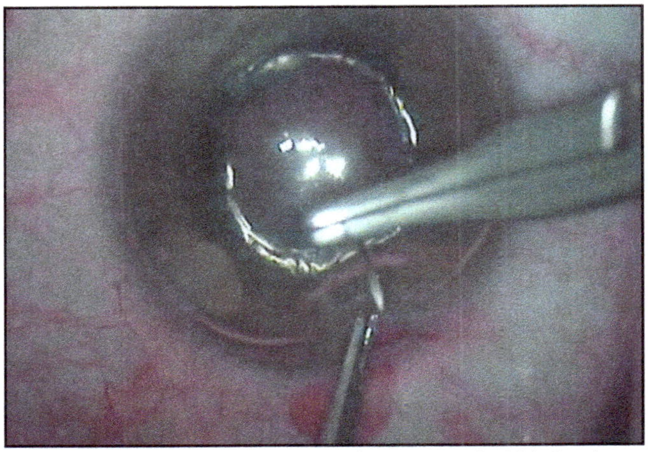

Figure 18-9. The incision is sutured once an air bubble has been injected to control the complete absence of vitreous. (Reprinted with permission from Dr. V. Orfeo and Dr. D. Boccuzzi.)

Suggested Readings

Amino K, Yamakawa R. Long-term results of out-of-the-bag intraocular lens implantation. *J Cataract Refract Surg*. 2000;26(2):266-270.

Gimbel HV, DeBroff BM. Intraocular lens optic capture. *J Cataract Refract Surg*. 2004;30(1):200-206. Review.

Holladay JT. International intraocular lens and implant registry 2004. *J Cataract Refract Surg*. 2004;30(1):207-229.

LeBoyer RM, Werner L, Snyder ME, Mamalis N, Riemann CD, Augsberger JJ. Acute haptic-induced ciliary sulcus irritation associated with single-piece AcrySof intraocular lenses. *J Cataract Refract Surg*. 2005;31(7):1421-1427.

Petternel V, Menapace R, Findl O, et al. Effect of optic edge design and haptic angulation on postoperative intraocular lens position change. *J Cataract Refract Surg*. 2004;30(1):52-57.

Suto C, Hori S, Fukuyama E, Akura J. Adjusting intraocular lens power for sulcus fixation. *J Cataract Refract Surg*. 2003;29(10):1913-1917.

19

Tear or Damage of the Intraocular Lens

Lucio Buratto, MD; Stephen F. Brint, MD, FACS; and Domenico Boccuzzi, MD, PhD

The intraocular lens (IOL) insertion process is an extremely delicate part of the procedure; incorrect handling of the lens may cause irreversible alterations or damage. Injector implantation has reduced the incidence of these complications as IOL insertion is much more delicate compared to the previous "holder and folder" methods. Nevertheless, incorrect loading of the lens into the cartridge, repeated attempts to fold the lens, or prolonged folding may lead to minor alterations, fractures, or tears of the lens itself. If the lens is positioned incorrectly in the cartridge, the progression of the plunger may be altered, causing a folding or tear of a haptic during insertion, with subsequent alteration of the stability of the lens in the bag. The optic may be damaged. Small alterations of the surface or small scratches induced by the handling of the IOL may be visible, particularly on the first postoperative days. These may not be responsible for deterioration of vision or any reduction in modulation transfer function (MTF).[1]

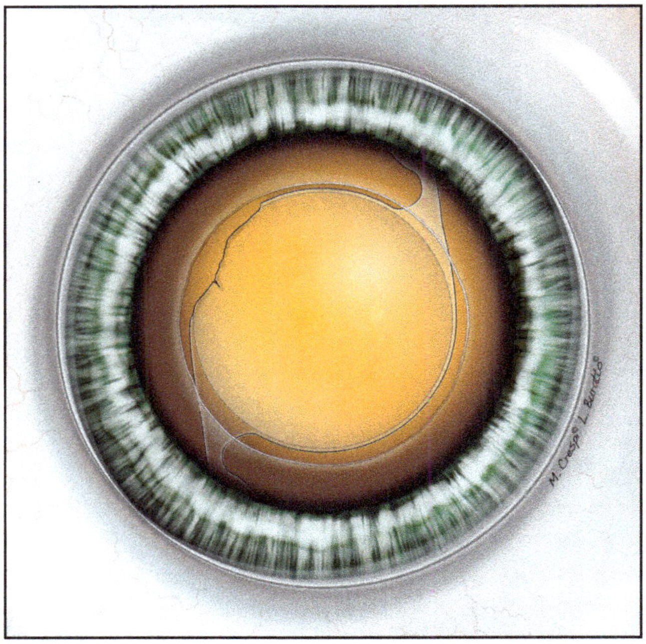

Figure 19-1. Peripheral damage to the lens optic. This type of alteration will not change the MTF.

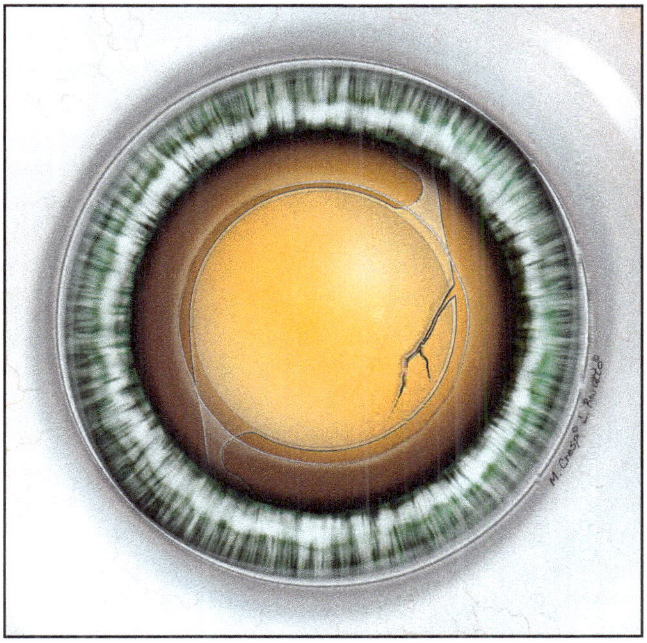

Figure 19-2. A visible crack around the optic of the silicone lens.

Buratto L, Brint SF, Boccuzzi D.
Cataract Surgery and Intraocular Lenses (pp 161–162).

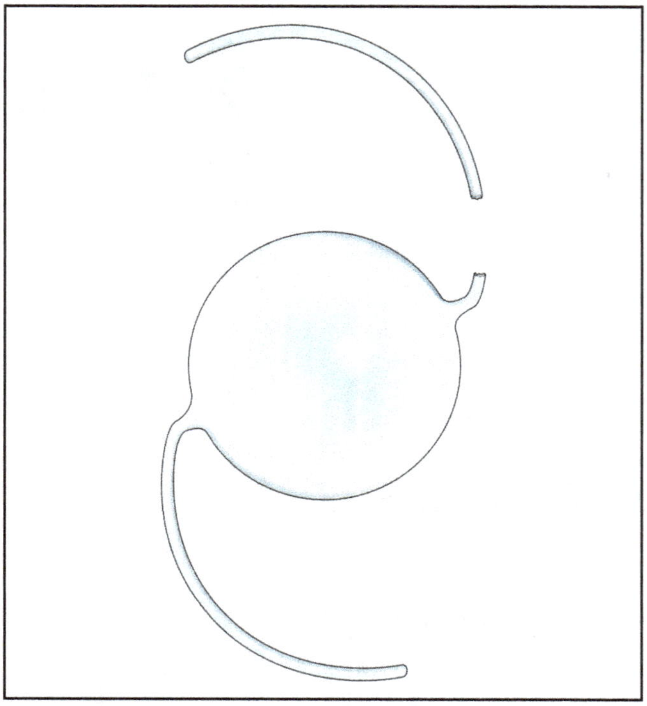

Figure 19-3. One-piece polymethylmethacrylate IOL. One of the haptics has been torn during the insertion process.

These alterations will be more obvious when the lens has been preheated. Cracks in the optic can compromise good functional outcome of the surgery, creating marked reduction in visual acuity. All of these phenomena can also appear during the steps of manual lens insertion with the use of the holder and folder (Figures 19-1 through 19-3).[2]

Peripheral optic tears that are far from the visual axis and from the pupil are not responsible for a reduction in the quality of sight. Structural alterations that are responsible for IOL decentration or tilting (haptic rupture) and central optic damage that interferes with vision require IOL exchange.

References

1. Erie JC, Newman B, Mahr MA, Khan AR, McIntosh M. Acrylic intraocular lens damage after folding using a forceps insertion technique. *J Cataract Refract Surg.* 2010;36(3):483-487.
2. Oshika T, Shiokawa Y. Effect of folding on the optical quality of soft acrylic intraocular lenses. *J Cataract Refract Surg.* 1996;22(suppl 2):1360-1364.

20

Irrigation/Aspiration Post Implantation

Lucio Buratto, MD; Stephen F. Brint, MD, FACS; and Domenico Boccuzzi, MD, PhD

Following insertion of the intraocular lens (IOL), prior to concluding the procedure, the surgeon must aspirate the viscoelastic substance (VES) from the anterior chamber and from the capsular bag, and in particular from behind the IOL.

As described previously, cohesive VES consists of large molecules; this type of VES will be aspirated in a single mass but it is essential to remove it completely to avoid postoperative pressure spikes. There are 2 types of surgical instruments necessary for this and for aspiration of the cortex following phaco. These dictate the surgical technique from the outset. On the basis of his or her experience and preferences, the surgeon can opt for monomanual or bimanual irrigation/aspiration (I/A). With the monomanual technique, the surgeon will need to create a small side-port incision to allow the insertion of small surgical instruments (eg, such as the chopper or a spatula). With the bimanual technique on the other hand, 2 larger side-port incisions are required to allow the insertion of the 2 I/A handpieces.

Instruments for Monomanual Irrigation/Aspiration

With monomanual I/A, the surgeon uses a one-way aspiration handpiece positioned at the end of the tip; there are 2 lateral irrigation openings in the sleeve, which may be silicone or metal like the remainder of the handpiece (silicone sleeve is normally used). The tip may have 1 of 3 designs: straight or angled at an angle of 45 or 90 degrees. The angled tips are preferable to the straight ones, particularly when used for aspiration of cortex, or to remove subincisional fragments, an area that is difficult to access with a straight tip. The tip is rounded, different from the phaco tip, and this reduces the risk of rupturing the posterior capsule during aspiration (Figure 20-1). The diameter of the aspiration opening is variable; however, a 0.3-mm diameter is preferable—this is the diameter necessary to allow good aspiration, without compromising the stability of the anterior chamber.

Disposable polycarbonate tips were recently released (eg, the Intrepid by Alcon Surgical). This has a capsule-friendly surface and can be fitted to the handpiece (Figures 20-2 and 20-3). By modifying the sleeve to different diameters, this tip can be used with incisions that vary between 2.75 and 2.2 mm (Figure 20-4). The tip of the handpiece can be straight, curved, or at an angle of 35 degrees and can be selected on the basis of the surgeon's requirements and preferences (Figure 20-5).

Bimanual (Buratto Technique)

The bimanual I/A technique involves the use of 2 handpieces. The infusion handpiece has a 0.8-mm cannula; at one end, there are 1 or 2 openings of variable diameter. Generally speaking, the diameter is 0.45 mm when there are 2 openings or 0.5 or 0.6 mm when there is a single opening. Actually, there are numerous different combinations with variations in the number and diameter of openings; there are variations in the position of the openings (at the tip or on the sides), its shape (round or oval), the shape of the tip (round or oval), and even the direction of the jet of fluid (frontal or downward).

Buratto L, Brint SF, Boccuzzi D.
Cataract Surgery and Intraocular Lenses (pp 163-166).

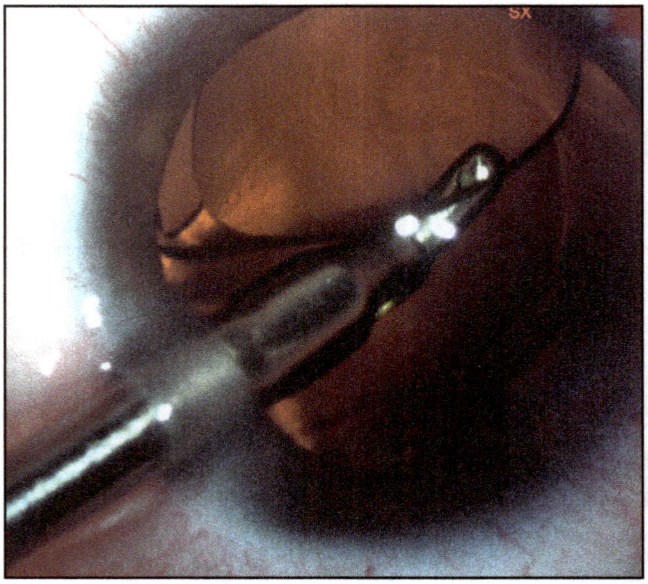

Figure 20-1. Steel handpiece for monomanual aspiration. The tip of the handpiece has a curve of 90 degrees to facilitate aspiration of the cortex located below the surgical access wound. Note that the lateral infusion openings are positioned perpendicular to the aspiration hole on the tip. This arrangement also prevents capturing the posterior capsule during the aspiration procedure to remove the viscoelastic behind the IOL. The tip of the handpiece is placed in a higher position with respect to the infusion channels to avoid capturing the capsule. (Reprinted with permission from Dr. V. Orfeo.)

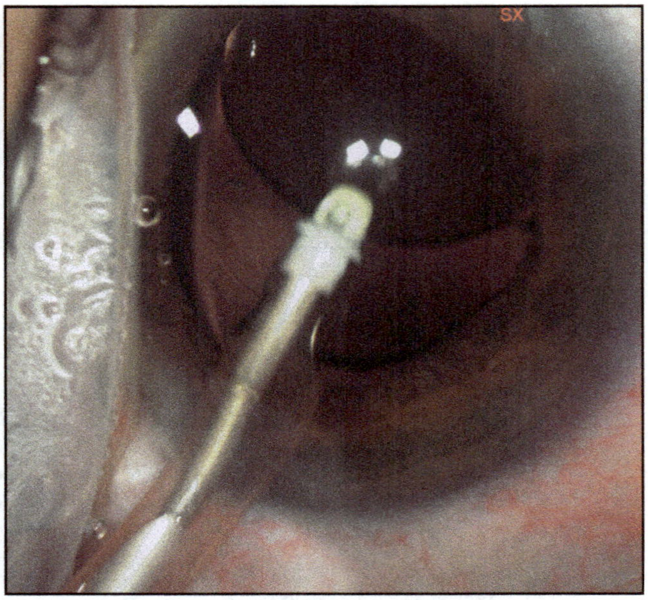

Figure 20-2. Handpiece with a polycarbonate tip for monomanual aspiration (Intrepid, Alcon Surgical).

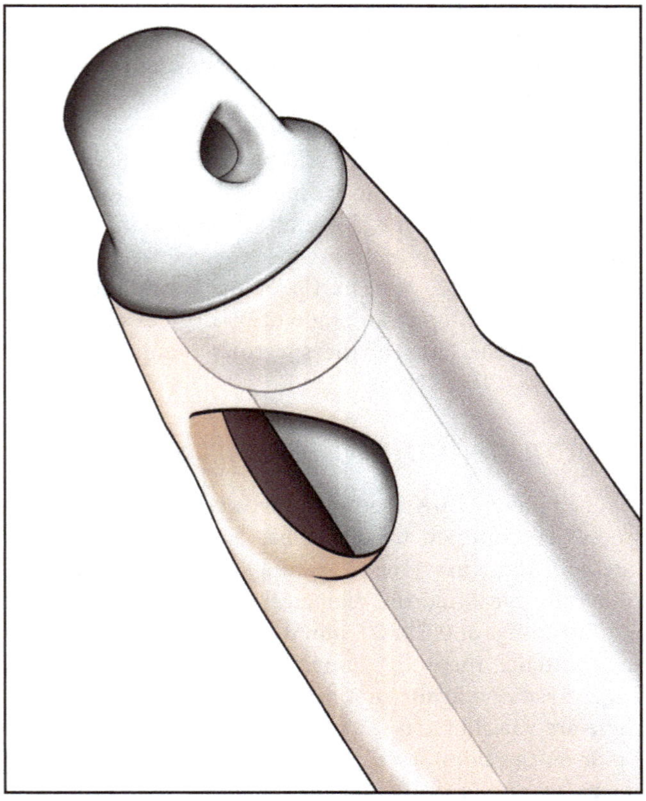

Figure 20-3. Magnification of the polycarbonate tip of the handpiece Intrepid.

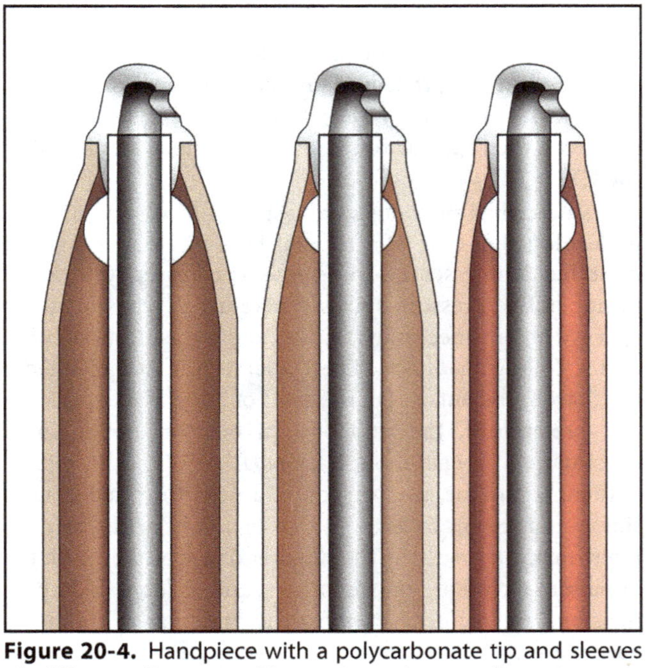

Figure 20-4. Handpiece with a polycarbonate tip and sleeves of different diameters. The various sleeves allow the one-channel handpiece to adapt to the different incision diameters of between 2.2 and 2.75 mm.

There are also a number of aspiration cannulas; however, the diameter of the opening is always 0.35 mm. The aspiration cannula is also available with a sanded tip that can be used to scratch the posterior capsule to remove small fragments that are adhered to the surface. It is important to remember that the action of the I/A handpieces must be matched; that is, they must supply the same amount of

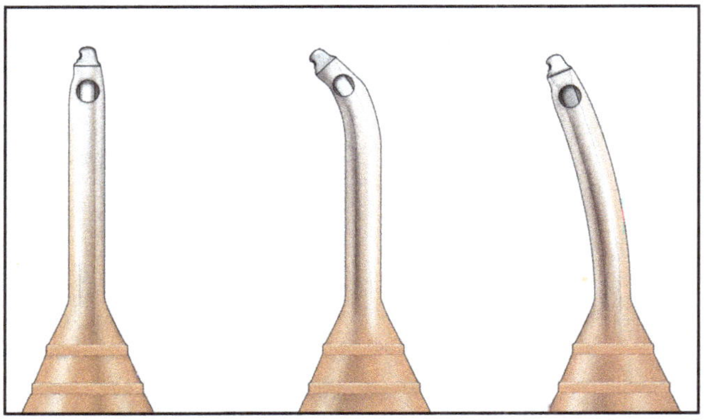

Figure 20-5. Disposable monomanual handpiece, Intrepid model in its 3 variations: straight, curved, and at an angle of 35 degrees.

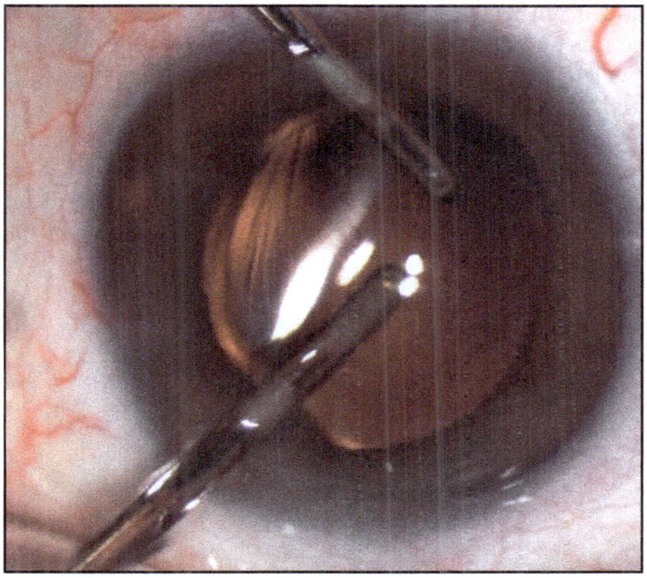

Figure 20-6. Bimanual aspiration method using an infusion handpiece and an aspiration handpiece.

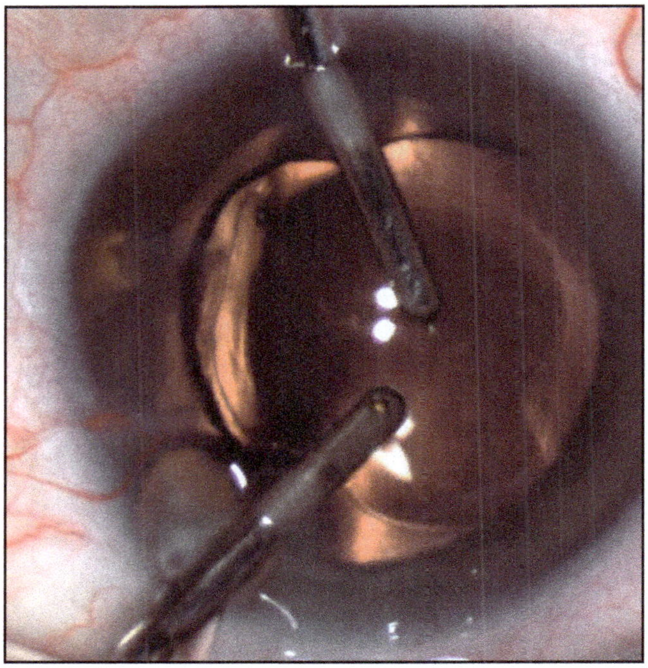

Figure 20-7. Aspiration method for removing the viscoelastic. Note that VES persists in the anterior chamber close to the irido-corneal angle.

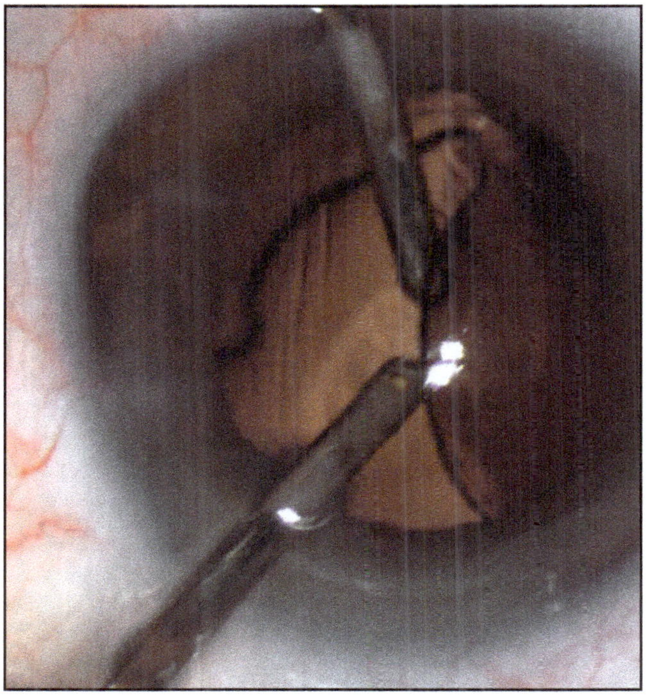

Figure 20-8. Aspiration of the VES behind the IOL using the bimanual technique. The infusion tip penetrates deeper than the aspiration tip to mobilize the VES and avoid capturing the posterior capsule.

infusion and aspiration, to avoid any variations in stability and maintenance of the anterior chamber (Figure 20-6).

Surgical Technique

Once the IOL has been carefully positioned in the bag, the surgeon proceeds with aspiration of the VES. He or she can enter the eye without penetrating too deeply, as the anterior chamber is filled with VES (Figure 20-7). For more experienced surgeons, during this step it is possible to position the coaxial device or the 2 I/A cannulas inside the eye, behind the IOL, taking care to slightly luxate the optic of the IOL upward, passing approximately 90 degrees from the haptic junction points (Figure 20-8). In order to avoid aspirating the posterior capsule, the coaxial I/A, is positioned with the aspiration tip facing upward, ensuring that the lateral fluid flow pushes the capsule backward (see Figure 20-1). On the other hand, with 2 cannulas, the infusion handpiece will be positioned in a slightly inferior position. This maneuver is not recommended for learning or less experienced surgeons; however, it allows total removal of VES from behind the lens. Alternately, the surgeon can enter the anterior chamber above the IOL and begin aspiration. When the upper portion has been completely cleaned, the VES can be removed from behind the lens by exerting mild pressure on the edges of the IOL, and this facilitates anterior passage of the VES. Here, high aspiration can be set on the phacoemulsification machine, between 450 and 550 mm Hg with the bottle of BSS at 80 to 100. The flow rate should be set at values not greater than 27 to 28 cm^3/min, to avoid sudden shallowing of the anterior chamber.

Suggested Readings

Buratto L. Zanini M, Savini G. Irrigation/aspiration. In: Buratto L, Werner L, Zanini M, Apple D, eds. *Phacoemulsification Prinicples and Techniques*. Thorofare, NJ: SLACK Incorporated; 2003:159-172.

Buratto L, et al. *Chirurgia della cataratta*. Vol 1, 2, 3. Fogliazza; 1998.

21

Closure of the Incision

Lucio Buratto, MD; Stephen F. Brint, MD, FACS; and Domenico Boccuzzi, MD, PhD

There are a number of techniques for creating the primary incision into the anterior chamber with cataract surgery. The most modern and most used is in clear cornea.

When this has been created correctly and is of appropriate size, the incision in clear cornea allows the creation of a self-sealing incision (Figures 21-1 through 21-3). At the end of the procedure, the surgeon uses a hydrodissection cannula (27 gauge) and a disposable syringe with balanced salt solution (BSS) to inject fluid into the corneal stroma at the sides of the tunnel, producing corneal edema that closes the incision (Figures 21-4 through 21-6).

Once the corneal stroma of the tunnel and the side-port incision have been hydrated, the surgeon should inject BSS into the anterior chamber to raise the intraocular pressure (IOP) slightly, while always ensuring that the pressure is not excessive. The pressure can be checked simply by compressing the eye with the tip of the hydrodissection cannula (Figure 21-7) or with a Merocel sponge tip to ensure the eye is not excessively hard and distended. It is recommended the patient be asked whether he or she can still see the light of the microscope. If not, it means that the pressure is excessively high and the central retinal vessels are being compressed. In this maneuver, special attention must be paid to severely myopic patients with extremely large eyes or staphylomas. Under these circumstances, the surgeon will never be convinced he or she has achieved the right pressure, due to the increased dimensions of the eye.

Once this has been completed, in addition to checking correct closure of the anterior chamber, it is advisable to check that the incisions are closed by exerting moderate pressure close to the opening with a dry sponge tip (Figure 21-8). If the surgeon sees liquid escaping from the anterior chamber (the sponge tip will become wet), it means that the tunnel is not sufficiently sealed and is unlikely to have good closure. The surgeon must hydrate the edges further or add a suture. It is extremely important that all of the incisions at the end of surgery are perfectly closed; in addition to ensuring good postoperative results, it will avoid the consequent drop in eye pressure that facilitates intraocular penetration of contaminated material.

If the incision is not self-sealing for whatever reason—incorrect creation of the tunnel, excessive stress of the tunnel during surgery, the need to enlarge the tunnel, or because of the deliberate modification of the radius of curvature of the specific meridian—the surgeon will have to add 1 or more 10/0 nylon sutures (Figures 21-9 through 21-11).

For tunnels of up to 3.2 mm, a single radial suture is sufficient; this should be positioned by inserting the tip of the needle into the central point of the incision, at approximately 1.5 mm toward the center of the cornea; with a single pass of the needle holder, the needle passes approximately 1.5 to 2 mm below the second corneal edge.

If the incision is larger, and a single suture is not sufficient to close the tunnel, the incision should be split into 3 or 4 parts depending on its length and sutured at these points. The sutures must be radial, meaning that they connect an imaginary line between the corneal vertex and the outer edges. A continuous suture, on the other hand, differs from individual sutures; it has a "∞" shape (the symbol for infinity) starting from the left edge and proceeding to the right. The nylon suture is created by crossing over and creating a perfect "8" shape.

Buratto L, Brint SF, Boccuzzi D.
Cataract Surgery and Intraocular Lenses (pp 167-170).

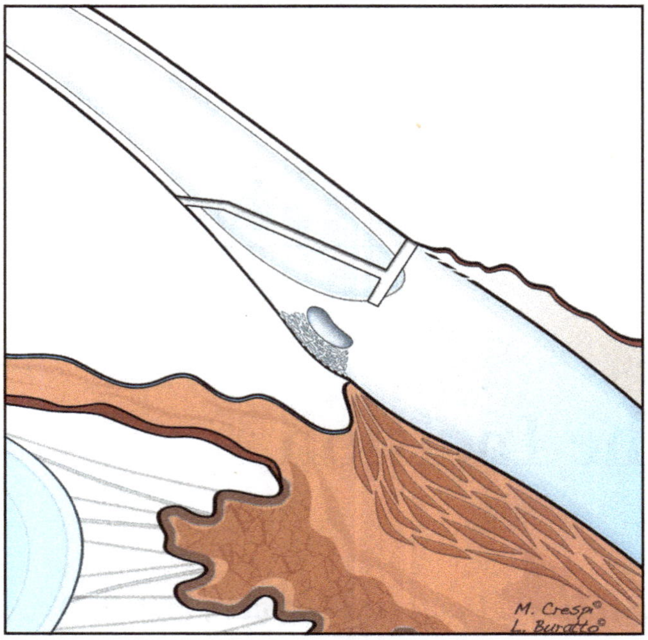

Figure 21-1. Incision in clear cornea on 3 planes with a deep precut.

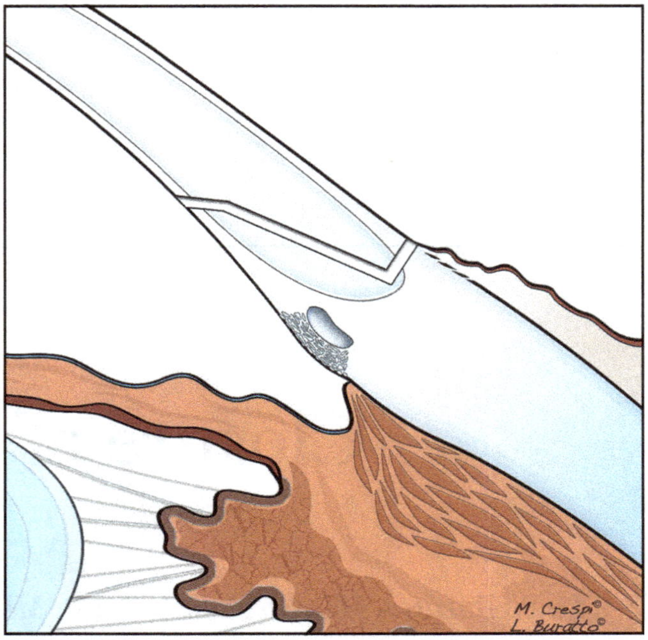

Figure 21-2. Incision in clear corneal on 3 planes with a superficial precut.

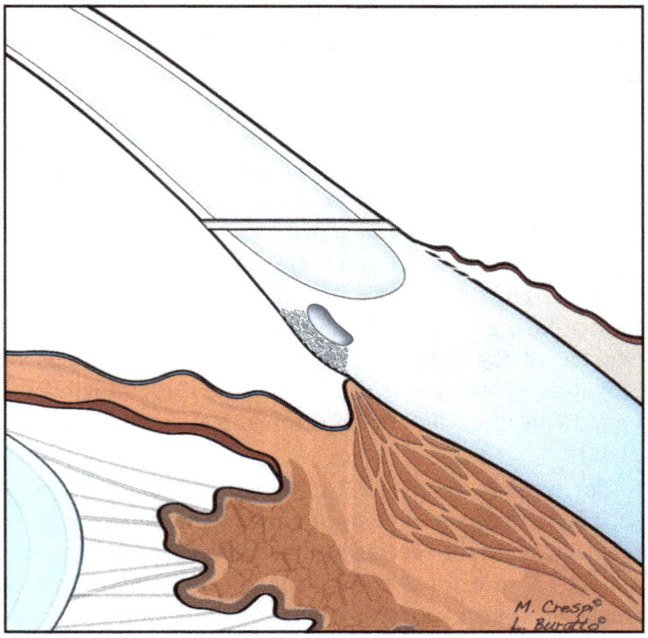

Figure 21-3. Incision in clear cornea with no precut.

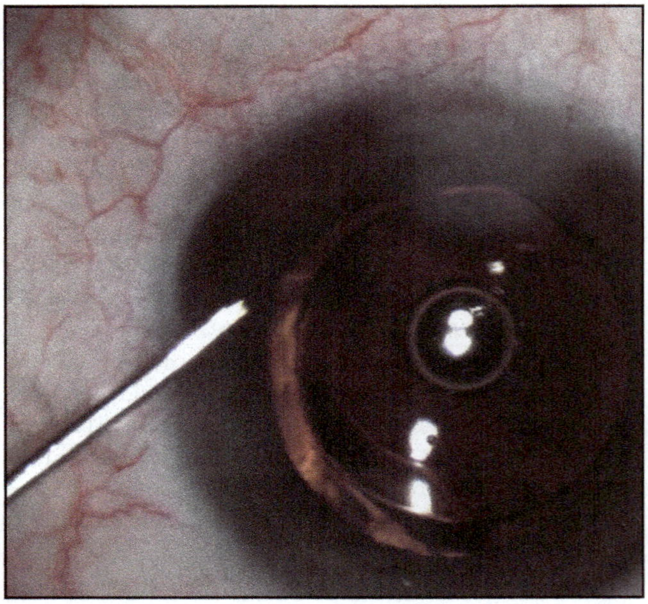

Figure 21-4. Hydration and closure of the main entrance; using a 27-gauge cannula to inject BSS into the corneal stroma of the edges of the main incision. Hydration of the stroma leads to whitening of the cornea.

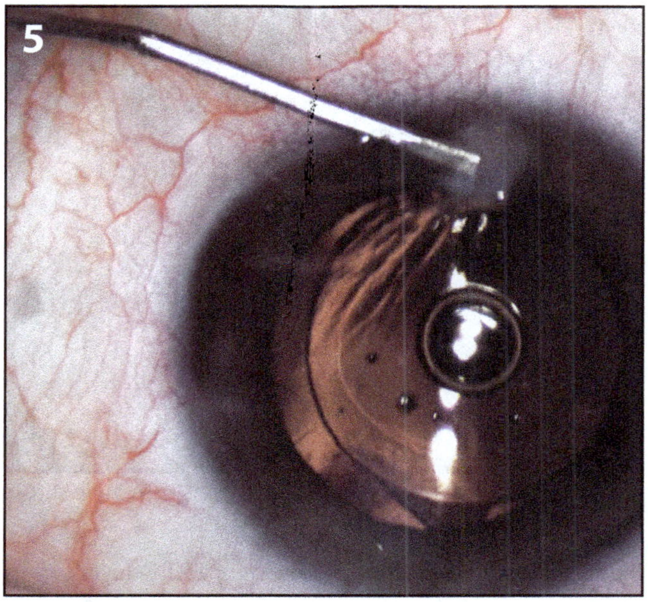

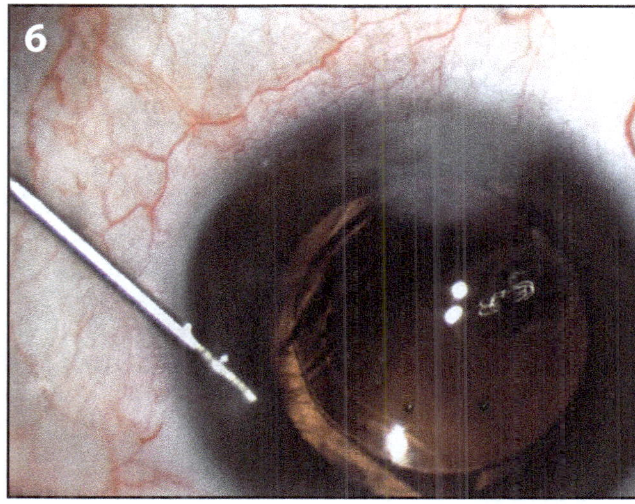

Figures 21-5 and 21-6. The side-port incision is closed by injecting BSS into the corneal stroma with a 27-gauge cannula. Hydration of the cornea will close the incisions.

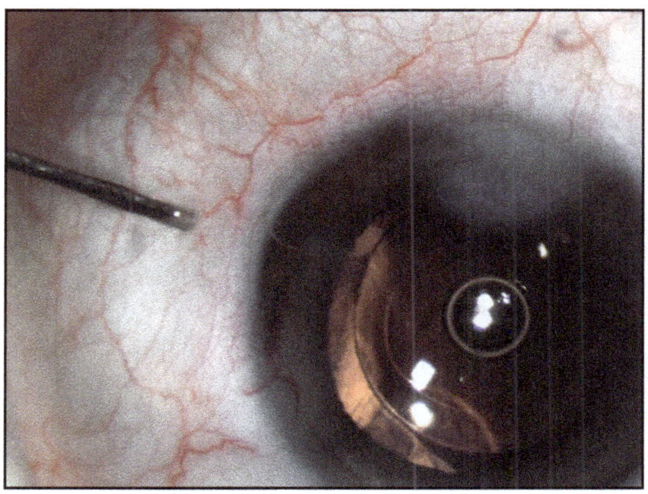

Figure 21-7. Examination of the ocular tone once the anterior chamber has been filled with BSS. This can be checked by pressing the eye with the tip of the cannula or a Merocel sponge tip.

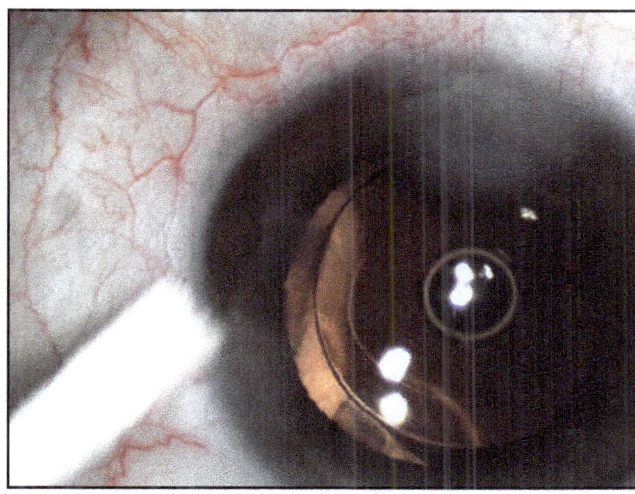

Figure 21-8. The surgeon must check the perfect closure of the incisions once the corneal incisions have been hydrated; he or she can do this by gently compressing the eye close to the incision with a dry Merocel tip.

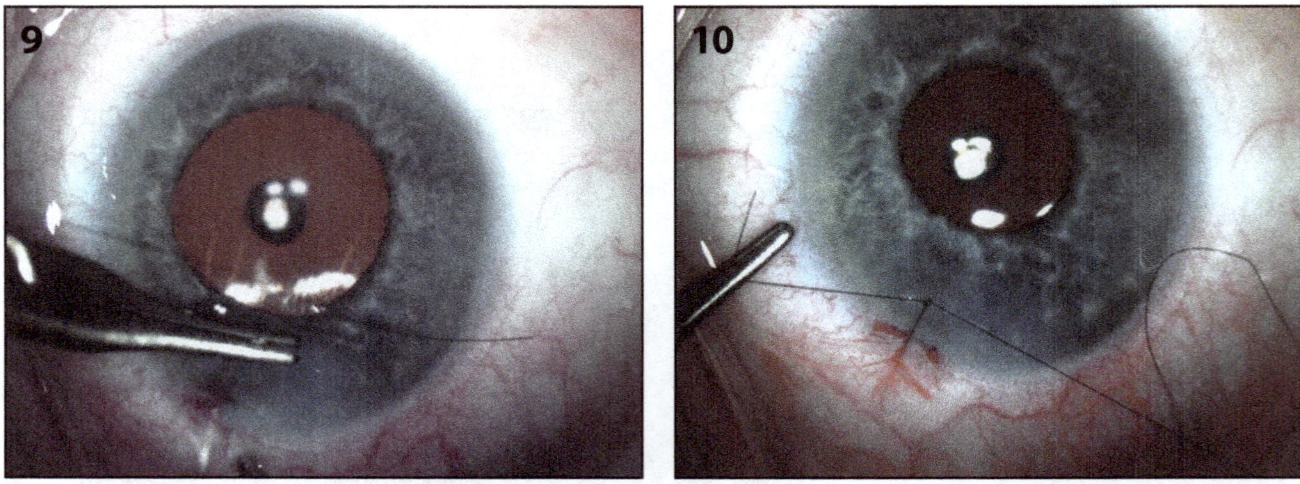

Figures 21-9 and 21-10. In the event the incision is not sealed perfectly, the surgeon should close the incision with a single suture or more of 10/0 nylon.

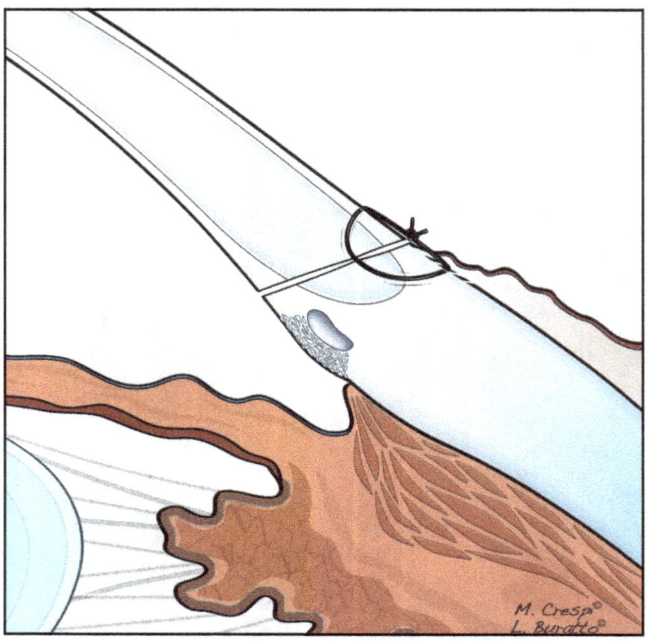

Figure 21-11. Diagram showing the correct positioning of the intrastromal corneal suture.

The continuous suture differs from individual sutures in that distribution of force is equal over the cornea. It will be astigmatically neutral. It is essential that the sutures are tightened with the correct amount of tension, that they correctly close the incision but do not induce astigmatism.

Suggested Reading

Buratto L, Zanini M, Savini G. Sutures. In: Buratto L, Werner L, Zanini M, Apple D, eds. *Phacoemulsification Prinicples and Techniques*. Thorofare, NJ: SLACK Incorporated; 2003:203-206.

22

Drugs and Fluids for Intraocular Use

Lucio Buratto, MD; Stephen F. Brint, MD, FACS; and Domenico Boccuzzi, MD, PhD

A number of fluids and substances for intraocular injection are used in modern cataract surgery: viscoelastic substance (VES), drugs, and irrigating solutions. These maintain the volume of the anterior chamber constant and also cool the phaco tip. The surgeon must fully understand the importance and properties of the substances he or she introduces into the eye to avoid damaging the endothelial cells or the sudden appearance of toxic anterior segment syndrome.

Irrigation Fluids

In the past, lactated Ringer was used as an irrigating solution; presently, balanced salt solution (BSS) and BSS Plus are most commonly used.

BSS, as its name would suggest, is a balanced sterile saline solution containing sodium chloride, calcium chloride, magnesium chloride, sodium acetate, and sodium citrate. This solution does not leave any residue, is isotonic with the ocular tissues, and contains ions essential for normal cell metabolism.

BSS Plus has a different concentration of the various ions with osmolarity that is slightly higher (305 mOsm/L as opposed to the 298 mOsm/L of BSS); the most important difference between the 2 solutions is the presence of glutathione, sodium bicarbonate, and glucose in BSS Plus (Table 22-1).

Glutathione (GSH and GSSG) is one of the body's natural antioxidants; it maintains the junctional complexes of the corneal endothelial cells and can preserve the integrity of the blood–ocular barrier. The absence of endocellular glutathione can lead to cellular apoptosis.[1-3]

Sodium bicarbonate is a natural physiological buffer in the human body. It is the principal molecule in the formation of aqueous humor and is essential for maintaining the blood–eye barrier. It is also essential for good function of the retina.[4,5]

Glucose is the main source of cell energy; it contributes to maintaining corneal transparency and is essential for correct retinal function.

Table 22-1 compares the compositions of the various solutions. Despite the fact that BSS Plus is unquestionably an innovative formulation and a more complete solution compared to normal BSS, studies have shown that when used in uncomplicated cataracts, there is no significant difference in the efficacy between the 2 solutions, in terms of the ocular response to surgery However, BSS Plus is preferable in eyes in which the cornea is already compromised (eg, Fuchs' dystrophy or in complicated cataracts). This is because with standard surgery, during an uncomplicated procedure, VES will adequately protect the corneal endothelium from the effects of fluid turbulence, ultrasound, and particles floating in the anterior chamber.

However, when the surgeon expects surgery to be prolonged, or when he or she recognizes reduced endothelial vitality, he or she should use enriched solutions such as BSS Plus to minimize surgical stress.

Some in vivo studies have demonstrated that postoperative corneal thickness and endothelial cell counts do not depend on the length of surgery or on the volume of irrigating substance selected, but on the chemical composition of the solution itself.

Cell density measured was unchanged both short term (15 to 30 minutes) and middle term (1 to 2 hours) following irrigation with BSS and BSS Plus.

Buratto L, Brint SF, Boccuzzi D.
Cataract Surgery and Intraocular Lenses (pp 171-173).

TABLE 22-1

Composition of Human Aqueous Humor, BSS Plus, BSS, S-MA2, and Hartmann's Lactated Ringer

INGREDIENT	HUMAN AQUEOUS HUMOR	BSS PLUS	BSS	S-MA2	HARTMANN'S LACTATED RINGER
Sodium	162.9	160.0	155.7	145.7	131
Potassium	2.2-3.9	5.0	10.1	4.8	5
Calcium	1.8	1.0	3.3	1.2	2
Magnesium	1.1	1.0	1.5	-	-
Chloride	131.6	130.0	128.9	120.1	111
Bicarbonate	20.15	25.0	-	25.0	-
Phosphate	0.62	3.0	-	-	-
Lactate	2.5	-	-	-	29
Glucose	2.7-3.7	5.0	-	8.3	-
Ascorbate	1.06	-	-	-	-
Glutathione	0.0019	0.3	-	-	-
Citrate	-	-	5.8	3.4	-
Acetate	-	-	28.6	4.4	-
pH	7.38	7.4	7.6	7.3	6.4
Osmolality (mOsm)	304	305	298	290	258

Compared to BSS Plus, BSS causes a significant increase in the coefficient of variation of the cell area (polymegathism) and a reduction in the percentage of hexagonal cells (pleomorphism). These changes are much more obvious following prolonged irrigation.

The corneal thickness, on the other hand, increases quite significantly 1 hour from irrigation with BSS compared to when BSS Plus is used.[6-10]

The temperature of the irrigation solutions (BSS, BSS Plus, or lactated Ringer) must be constant at 23°C—the same temperature as the operating room.[11] According to some authors, intraocular irrigation liquids used at a temperature of 10°C can reduce immediate postoperative inflammation.[12]

However, other studies indicate that the anti-inflammatory effect of cooled solutions only has a short-term action, and there is no long-term difference in the development of ocular inflammation when fluids at room temperature are used as opposed to solutions at a lower temperature.[13]

Drugs Contained in the Irrigation Fluids

It is extremely important that any drug added to the irrigation solution or any of the fluids to be injected into the anterior chamber (eg, for hydrodissection, closure of the incisions, filling the eye) are preservative free. The additive benzalkonium chloride is extremely toxic. The drugs must also be free from stabilizing agents such as bisulfite and metabisulfite. It should also be remembered that 6.5 is the minimum pH tolerated by the corneal endothelium.

There are a number of substances that can be injected into the anterior chamber—anesthetic agents, antibiotics, and epinephrine. Epinephrine is used to improve and maintain pupil dilation when the surgery induces miosis or under other surgical conditions such as intraoperative floppy iris syndrome with tamsulosin or other alpha antagonists.

Anesthetics for the Anterior Chamber

When topical anesthesia is used in cataract surgery using an incision in clear cornea, the surgeon may find it useful to inject an anesthetic agent into the anterior chamber to improve the analgesic effect. Preservative-free 4% lidocaine is the most commonly used anesthetic agent; it should be diluted 1:3 with BSS. This will produce a 1% lidocaine solution with a pH of 7 that is ideal for the corneal endothelium. The solution is called Shugarcaine because it was described by Joel K. Shugar.

In order to avoid intraoperative floppy iris syndrome in patients using tamsulosin or other alpha-antagonists, studies have shown the efficacy of epi-Shugarcaine—a solution consisting of 9 mL of BSS, 3 mL of preservative-free 4% lidocaine, and 4 mL of bisulfite-free epinephrine (1:1000 dilution). Epinephrine can antagonize the alpha-antagonist effect of tamsulosin and can compete with the α1c receptors targeted by the drug itself; mydriasis will therefore be improved.[14,15]

According to Dr. Shugar, this formulation has greater efficacy when it is injected into the eye prior to using VES, and when tropicamide has been used to dilate the patient.

Intracameral Antibiotics

In an article published in 2006,[16,17] the European Society of Cataract & Refractive Surgeons (ESCRS) reported the results of a multicenter, prospective, randomized study on almost 16,000 patients. The study showed that the intracameral use of cefuroxime at the end of the cataract procedure significantly reduced the incidence of postoperative endophthalmitis. The dosage of cefuroxime was 1 mg in 0.1 mL of saline solution, to be injected at the end of surgery. The objective of this study was not to demonstrate the efficacy of cefuroxime with respect to other antibiotics or with respect to other preventative practices—such as the use of povidone iodine pre- and postoperative, or with respect to postoperative topical antibiotic therapies. It simply attempted to demonstrate the importance and efficacy of intracameral antibiotics at the end of the surgical procedure in the prevention of endophthalmitis.

In a study conducted by ESCRS, researchers observed a 5-fold reduction in the number of endophthalmitis as opposed to 0.3% of patients not injected with cefuroxime.

Other antibiotics are also suitable for the prevention of postoperative infections, for example, gatifloxacin and moxifloxacin (fourth-generation fluoroquinolones), cephalosporins (cefuroxime[18] and cefazolin[19]), and vancomycin (glycopeptide antibiotics).

References

1. Araie M, Shirasawa E, Hikita M. Effect of oxidized glutathione on the barrier function of the corneal endothelium. *Invest Ophthalomol Vis Sci.* 1988;29:1884-1887.
2. Araie M, Shirasawa E, Ohashi T. Intraocular irrigating solutions and permeability of the blood-aqueous barrier. *Arch Ophthalmol.* 1990;108:882-885.
3. Ghibelli L, Fanelli C, Rotilio G, et al. Rescue of cells from apoptosis by inhibition of active GSH extrusion. *FASEB J.* 1998;12:479-486.
4. Winkler BS, Simson V, Benner J. Importance of bicarbonate in retinal function. *Invest Ophthalmol Vis Sci.* 1977;16:766-768.
5. Winkler BS. Comparison of intraocular solutions on glycolysis and levels of ATP and glutathione in the retina. *J Cataract Refract Surg.* 1988;14:633-637.
6. Matsuda M, Kinoshita S, Ohashi Y, et al. Comparison of the effects of intraocular irrigating solutions on the corneal endothelium in intraocular lens implantation. *Br J Ophthalmol.* 1991;75:476-479.
7. Araie M, Shirasawa E, Hikita M. Effect of oxidized glutathione on the barrier function of the corneal endothelium. *Invest Ophthalmol Vis Sci.* 1988;29:1884-1887.
8. Whikehart DR, Edelhauser HF. Glutathione in rabbit corneal endothelia: the effects of selected perfusion fluids. *Invest Ophthalmol Vis Sci.* 1978;17:455-464.
9. Matsuda M, Tano Y, Edelhauser HF. Comparison of intraocular irrigating solutions used for pars plana vitrectomy and prevention of endothelial cell loss. *Jpn J Ophthalmol.* 1984;28:230-238.
10. Glasser DB, Matsuda M, Ellis JG, Edelhauser HF. Effects of intraocular irrigating solutions on the corneal endothelium after in vivo anterior chamber irrigation. *Am J Ophthalmol.* 1985;99(3):321-328.
11. Vasavada V, Vasavada Vaishali, Dixit NV, Raj SM, Vasavada AR. Comparison between Ringer's lactate and balanced salt solution on postoperative outcomes after phacoemulsification: a randomized clinical trial. *Indian J Ophthalmol.* 2009;57(3):191-195.
12. Findl O, Amon M, Kruger A, Petternel V, Schauersberger J. Effect of cooled intraocular irrigating solution on the blood-aqueous barrier after cataract surgery. *J Cataract Refract Surg.* 1999;25:566-568.
13. Praveen MR, Vasavada AR, Shah R, Vasavada VA. Effect of room temperature and cooled intraocular irrigating solution on the cornea and anterior segment inflammation after phacoemulsification: a randomized clinical trial. *Eye (Lond).* 2009;23(5):1158-1163. Epub 2008 Jun 27.
14. Myers WG, Shugar JK. Optimizing the intracameral dilation regimen for cataract surgery: prospective randomized comparison of 2 solutions. *J Cataract Refract Surg.* 2009;35(2):273-276.
15. Schulze R Jr. Epi-Shugarcaine with plain balanced salt solution for prophylaxis of intraoperative floppy-iris syndrome. *J Cataract Refract Surg.* 2010;36(3):523.
16. Seal DV, Barry P, Gettinby G, et al. ESCRS study of prophylaxis of postoperative endophthalmitis after cataract surgery: case for a european multicenter study. ESCRS Endophthalmitis Study Group. *J Cataract Refract Surg.* 2006;32(3):396-406.
17. Barry P, Gardner S, Seal D, et al. Clinical observations associated with proven and unproven cases in the ESCRS study of prophylaxis of postoperative endophthalmitis after cataract surgery. ESCRS Endophthalmitis Study Group. *J Cataract Refract Surg.* 2009;35(9):1523-1531, 1531.e1.
18. Montan PG, Wejde G, Koranyi G, Rylander M. Prophylactic intracameral cefuroxime. Efficacy in preventing endophthalmitis after cataract surgery. *J Cataract Refract Surg.* 2002;28(6):977-981.
19. Romero-Aroca P, Méndez-Marin I, Salvat-Serra M, Fernández-Ballart J, Almena-Garcia M, Reyes-Torres J. Results at seven years after the use of intracamerular cefazolin as an endophthalmitis prophylaxis in cataract surgery. *BMC Ophthalmol.* 2012;12:2.

Suggested Reading

Hejny C, Edelhauser HF. Surgical pharmacology: intraocular solutions and drugs for cataract surgery. In: Buratto L, Werner L, Zanini M, Apple D, eds. *Phacoemulsification Prinicples and Techniques.* Thorofare, NJ: SLACK Incorporated; 2003:219-246.

Section II

23

Latest Generation Multifocal Intraocular Lenses and Emerging Accommodative Intraocular Lenses

Jorge L. Alió, MD, PhD, FEBO; Felipe Soria, MD; and Ghassan Zein, MD, PhD, FRCS (Ophth) UK

Multifocal intraocular lenses (IOLs)[1-3] were developed with the intention to solve the visual limitation at near and intermediate distances that occur with monofocal IOLs. A multifocal IOL is a lens that, due to its optical design, is capable of creating different foci by dispersing the incoming light to the eye; this may be achieved through different optical principles, the main ones being the so-called refractive and diffractive ones.

Multifocal IOLs and other presbyopic IOLs exist to compensate 2 aging natural processes: phakic presbyopia and presbyopic cataract. They are considered today as premium IOLs, and aim to increase the visual functional performance of the pseudophakic patient, to allow the eye to be focused at all distances including intermediate and near, hence improving the quality of life.

If we could strive for perfection in achieving the perfect multifocal IOL, the following optical principles should be considered:

- Focus dominant for far vision: Our brain's dominant need is for distance vision; it also decreases the effect of focus overlapping that is typical of multifocal optical design and reduces glare and haloes.
- Adequate disparity between near and far foci: In order to produce intermediate vision, some multifocal IOLs produce overlapping of foci, creating haloes and glare. When less than 3.00 D of near vision add exists, the incidence of haloes increases due to superposition of the different foci.
- Aspheric design: In order to compensate for corneal spherical aberration and to improve the quality of the image.
- Available toric model: If an eye is left with more than 1.00 D of astigmatism, laser touch-up is required; 70% of the population has more than 1.00 D of cylinder.
- Pupil-independent mechanism: Pupil size after surgery is unpredictable, so increasing the depth of focus should not depend on pupil size.
- Good optical performance: Once an IOL is implanted, intraocular conditions may affect its optical performance and this can decrease by more than 50% from what has been demonstrated on the optical bench.
- Good capsular stability: Stability should be guaranteed by the design of the IOL and the quality of its biomaterial. Capsule contraction is an important issue that can cause tilt, decentration, or displacement of the IOL.
- Low rate of posterior capsular opacification (PCO): Lens design and biomaterial should aim to keep the posterior capsular transparent. Neodymium:yttrium-aluminum-garnet (Nd:YAG) capsulotomy may be followed by significant complications.
- Implantable through a sub-2-mm incision: With this kind of incision, there is no change of preoperative astigmatism or aberrometric profile. Microincision cataract surgery (MICS) is a concept that helps the surgeon to control this variable for optimal performance of the IOL.[4-12]
- Evidence of good visual outcomes for far, intermediate, and near vision that can be adapted to the lifestyle of the patient: The main goal should be the provision of excellent quantity and quality of vision for all distances. Today, intermediate vision is increasingly necessary.

Buratto L, Brint SF, Boccuzzi D.
Cataract Surgery and Intraocular Lenses (pp 177-188).

On the other hand, in cataract surgery, capsulorrhexis, a critical and essential step, especially when implanting "premium lenses," requires an exact diameter and centration to achieve optimum effect on the stability of the lens, and thus contribute to the success and performance of these lenses with accommodative, multifocal, and toric characteristics. In the era of femtosecond laser technology, one can achieve an accurate and predictable size, shape, and centration,[13] and also a more resistant capsulorrhexis, giving stronger support during lens removal and IOL implantation.[14-16]

Femtosecond laser-assisted cataract surgery followed by MICS concept and associated with a premium IOL achieves the best of both worlds.

If we could accomplish a perfect optical design in a multifocal IOL followed by a perfect surgery, this is not enough to guarantee success. The beginning and the success fall in correct patient selection. Several multifocal IOLs are currently available and we are presenting the technologies available so that the surgeon can choose the best IOL for his or her patient. We repeat—the perfect multifocal IOL does not exist.

Criteria for Multifocal Intraocular Lens Implantation

The following considerations should be analyzed in order to select a good candidate and a satisified patient:

A. Major criteria

1. Normal, good visual potential
2. Good contrast sensitivity potential
3. Appropriate age: Advanced senility is not successful for multifocal IOLs
4. Normal quality of the cornea (not in significantly aberrated corneas)
5. Exclude comorbidities (amblyopia, glaucoma, and macular disease)
6. Educate and manage patient expectations: Assess individual lifestyle, motivation, or determination to function without glasses

B. Minor criteria

1. Personality type: Obsessive and perfectionist patients are not good candidates (eg, patients who cannot afford having a floater)
2. Profession: Multifocal IOLs have the disadvantage of creating haloes, glare, and reduction of contrast sensitivity, so they are not recommended in patients who have a profession related to night activitites (eg, pilots, drivers)

Multifocal Intraocular Lenses

A multifocal IOL is a lens that is capable, due to its optical design, of creating different foci by dispersing incoming light to the eye. Principally, there have been 2 main multifocal IOL designs: refractive and diffractive.

Refractive MFIOLs consist of a series of concentric rotational radially symmetric zones with differing focal lengths. Zones may be spherical or aspheric, with spherical zones providing one focal length and aspheric zones providing multiple focal lengths. Hence, IOLs with spherical zones produce alternating multifocality between zones, whereas IOLs with aspheric zones produce a uniform distribution of multifocality over the IOL surface.[15,16] There is a new generation of refractive lenses with rotational assymetryical profiles with a sector of the near vision VDD.

Diffractive MFIOLs function via the principle of a phase zone plate with gratings along the IOL surface. Each grating diffracts light away from the primary (distance) focus toward a secondary (near) focus. The grating width decreases as the distance from the center of the IOL increases, which provides greater angles of diffraction. The relative distribution of light energy and the focal point locations can be adjusted by varying the size and pattern of the rings.[17]

Presbyopic IOLs existing today include the following:

Multifocal IOLs

- Refractive IOLs
  - Rotational symmetrical
    - ReZoom
    - Rayners
  - Rotational asymmetrical (Sectorial)
    - Mplus+3, +1.5
- Diffractive IOLs: AcrySof IQ ReSTOR (+4, +3, +2.5), Acri.LISA (Carl Zeiss Meditec AG), Tecnis (Abbott Medical Optics [AMO]), SeeLens

Inside the capsular bag accommodative IOLs

- Mechanical single optic: Crystalens HD (Bausch + Lomb)
- Mechanical double optic: Synchrony (AMO)

Sulcus-placed accommodative IOLs

- AkkoLens
- NuLens

AcrySof Restor SN6AD3 , SN6AD1 (Alcon Laboratories)

These 3 IOLs have the same multifocal, symmetric, biconvex, apodized, difractive optic.

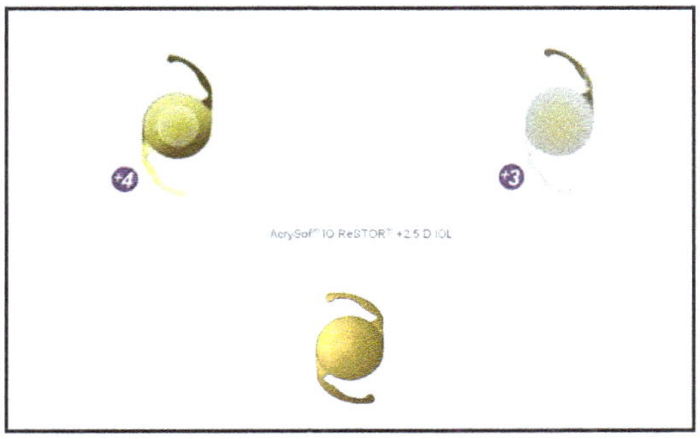

Technical Specifications[18]

Multifocal optic	Proprietary symmetric biconvex apodized diffractive optic
Compensation for positive corneal spherical aberration	Aspheric optic
Add power	+3.0 D
Add power at spectacle plane	+2.5 D
Number of steps	9
Diopter range	+6.0 to +34.0 D
Optic diameter	6.0 mm
Overall length	13.0 mm
IOL design	Single-piece
Haptic design	Stableforce modified-L
Optic/haptic material	Hydrophobic acrylic
Suggested A-constant*	118.9
Haptic angulation	0 degrees
Filtration	UV and high-energy blue light

The central optic has a 3.5 mm apodized diffractive structure, and centrifugally, there is a decrease in the step heights from 1.3 to 0.2 µm. In the outer part of the lens, a refractive zone is present.

The main differences between both the types of IOLs are as follows:

- An add power of +4 D for the SN6AD3 and –3 D for the SN6AD1.
- The explanation of this is found in the characteristics of the optical designs where 12 refractive rings compose the +4 D and 9 refractive rings compose the +3 D IOL. The space between 9 rings is greater, resulting in the modification of the power.
- Spectacle plane of 3.2 D add for the SN6AD3 and 2.4 D for the SN6AD1.

Clinical Studies

Evaluating Vision

The ReSTOR +3.00 D add has performed better than the ReSTOR +4.00 D add at all intermediate distances studied, with similar performance for distance and near visual acuity, contrast sensitivity, and quality of life.[19] Uncorrected near visual acuity (UNVA) and distance-corrected near visual acuity (DCNVA) is better with the Restor SN6AD3, than with the Lentis Mplus LS-312 IOL, whereas intermediate visual acuity is better with the Lentis Mplus LS-312 IOL.[20]

Evaluating Reading Performance

ReSTOR SN6AD3 has significantly better uncorrected reading acuity than monofocals and refractive multifocal IOLs.[21]

The AcrySof ReSTOR SN6AD3 and Acri.LISA 366D had significantly better uncorrected reading acuity than theAcriSmart 48S and ReZoom at 1 and 6 months postoperatively ($P < .01$).[21]

Same results were obtained by Gil et al.[22]

Evaluating Photic Phenomena

Patients with ReSTOR SN6AD3 can perform most daily tasks at near and intermediate distances, with more night-driving limitation than with a full diffractive IOL.[23]

Contrast sensitivity is better with the ReSTOR SN6AD1 at 12 cycles per degree (cpd) and 18 cpd under photopic conditions than with the Lentis Mplus LS-312. No significant differences were found under mesopic conditions.[24] The ReSTOR +3.00 D and the ReSTOR +4.00 D are performed similarly with respect to contrast sensitivity, quality of life, and spectacle independence rates.[25]

Conclusion

Patients implanted with a multifocal IOL with lower addition (ReSTOR +3.00 D) had better performance at intermediate distances compared with the ReSTOR +4.00 D add IOL with similar performance for distance and near visual acuity, contrast sensitivity, and quality of life. Still, intermediate vision is not as good as distance and near. Multifocal IOLs with a diffractive component provided a comparable reading performance that was significantly better than the one obtained with refractive multifocal and monofocal IOLs. Photopic contrast sensitivity is better with the ReSTOR +3.00 D than with the multifocal Lentis Mplus LS-312 at high spatial frequencies and comparable between both at low frequencies and under mesopic conditions.

AcrySof ReSTOR +2.5 D IOL was launched at the annual meeting of the European Society of Cataract and Refractive Surgeons (ESCRS) in Milan, Italy, in 2012. According to company literature, this multifocal IOL received the Conformité Europėene (CE) Mark approval in February 2012, and is designed for patients with distance-dominant lifestyles who desire the opportunity for decreased dependence on spectacles. Currently, we are evaluating the efficacy of this new multifocal IOL in our center.

AT LISA 809M (Formerly Known as Acri.LISA 366D) (Carl Zeiss Meditec AG)

The AT LISA 809M is an aspheric bifocal biconvex refractive-diffractive IOL.

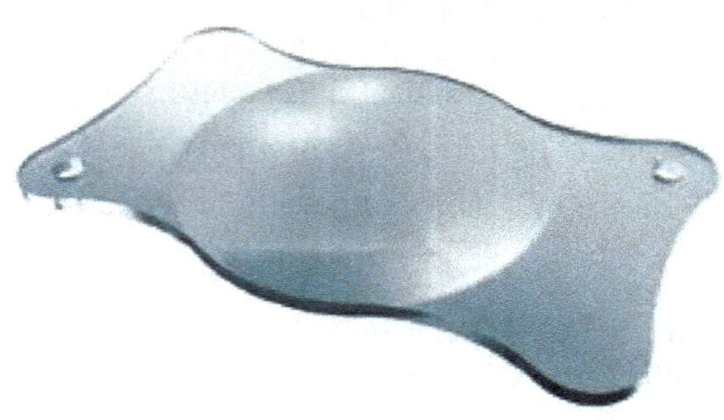

Technical Specifications[26]

Model name (type)	
Dimensions	Optic diameter 6 mm, total diameter 11 mm
Optic material	Hydrophylic acrylic (25%) with hydrophobic surface
Optic design	Multifocal (diffractive +3.75 D at the IOL plane), aspheric (abberation correcting)
Haptic material, design, angulation	Single-piece IOL, no angulation
Available powers	+10 to +30 D by 0.5 D (0 to +9.5 D by 0.5 D upon request)
Suggested A-constant	117.8
Features	Multifocal, aspheric MICS IOL. Light distributed asymmetrically between distance (65%) and near focus (35%). SMP technology (lens surface without sharp angles) ideal for optical imaging quality with reduced light scattering. Patients' satisfaction rate is very high as they achieve excellent near and distance vision, as well as very good intermediate vision.
Availability	Available outside the US only

Clinical Studies

Evaluating Vision

Acri.LISA 366D has significantly better uncorrected reading acuity than monofocal and refractive multifocal IOLs at 1 and 6 months postoperatively.[21]

Significantly better values of UNVA ($P<.01$) and DCNVA ($P<.04$) were found in Acri.LISA, comparing it with Lentis Mplus LS-312. In the defocus curve, significantly better visual acuities were present in eyes in Lentis Mplus LS-312 for intermediate vision levels of defocus ($P\leq.04$) compared with Acri.LISA.[27]

Evaluating Photic Phenomena

Contrast sensitivity improves significantly at all spatial frequencies under photopic and scotopic conditions after surgery.[28] Significantly better values are observed in photopic contrast sensitivity for high spatial frequencies in Lentis Mplus LS-312 versus Acri.LISA.[27]

Evaluating Reading Performance

It provides a comparable reading performance that is significantly better than the one obtained with refractive multifocal and monofocal IOLs.[21] The quality-of-life index related to reading ability improves significantly at 3 months. Implantation of the multifocal diffractive IOL significantly improved reading performance, which had a positive effect on the patient's quality of life postoperatively.[28]

Conclusion

Acri.LISA design provides excellent distance and near visual outcomes and intraocular optical performance parameters. Multifocal IOLs with a diffractive component provided a comparable reading performance that was significantly better than the one obtained with refractive multifocal and monofocal IOLs, thus improving the quality of life. Decreased contrast sensitivity and glare and haloes are common.

ReZoom (Abbott Medical Optics)

The ReZoom is a second-generation refractive multifocal lens. The optic is composed of 5 optical zones. Odd zones 1, 3, and 5 are adjusted for far vision and even zones 2 and 4 are for near vision.

It is a pupil-dependent IOL, where the light going through a 2.0-mm pupil is distributed as follows: 83% for distant focus, and 17% for intermediate focus. In a 5.0-mm pupil, the light is distributed as 60% for distant focus, 10% for intermediate focus, and 30% for near focus.[27]

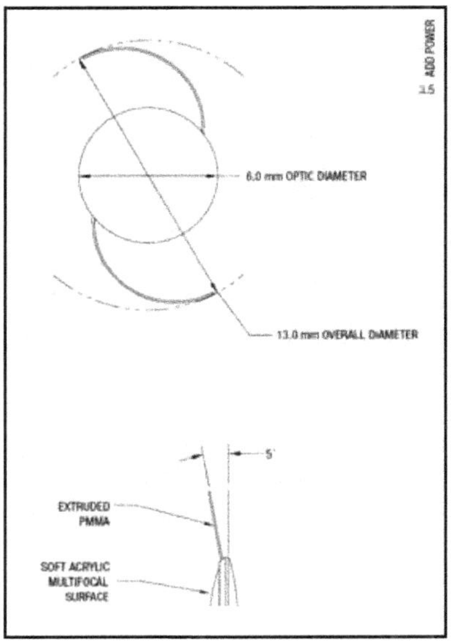

Technical Specifications[29]

Description	NXG1
Optic characteristics	
Diameter	6.0 mm
Shape	Biconvex
Material	Acrylic/UV
Manipulation holes	None
Powers	6.0 to 30.0 D 0.5-D increments
A-constant	118.4
Theoretical AC depth	5.2 mm
Surgeon factor	1.45
Haptic characteristics	
Overall length	13.0 mm
Style	Modified C
Material	60% blue core Polymethylmethacrylate monofilament
Angle	5 degrees
Compressibility	
11 mm	106 mg
10 mm	193 mg
Average weight in air	22.8 mg
Recommended folding instruments	
Unfolder Emerald Series Handpiece	EMERALDT
Unfolder Emerald Series Cartridge	EMERALDC

Clinical Studies

Evaluating Vision

There is dependence on spectacles for near tasks. Intermediate vision is spectacle independent.[30]

Distant visual performance was excellent under photopic conditions, but was reduced under mesopic levels.[31]

Mixing and matching multifocal IOLs in selected cataract patients provides an excellent visual outcome, a high level of patient satisfaction, and spectacle-free visual function. A period of neuroadaptation lasting at least 6 months is necessary to obtain better visual function results.[32]

Evaluating Reading Performance

Multifocal IOLs with a diffractive component provided a comparable reading performance that was significantly better than the one obtained with refractive multifocal and monofocal IOLs.[21]

Evaluating Photic Phenomena

Photic phenomena were present in all IOLs, albeit more frequently in ReZoom IOLs.[30]

Tecnis (Abbott Medical Optics) One-Piece ZMB00 and Three-Piece ZMA00

Each of these models is designed with a full diffractive posterior surface that makes it pupil independent and the light is distributed equally for near and distance focus retaining high quality of near vision even with pupil expansion in low-light conditions. The anterior aspheric surface corrects spherical aberration to essentially zero.[33] Full diffractive surface and +4.0 D add power correct chromatic aberration at near. The light distribution between the distance and near focus is approximately 50/50.[34] The lens blocks UV radiation but allows the passage of blue light, which is fundamental to good scotopic sensitivity.[35]

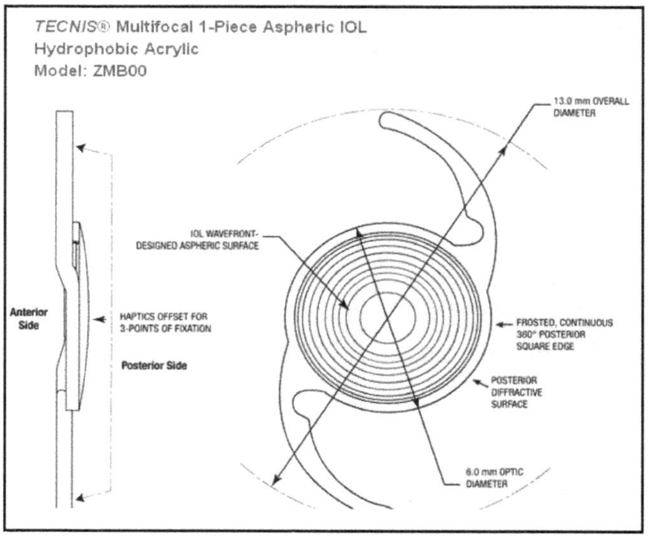

Technical Specifications[36]

Optic characteristics	
Powers	+5.0 to +34.0 D in 0.5-D increments
Diameter	6.0 mm
Optic design	Biconvex Anterior aspheric surface Posterior diffractive surface
Near add	+4.0 D
Material	UV-blocking hydrophobic acrylic
Refractive index	1.47
Edge design	ProTEC frosted, continuous 360-degree posterior square edge
A-constant*	118.8
Haptic characteristics	
Overall length	13.0 mm
Haptic design	C, offset from optic

*Based on Contact Ultrasound Biometry. Value theoretically derived for a typical 20.0 D lens. AMO recommends that surgeons personalize their A-constant based on their surgical techniques and equipment, experience with the lens model, and postoperative results.

Clinical Studies

In a study, a sample of 70 eyes were implanted with Tecnis ZMB00; 90% of the patients rated their monocular distance vision without correction as good to very good at 60 days postoperatively, and 97.1% had the same opinion of their monocular near vision at 60 days postoperatively. Also, there was a minimal perception of photic phenomena, the presence of postoperative optimized intraocular optics, and an excellent contrast sensitivity outcome.[35] The aspheric diffractive multifocal IOL Tecnis ZMB00 provides a restoration of the far and near visual function after phacoemulsification surgery for cataract removal or presbyopia correction.[34]

SeeLens MF (Hanita)

A new model of apodized diffractive IOLs has been introduced into clinical practice, with an asymmetrical light distribution—the SeeLens MF (Hanita Lenses) is an aspheric apodized diffractive multifocal IOL. This lens is a single-piece IOL with an optic diameter of 6.0 mm and an overall diameter of 13.0 mm. The incident light is distributed with 65% to distance and 35% to near for a 3-mm diameter pupil. This IOL is made from hydrophilic Acrylic HEMA/EOEMA copolymer and has a UV blocker and violet light filter. The near vision add of this lens is +3.00 D over the distance power. The new design offers square edge haptics that reduce possible PCO.

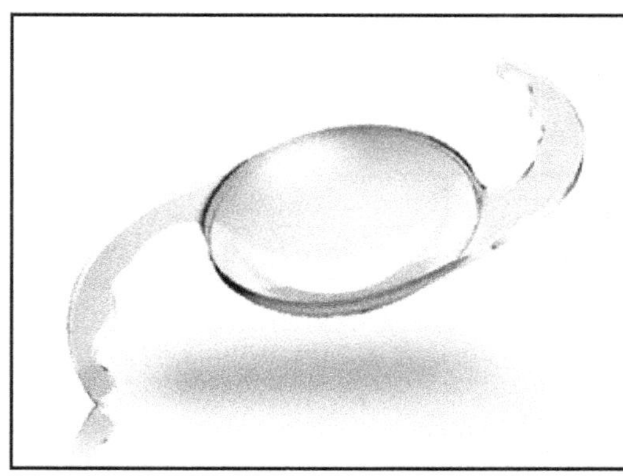

Technical Specifications[37]

Overall length	13.0 mm
Optic diameter	6.0 mm
Power range	0.00 to +7.00 D (1.0-D increments) +7.50 to +30.00 D (0.5-D increments) +31.00 to +40.00 (1.0-D increments)

Optic design	Biconvex
Edge	360-degree square edge design
Haptic angulation	5 degrees
Material	Hydrophilic acrylic UV
Filtration	UV blocker and violet light filter
Refractive index	1.462 (35°C)
YAG laser	Compatible
A-constant	118.6* for IOL Master, SRK/T 118.26* for US Biometry, SRK/T
Placement	Capsular bag
CE Approved	

*It is recommended that surgeons personalize their A-constant based on their surgical techniques and equipment experience, and postoperative results. For more information, please visit Hanita Lenses web.

Clinical Studies[38]

Visual and Refractive Outcomes

No significant change in the DCNVA was detected between 1 and 3 months after surgery, but a significant improvement was found between 3 and 6 months after surgery. The uncorrected intermediate visual acuity (UIVA) at 63 cm was 0.20 ± 0.13, 0.24 ± 0.14, and 0.27 ± 0.15 at 1, 3, and 6 months after surgery, respectively, and distance z-corrected intermediate visual acuity (DCIVA) at 63 cm was 0.23 ± 0.10, 0.25 ± 0.14, and 0.24 ± 0.10 at 1, 3, and 6 months postoperatively, respectively.

Defocus Curve

This multifocal IOL provided 2 peaks of maximum vision, one at distance (around 0 defocus level) and 1 at near (around –2.5 D defocus level). Between these 2 peaks, defocus of approximately –1.5 D was felt to provide acceptable intermediate vision (greater than 0.3 LogMAR).

Evaluating Contrast Sensitivity

A significant increase in scotopic contrast sensitivity was seen for 6 cycles of spatial frequency during follow-up, but no significant changes were found for the rest of spatial frequencies.

Optical Quality Outcomes

Measurement of intraocular aberrations demonstrated a significant reduction in intraocular higher-order aberrations and in the asymmetric aberrations (coma and coma-like aberrations). The patients achieved better levels of Strehl ratio from the ones seen preoperatively. In addition, the mean postoperative Strehl ratio was better than those seen in a normal population of the same age and was comparable to values in young, healthy patients.

Conclusion

The new diffractive SeeLens MF IOL can successfully restore distance, intermediate, and near vision after cataract surgery. The double-edge design of the optic may reduce the rate of PCO, although further long-term follow-up of the patients should be performed in order to address this matter. Contrast sensitivity function in photopic conditions shows better results than those obtained with other diffractive platforms. The defocus curve for the near, intermediate, and distance vision demonstrated excellent results. Furthermore, long-term investigations with larger samples of patients are required in future studies with the SeeLens MF IOL.

Lentis Mplus LS-312 (Oculentis GmbH) (+3, +1.5)

This is the first multifocal IOL with a rotational asymmetrical concept. The asymmetry comes due to the different sectors where the light is refracted in a specific foci; in other words, there is an asymmetric distance-vision dominant zone.

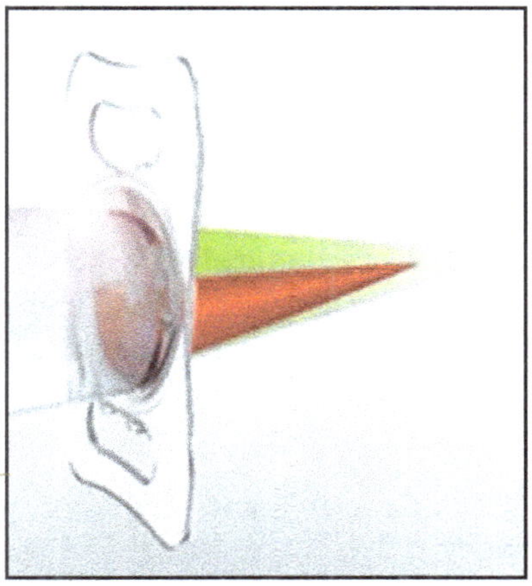

Technical Specifications[39]

Product	Lentis Mplus LS-313 MF30
Type	Foldable 1-piece multifocal acrylic IOL
Optic size	6.0 mm
Overall length	11.0 mm
Haptic angulation	0 degrees

Clinical Studies

Evaluating Vision

Lentis Mplus LS-312 MF30 IOL has statistically significantly better UNVA and DCNVA than Lentis Mplus LS-312 MF15 IOL. Instead, Lentis Mplus LS-312 MF 30 has significantly better UIVA at 3 months.[40]

It provides adequate distance, intermediate, and, to a lesser extent, near vision with high rates of spectacle freedom.[41]

DCNVA is significantly better with the Lentis Mplus versus Crystalens HD.[42]

Refractive predictability and intermediate visual outcomes with the Lentis Mplus LS-312 IOL improved significantly when implanted in combination with a capsular tension ring.[43]

UNVA and DCNVA are better with the ReSTOR SN6AD3 IOL than with Lentis Mplus LS-312 IOL, but intermediate visual acuity is better with the Lentis Mplus.[44]

In the defocus curve, significantly better visual acuities are present in eyes with the Lentis Mplus IOL for intermediate vision levels of defocus versus Acri.LISA 366D.[27]

Evaluating Contrast Sensitivity

There are no significant differences in contrast sensitivity between the Lentis Mplus versus Acri.Smart 48S monofocal IOL.[45]

The Crystalens HD has better contrast sensitivity under photopic conditions at all spatial frequencies than Lentis Mplus.[42]

Photopic contrast sensitivity is significantly better with Lentis Mplus IOL than with the ReSTOR SN6AD3 IOL.[38]

Significantly better values were seen in photopic contrast sensitivity for high spatial frequencies in the Lentis Mplus versus Acri.LISA 366D.[27]

Evaluating Photic Phenomena

Moderate haloes, glare, and night vision problems are reported by 6.2%, 12.5%, and 15.6% of patients, respectively.[39]

Diffractive Trifocal: FineVision

This is a trifocal, single-piece, foldable, and aspheric IOL with 2 fully diffractive structures, one with +1.75 D addition and another one with +3.5 D addition connected by a spring system. It is made of 25% hydrophilic material with yellow chromophore embedded in the matrix polymer.[46] The light is divided in 43% for far vision, 15% for intermediate vision, and 28% for near vision. The remaining 14% of light energy is lost by other diffractive patterns.[46,47]

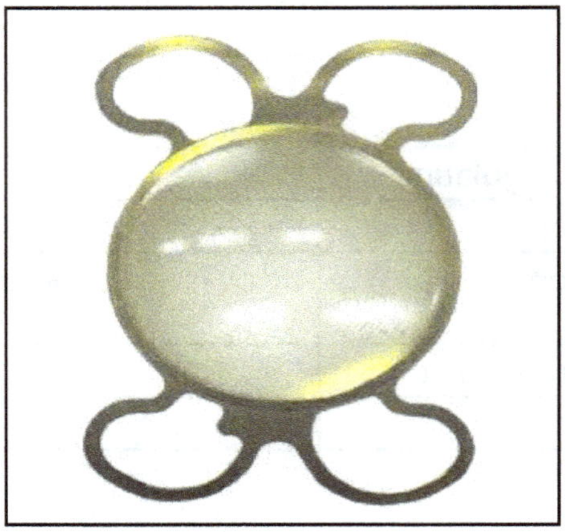

Technical Specifications[48]

Material	25% hydrophilic acrylic
Overall diameter	10.75 mm
Optic diameter	6.15 mm
Optic	Aspheric trifocal diffractive FineVision
Filtration	UV and blue light
Angulation	5 degrees
Injection system	Microincision injection
Incision	≥1.8 mm
Power	+10 to +35 D (0.5-D steps)
Suggested constants*	Hoffer Q: pACD = 5.35 (interferometry), 5.26 (US) Holladay 1: Sf = 1.60 (interferometry), 1.48 (US) SRK II: A = 119.1 (interferometry), 118.9 (US) SRK/T: A = 118.8 (interferometry), 118.6 (US) Haigis**: a0 = 1.36, a1 = 0.4, a2 = 0.1 (interferometry)

*Estimates only; surgeons are recommended to use their own values based upon their personal experience. Release date: 25.06.12. Refer to our website for updates.

**Not optimized.

Clinical Studies

Evaluating Vision

In a follow-up of 3 months in a study conducted by the author, the distance UCVA and BCVA improved significantly, as well as the near UCVA, and that total stability was found in both manifest sphere and cylinder. Additionally, the efficacy and safety indexes were 1.58 and

1.93, respectively, indicating that the lens is safe and effective in patients.[49]

Conclusion

Patients achieve a good quality of vision for far, intermediate, and near vision without the presence of glare, halos, and ghost images. As the first trifocal diffractive IOL on the market, it represents a new trend in visual quality after cataract surgery.

In-the-Bag Accommodative Intraocular Lenses

One of the main issues of multifocal IOLs is that they divide the light entering the eye into near and distance foci; the near vision provided is at the expense of reducing contrast sensitivity and causing photic visual phenomena, such as increased haloes and glare (1 to 6 near visual outcomes with single optic and dual optic accommodating IOLs). A way to achieve pseudoaccommodation without this phenomenon is to design accommodating IOLs. The concept is using a single optic that is based on the forward movement of the optic with ciliary muscle contraction to provide near focus. Actually there are 2 main types as follows:

- Single optic: Crystalens HD
- Dual optics: Synchrony

Crystalens HD (Bausch + Lomb)

The Crystalens HD is a biconvex single optic accommodating IOLs of a biocompatible third-generation silicone (Biosil) with a refractive index of 1.428.

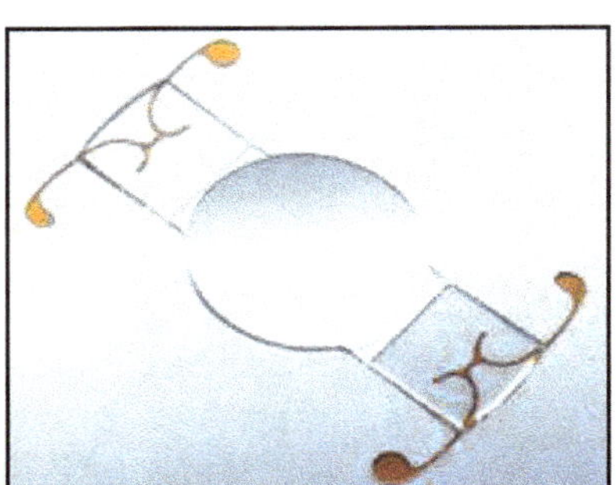

Technical Specifications[50]

Material	Biosil
Refractive index	1.427
Optic	Biconvex with central anterior surface modification
Optic size	50 mm
Haptics	Polyimide
Overall diameter	Plate: 10.5 mm Haptics: 11.5 mm (17.0 to 33.0 D) 12.0 mm (10.0 to 16.75 D)
Diopter range	10.0 to 33.0 in half D steps 18.0 to 22.0 in quarter D steps
A-constant*	118.3
ACD*	5.43 mm
Surgeon factor*	N/A
Product order code	HD520 (10.0 to 16.75 D) HD500 (17.0 to 33.0 D) CI-23A Crystalsert Single Use Injection System

*A-constant, ACD, and Surgeon Factor are estimates only. It is recommended that each surgeon develop his/her own values.

Synchrony (Visiogen)

The Synchrony IOL is a dual-optic accommodating IOL consisting of a single-piece, dual-optic, foldable silicone IOL with a high-plus power moving optic coupled to a low-power static minus-lens joined by spring haptic.

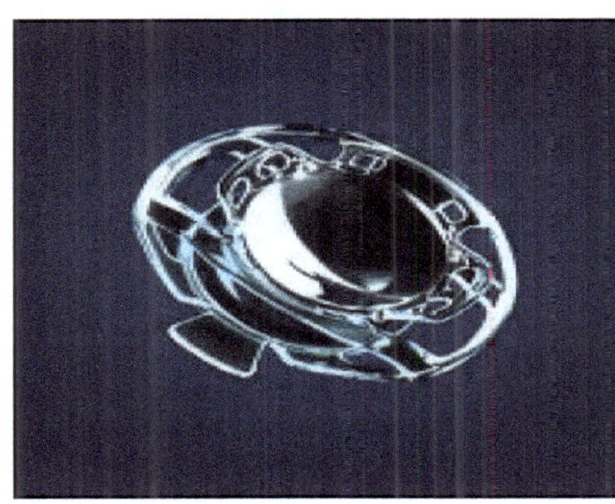

Crystalens HD Versus Synchrony[51]

Clinical Studies

Evaluating Vision

Comparing single-optic (Crystalen HD) versus dual-optic (Synchrony): No significantly better differences were found in near and intermediate visual outcomes. Significantly better uncorrected distance visual acuity

(UDVA) and corrected distance visual acuity (CDVA) were found for the dual-optic group.

Evaluating Contrast Sensitivity

Contrast sensitivity values were significantly better for the dual-optic IOL than for the single-optic IOL.

Evaluating Ocular Aberrations

The ocular Strehl ratio was significantly better for the dual-optic IOL. Higher values of postoperative total and higher root-mean-square (RMS) aberrations were observed in the single-optic group.

Evaluating Posterior Capsular Opacification

A PCO rate of 40% was observed in the group with the single-optic design and a 8% with the dual-optic design.

Sulcus-Placed Accommodative Intraocular Lenses

AkkoLens Lumina

Accommodating IOLs use small ciliary movements to mechanically move the IOL hinges in order to place the optic more anterior or posteriorly. In contrast, AkkoLens has an anterior element with a spherical lens to correct the overall refraction of the eye, and a cubic optical surface for varifocal effects. These optical elements move relative to each other perpendicularly to the optical axis, in the same plane with the movement of the ciliary muscle.

The lens is injected through a 2.8-mm incision and is positioned in the sulcus of the eye to ensure emmetropia and to avoid problems generally associated with the lens-less, capsular bag.

Clinical Studies

In a study executed by our group,[52] a comparison of accommodation amplitude and visual acuity of the AkkoLens Lumina with a monofocal IOL (AcrySof SN60AT) was performed. The preliminary results show that the AkkoLens Lumina successfully restores visual acuity for far and for near and also provides sufficient accommodation to allow sharp vision up to a reading distance of 33 cm.

Dynacurve, NuLens[53]

The NuLens accommodating IOL has polymethylmethacrylate (PMMA) haptics that are secured by internal scleral fixation to the sulcus without sutures; a PMMA anterior reference plane, which also provides basic vision correction for distance; a small chamber containing a solid silicone gel; and a posterior piston with an aperture at the center.

Ten eyes of 10 patients were evaluated. The mean number of lines patients could read increased from 1.0 preoperatively to 3.8 lines 6 months postoperatively, indicating improvement in UNVA after IOL implantation. The mean change in cross-section measurements of the IOL was 0.06 mm at 1 month; the value peaked at 3 months (0.21 mm), after which it decreased steadily, becoming stable at 9 months (0.09 mm, which is equivalent to 10.00 D of accommodation). Corrected near visual acuity improved slightly (0.7 Jaeger lines) at 12 months, with the best reading distance at 10 cm. These results suggest that the near and distance visual acuities were approximately equal, and therefore the IOL can produce accommodation of 10.00 D.

The principal mode of accommodation seems to be functional and provides accommodation up to 10.00 D. Patients' near visual acuity improved without compromising distance visual acuity. Low-vision patients gained angular magnification and could read at a distance of 10 cm.

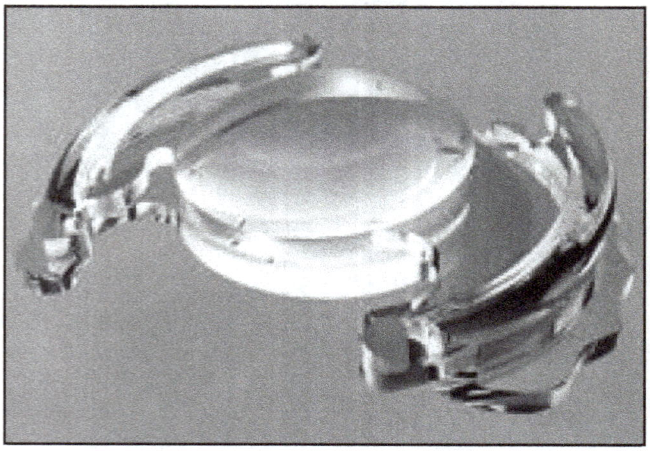

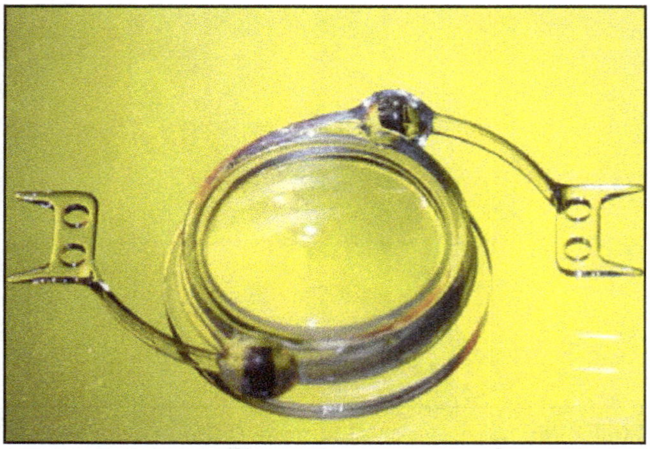

WIOL-CF[54,55]

The WIOL-CF is designed as a full-disc overall optic, approximately 9 mm in diameter and 1 to 1.5 mm in thickness, to completely fill the posterior capsule. It has a meniscoid anterior surface and a hyperboloid posterior surface contacting the posterior capsule. The WIOL-CF can be inserted through a 2.8-mm incision. Of course, in order to achieve optimum results it is important to educate the patient that near vision accommodation requires effort and time. Patients should be trained to utilize the accommodative features of the lens, which will allow them to lead an active life without being spectacle dependent. The mean UDVA improved from 0.45 to 0.66 D postoperatively. The mean CDVA improved from 0.57 D preoperatively to 0.75 D at the last follow-up. No eyes lost any lines of CDVA, and 71% of eyes gained lines of distance-corrected visual acuity. Approximately 65% of patients achieved J1 near vision without any spectacle aid. Putting the results into context, Dr. Portaliou said that the WIOL-CF seems to represent a promising solution for patients who lead an active life and require good near, intermediate, and far vision. However, the nature of the lens means that postoperative patient training is critical in order to achieve the maximum degree of pseudoaccommodation and provide high-quality near vision without the use of glasses.

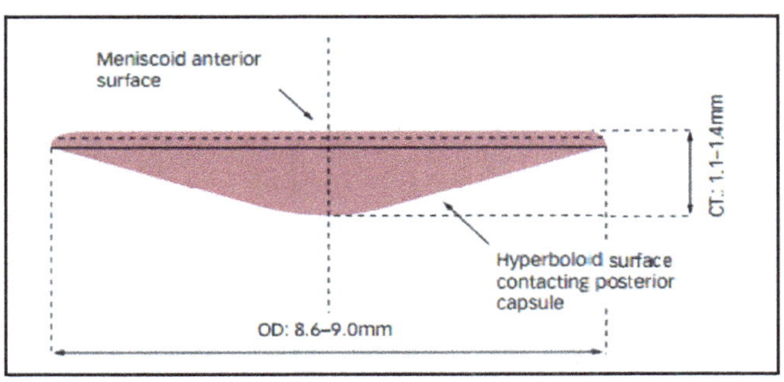

References

1. Bellucci R. Multifocal intraocular lenses. *Curr Opin Ophthalmol.* 2005;16:33-37.
2. Keates RH, Pearce JL, Schneider RT. Clinical results of the multifocal lens. *J Cataract Refract Surg.* 1987;13:557-560.
3. Duffey RJ, Zabel RW, Lindstrom RL. Multifocal intraocular lenses. *J Cataract Refract Surg.* 1990;16:423-429.
4. Yu JG, Zhao YE, Shi JL, et al. Biaxial micro incision cataract surgery versus conventional coaxial cataract surgery: meta-analysis of randomized controlled trials. *J Cataract Refract Surg.* 2012;38:894-901.
5. Can İ, Bayhan HA, Çelik H, Ceran BB. Comparison of corneal aberrations after biaxial microincision and microcoaxial cataract surgeries: a prospective study. *Curr Eye Res.* 2012;37:18-24.
6. Can I, Takmaz T, Bayhan HA, Ceran B. Aspheric microincision intraocular lens implantation with biaxial microincision cataract surgery: efficacy and reliability. *J Cataract Refract Surg.* 2010;36:1905-1911.
7. Alió JL, Elkady B, Ortiz D. Corneal optical quality following sub 1.8 mm micro incision cataract surgery vs. 2.2 mm mini-incision coaxial phacoemulsification. *Middle East Afr J Ophthalmol.* 2011;17:94-99.
8. Tong N, He JC, Lu F, Wang Q, Qu J, Zhao YE. Changes in corneal wavefront aberrations in micro incision and small incision cataract surgery. *J Cataract Refract Surg.* 2008;34:2085-2090.
9. Denoyer A, Denoyer L, Marotte D, Georget M, Pisella PJ. Intraindividual comparative study of corneal and ocular wavefront aberrations after biaxial microincision versus coaxial small-incision cataract surgery. *Br J Ophthalmol.* 2008;92:1679-1684.
10. Elkady B, Alió JL, Ortiz D, Montalbán R. Corneal aberrations after microincision cataract surgery. *J Cataract Refract Surg.* 2008;34:40-45.
11. Kurz S, Krummenauer F, Thieme H, Dick HB. Contrast sensitivity after implantation of a spherical versus an aspherical intraocular lens in biaxial micro incision cataract surgery. *J Cataract Refract Surg.* 2007;33:393-400.
12. Yao K, Tang X, Ye P. Corneal astigmatism, high order aberrations, and optical quality after cataract surgery: microincision versus small incision. *J Refract Surg.* 2006;22:1079-1082.
13. Werner L, Olson RJ, Mamalis N. New technology IOL optics. *Ophthalmol Clin North Am.* 2006;19:469-483.
14. Lichtinger A, Rootman DS. Intraocular lenses for presbyopia correction: past, present, and future. *Curr Opin Ophthalmol.* 2012;23:40-46.
15. Slade S. US experience and results. In: Slade, S, ed. *Laser Refractive Cataract Surgery Science, Medicine and Industry.* Wayne: Bryn Mawr Communications LLC; 2012:164
16. Nagy Z, Takacs A, Filkorn T, Sarayba M. Initial clinical evaluation of an intraocular femtosecond laser in cataract surgery. *J Refract Surg.* 2009;25:1053-1060.
17. McAlinden C, Moore JE. Multifocal intraocular lens with a surface-embedded near section: short-term clinical outcomes. *J Cataract Refract Surg.* 2011;37:441-445.
18. Alcon surgical for professionals. AcrySof IQ ReSTOR IOL Product Specifications; 2012 Available from: http://www.alcon-surgical.com/Product-Specifications.aspx
19. Santhiago MR, Wilson SE, Netto MV, et al. Visual performance of an apodized diffractive multifocal intraocular lens with + 3.00-D addition: 1-year follow-up. *J Refract Surg.* 2011;27 899-906.
20. Alió JL, Plaza-Puche AB, Javaloy J, Ayala MJ. Comparison of the visual and intraocular optical performance of a refractive multifocal IOL with rotational asymmetry and an apodized diffractive multifocal IOL. *J Refract Surg.* 2012;28:100-105.
21. Alió JL, Grabner G, Plaza-Puche AB, Rasp M, Piñero DP, Seyeddain O, Rodríguez-Prats JL, Ayala MJ, Moreu R, Hohensinn M, Riha W, Dexl A. Postoperative bilateral reading performance with 4 intraocular lens models: six-month results. *J Cataract Refract Surg.* 2011;37:842-852.
22. Gil MA, Varon C, Rosello N, Cardona G, Buil JA. Visual acuity, contrast sensitivity, subjective quality of vision, and quality of life with 4 different multifocal IOLs. *Eur J Ophthalmol.* 2012 22:175-187.
23. Alió JL, Plaza-Puche AB, Piñero DP, Amparo F, Rodríguez-Prats JL, Ayala MJ. Quality of life evaluation after implantation of 2 multifocal intraocular lens models and a monofocal model. *J Cataract Refract Surg.* 2011;37 638-648.
24. Alfonso JF, Fernández-Vega L, Blázquez JI, Montes-Micó R. Visual function comparison of 2 aspheric multifocal intraocular lenses. *J Cataract Refract Surg.* 2012;38:242-248.

25. Santhiago MR, Wilson SE, Netto MV, et al. Visual performance of an apodized diffractive multifocal intraocular lens with + 3.00-D addition: 1-year follow-up. *J Refract Surg.* 2011;27:899-906.
26. IOLs by Carl Zeiss Meditec. Focusing on the future in surgical ophthalmology. Product Portfolio. Available from: http://download.zeiss.de/medical/acrilisa/IOL-Portfolio_FINAL.pdf
27. Alio JL, Plaza-Puche AB, Javaloy J, Ayala MJ, Moreno LJ, Piñero DP. Comparison of a new refractive multifocal intraocular lens with an inferior segmental near add and a diffractive multifocal intraocular lens. *Ophthalmology.* 2012;119:555-563.
28. Alió JL, Plaza-Puche AB, Piñero DP, et al. Optical analysis, reading performance, and quality-of-life evaluation after implantation of a diffractive multifocal intraocular lens. *J Cataract Refract Surg.* 2011;37:27-37.
29. ReZoom Multifocal IOL. Abbott Medical Optics Inc. Available from: http://www.amo-inc.com/products/cataract/refractive-iols/rezoom-multifocal-iol
30. Gil MA, Varon C, Rosello N, Cardona G, Buil JA. Visual acuity, contrast sensitivity, subjective quality of vision, and quality of life with 4 different multifocal IOLs. *Eur J Ophthalmol.* 2011;22:175-187.
31. Muñoz G, Albarrán-Diego C, Cerviño A, Ferrer-Blasco T, García-Lázaro S. Visual and optical performance with the ReZoom multifocal intraocular lens. *Eur J Ophthalmol.* 2012;22:356-362.
32. Lubiński W, Podboraczyńska-Jodko K, Gronkowska-Serafin J, Karczewicz D. Visual outcomes three and six months after implantation of diffractive and refractive multifocal IOL combinations. *Klin Oczna.* 2011;113:209-215.
33. Terwee T, Weeber H, van der Mooren M, Piers P. Visualization of the retinal image in an eye model with spherical and aspheric, diffractive, and refractivemultifocal intraocular lenses. *J Refract Surg.* 2008;24:223-232.
34. Friedrich R. Intraocular lens multifocality combined with the compensation for corneal spherical aberration: a new concept of presbyopia-correcting intraocular lens. *Case Report Ophthalmol.* 2012;3:375-383.
35. Bautista CP, González DC, Gómez AC. Evolution of visual performance in 70 eyes implanted with the Tecnis ZMB00 multifocal intraocular lens. *Clin Ophthalmol.* 2012;6:403-407.
36. TECNIS Multifocal 1-Piece Aspheric IOL Hydrophobic Acrylic Model: ZMB00. Available from: http://www.tecnismultifocal.com/us/healthcare-professionals/lens-specifications-zmb00.php
37. Hanita Lenses, Spheric IOLs, SeeLens. Available from: http://www.hanitalenses.com/product/seelens/
38. Alió JL, Vega-Estrada A, Plaza-Puche A. Clinical outcomes with a new diffractive multifocal IOL. *J Cataract Refract Surg.* In review.
39. Oculentis, LentisMplus IOL. Available from: http://www.oculentis.com/profLentisMplusDatasheets.html
40. Alió JL, Plaza-Puche AB, Piñero DP, Javaloy J, Ayala MJ. Comparative analysis of the clinical outcomes with 2 multifocal intraocular lens models with rotational asymmetry. *J Cataract Refract Surg.* 2011;37:1605-1614.
41. Muñoz G, Albarrán-Diego C, Ferrer-Blasco T, Sakla HF, García-Lázaro S. Visual function after bilateral implantation of a new zonal refractive aspheric multifocal intraocular lens. *J Cataract Refract Surg.* 2011;37:2043-2052.
42. Alió JL, Plaza-Puche AB, Montalban R, Javaloy J. Visual outcomes with a single-optic accommodating intraocular lens and a low-addition-power rotational asymmetric multifocal intraocular lens. *J Cataract Refract Surg.* 2012;38:978-985.
43. Alió JL, Plaza-Puche AB, Piñero DP. Rotationally asymmetric multifocal IOL implantation with and without capsular tension ring: refractive and visual outcomes and intraocular optical performance. *J Refract Surg.* 2012;28:253-258.
44. Alió JL, Plaza-Puche AB, Javaloy J, Ayala MJ. Comparison of the visual and intraocular optical performance of a refractive multifocal IOL with rotational asymmetry and an apodized diffractive multifocal IOL. *J Refract Surg.* 2012;28:100-105.
45. Alió JL, Piñero DP, Plaza-Puche AB, Chan MJ. Visual outcomes and optical performance of a monofocal intraocular lens and a new-generation multifocal intraocular lens. *J Cataract Refract Surg.* 2011;37:241-250.
46. Gatinel D, Pagnoulle C, Houbrechts Y, Gobin L. Design and qualification of adiffractive trifocal optical profile for intraocular lenses. *J Cataract Refract Surg.* 2011;37:2060-2067.
47. Cochener B, Vryghem J, Rozot P, et al. Visual and refractive outcomes after implantation of a fully diffractive trifocal lens. *Clin Ophthalmol.* 2012;6:1421-1427.
48. Physiol, FineVision. Available from: http://www.physiol.eu/medias/upload/files/FineVision_brochure_Oct2012.pdf
49. Alió JL. Early experience with the FineVision IOL. *Cataract & Refractive Surgery Today Europe.* 2012;Nov/Dec.
50. Crystalens HD Intraocular Lens. Bausch & Lomb. Available from: http://www.bausch.co.uk/en-GB/ECP/Our-Products/Cataract-Surgery/Lens%20Systems/Crystalens-HD
51. Alió JL, Plaza-Puche AB, Montalban R, Ortega P. Near visual outcomes with single-optic and dual-optic accommodating intraocular lenses. *J Cataract Refract Surg.* 2012;38:1568-1575.
52. Alio JL, Vega-Estrada A, Peña P, et al. Accommodation amplitude and visual acuity of the accommodative intraocular lens: the AkkoLens Lumina. Presented at the European Society of Cataract & Refractive Surgeons, October 2013.
53. Alió JL, Ben-nun J, Rodríguez-Prats JL, Plaza AB. Visual and accommodative outcomes 1 year after implantation of an accommodating intraocular lens based on a new concept. *J Cataract Refract Surg.* 2009;35:1671-1678.
54. Portaliou D, Kymionis G, Pallikaris I. The WIOL-CF accommodative intraocular lens. Available from: http://www.ivo.gr/files/items/2/257/the_wiol-cf_accommodative_intraocular_lens.pdf
55. McGrath, D. IOL shows promise. Available from: http://escrs.org/publications/eurotimes/11May/IOLshowpromise.pdf

24

Avoiding and Managing Patient Dissatisfaction After Intraocular Lens Implantation After Cataract Surgery

Johann A. Kruger, MMed Ophth, FCS (SA) Ophth, FRCS Ed Ophth

Intraocular lens (IOL) technology has evolved tremendously over the recent years, and so have marketing techniques. This has led patients to become more discerning and have higher expectations after cataract surgery. The advent of LASIK surgery has also raised patient expectations.

Is the patient always satisfied after phacoemulsification with an IOL implant? This is a question we often ask ourselves as surgeons after surgery—even when our surgery was done properly and without complications.

Unfortunately the answer is NO! This can lead to anxiety in both the surgeon and the patient. It is important to identify the cause of the dissatisfaction and try to resolve it. The incidence of dissatisfaction ranges from 2% to 8% and higher.[1-5]

Today, cataract surgery and IOL implantation requires a new approach. In the past, the patient received surgery without considering spectacle independence or necessarily a good refractive result. A lens was only implanted to resolve aphakia and the patient was satisfied even if only his or her sight was restored, ignoring spectacle independence.

Nowadays the patient presents for surgery and expects a functional and refractive result; the patient knows he or she has multiple solutions. The patient also knows that cataract surgery available today is cataract refractive surgery, which is safe and he or she can have a customized/premium IOL. Patients are aware that preoperative refractive defects can be corrected and they can obtain increased quality of vision.

Patients expect good surgical results, sharp and high-quality vision, and vision without spectacles for reading, computer use, and driving at night. In a Swedish study, it was found that postoperative ametropia is the most common cause of patient dissatisfaction after cataract surgery. The dissatisfaction incidence was 8% in 459 surgeries. In patients where there was maculopathy, there was a significantly higher dissatisfaction rate.[1]

In a Grecian study by Chatziralli and coworkers a small percentage of dissatisfied patients were found. They did a patient satisfaction survey in 397 patients who had undergone uneventful phacoemulsification cataract surgery. Best-corrected visual acuity (BCVA) was measured before and after cataract surgery. They found macular disease, diabetic retinopathy, and glaucoma, which were the main limiting factors. Thus, in cataract surgery, the preoperative examination is important and the patient with the above-mentioned pathologies needs to be warned preoperatively.[2]

Dissatisfaction after IOL implantation following cataract surgery can also be due to complications during surgery or postoperative lacrimal disorders, but most of the time problems are related to the IOL. Most commonly, there is a refractive error affecting the functional result and it could be due to the type of IOL used as well.

Dissatisfaction after monofocal IOL implantation is less common. In most cases, it is related to a refractive surprise. The surgeon can resolve this with laser vision correction or IOL exchange in extreme cases. In cases of toric IOLs, which are used more frequently nowadays, there may be residual astigmatism. This may be corrected with laser vision correction as well.

Other causes of dissatisfaction may also be where there was vitreous loss, an unstable or decentered IOL, or IOL tilt causing visual distortion.

Dissatisfaction in IOL patients is most frequently seen with multifocal IOLs. Multifocal IOLs have been used for

Buratto L, Brint SF, Boccuzzi D.
Cataract Surgery and Intraocular Lenses (pp 189-192).

TABLE 24-1

PATIENT SATISFACTION SURVEY

QUESTION POSED	YES OR GOOD OR NO PROBLEMS	UNDECIDED OR AVERAGE	NO OR POOR OR PROBLEMATIC
Are you satisfied with your DISTANCE vision?	76%	11%	13%
Are you satisfied with you INTERMEDIATE vision?	76%	11%	13%
Are you satisfied with you NEAR vision?	76%	11%	13%
Problems with glare/haloes/nighttime driving?	62%	25%	13%
Would you have this surgery again?	76%	22%	2%
Would you recommend this surgery to somebody else?	76%	22%	2%

years offering spectacle independence. But their optics have several disadvantages: loss of contrast sensitivity, haloes, and difficulty with night vision. Limited intermediate vision is also a drawback. One reason for higher dissatisfaction rate in multifocal IOLs as opposed to monofocal IOLs is directly linked to higher patient expectations.

N. E. de Vries reported that in the majority of dissatisfied patients after multifocal implantation, the cause of dissatisfaction can be treated successfully. They reported on 76 eyes in 47 patients and found that complaints in 72 eyes were most commonly due to photic phenomena (25 eyes) and unsatisfactory acuity (47 eyes). The leading causes were residual ametropia and astigmatism (49 eyes), posterior capsular opacification (12 eyes), and large pupil size. They were able to successfully manage the dissatisfaction in 82% of patients with photorefractive keratectomy (PRK) or yttrium-aluminum-garnet laser capsulotomy.[3]

In a study by the author of 50 eyes in 28 patients receiving a multifocal M-plus IOL after microincisional phacoemulsification procedure in cataract patients, only 2% of patients were dissatisfied and would not recommend the surgery. This was linked to a poor refractive outcome. Seventy-five percent of patients were very satisfied, 11% were somewhat satisfied, and 13% were not happy with their outcome (Table 24-1).

The key is that patients need to be educated preoperatively on the advantages and disadvantages of multifocal IOLs.

In case of dissatisfaction, the key is to dedicate time to the patient and follow a systematic approach. The patient must feel supported and it is necessary to identify and understand the reasons for the dissatisfaction.

Acknowledge that there is a problem and acknowledge the impact and any distress the patient has experienced, "Mr. Kruger, as you know, there has been a problem with your vision."

Express regret that he or she is not happy with his vision, "Mrs. Kruger, I'm sorry you are experiencing haloes. We spoke about this prior to the surgery." One must, however, be careful not to admit error on the surgeon's behalf.

The patient must explain his or her story or experience in terms of how it is affecting him or her, in his or her own words. The surgeon needs to know if the patient has knowledge or understanding and perspective of the problem he or she has. It also helps to understand what emotions the patient is experiencing. Once the patient has spoken, the surgeon should summarize the patient's story: "Can you tell me in your own words?"; "How do you feel about your vision and the surgery?"; then the surgeon can respond with "So let me see if I understand correctly." In this section, it is important to include in your story summary, for instance, that the informed consent was taken and the possible side effects were discussed. "Glare and haloes are encountered in some people as discussed with you before in the informed consent." The patient will normally agree with you that it was discussed beforehand and that he or she actually just needs reassurance that it is not abnormal or seeks a solution.

Encourage communication and seek questions the patient may further need to be answered. You can also ask to contact a colleague or to provide the information to further investigate a solution. For instance, "What other questions do have?" and "There are a few things that are important for you to know" and "I promise to get back to you with some answers."

The patient should be actively involved in the solution to the problem and one must seek the patient's ideas on going forward. Seek permission to propose some of your own thoughts. Also, negotiate an agreed plan. For instance, "Mr. Kruger, we can give you glasses or we can do laser vision correction to improve your vision as discussed prior to the surgery with you. Do you recall that?" and end by saying, "So it sounds like this may be the way forward for you."

Avoid abandonment and keep communication open with the patient. Specifically express your desire to continue care and even stay in contact with the patient (even if you are referring the patient to another colleague) by saying, "Mr. Kruger, I would like to continue caring for you and keep in contact so that I can make sure everything possible is done to reduce your symptoms. We are going to improve your vision with a laser procedure."

This approach is preferable and will also limit the patient from taking unnecessary legal steps against the surgeon for whatever reason. It gives time to the patient and the surgeon to overcome the dissatisfaction.

Questions that need to be answered in solving the problem are: Were the preop requirements fulfilled? Were the surgical prerequisites fulfilled? Was the eye free of pathology preoperatively? Was a refractive surgery approach taken? Was the appropriate IOL inserted in this specific patient? Was the patient appropriately selected for a multifocal IOL? What was the visual acuity potential? Does the patient have good bilateral vision? Is there good binocularity?

From here the surgeon must perform several examinations to identify the reason for compromised vision or an unhappy patient: examination of the capsular bag/IOL, fundus photography, and retinal optical coherence tomography; refraction, total, and corneal aberration wavescan; and pupil and IOL functionality (Figure 24-1).

Did the patient have realistic expectations of the surgery? Were the appropriate vision requirements determined for the patient specifically (various distance vision)? What work activity requirements are there? What are the general needs of this particular patient? What are the quality and lifestyle requirements to satisfy a patient with multifocal IOL? Precise postop refraction is a mandatory goal. Life and sight without spectacles—this is the desire of most patients entering into an operating room.

A multifocal IOL implant theoretically means a promise for emmetropia and spectacle freedom. However, in roughly 15% of patients, postoperative emmetropia is not obtained. (Explain before surgery in the informed consent!) Offer a bioptics package with every multifocal IOL implant, which includes a possible laser vision correction as an enhancement or a possible IOL change. (Explain before surgery!) This makes patients aware that the surgery is not perfect, and is especially mandatory in multifocal ICL patients.

Causes of dissatisfaction are residual refractive problems, quality disorders such as night vision problems (haloes and glare), blurred vision, intermediate vision problems, distance vision problems, and lacrimal disorders.

In cases of residual refractive problems, a spherical or astigmatic remnant causes problems with long distance and near vision and affects the overall result.

In cases of a small spherical or cylindrical error, the solution is laser vision correction (PRK or LASIK), as spectacles or contact lenses are not well accepted in most cases.

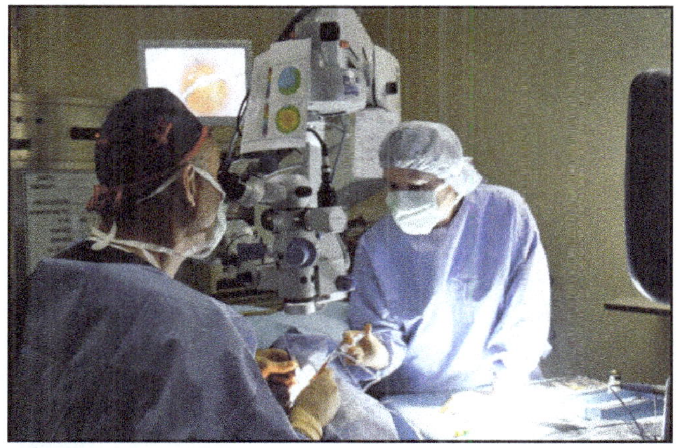

Figure 24-1. During surgery the Pentacam (Oculus) image is on hand to guide the surgeon during surgery.

Substantial spherical or cylindrical error may require LASIK or piggyback IOL or explanation and lens exchange.

LASIK or PRK is the preferable procedure as it has a quicker and less problematic visual recovery and wavefront higher-order aberrations can be corrected.

If an enhancement is considered, it should only be done after the implant for the second eye when the vision has stabilized (minimum 1 to 2 months for problems of 1 D or more, after 3 months or more for lesser problems)

Explanation and new implant should only be done after 3 months and only if the patient is truly dissatisfied and agrees to this. In this situation evaluate vision quality and decide to replace with a multifocal or monofocal IOL. If a multifocal IOL, which type? If other IOL issues (decentration, etc), is it best to use a monofocal IOL?

If there is dissatisfaction due to photic phenomena and night vision problems such as glare or haloes, a "wait and see" approach should be taken as the problems diminish over time. Specific spectacles for night driving and miotics (brimonidine or pilocarpine) should be used. Explantation should only be pursued if the problems are intolerable, but is seldom necessary as the patient may become more tolerant over time. Explantation must be tested by demonstrating to the patient what his or her near vision will be like by holding a –2 lens or –2.00 glasses in front of the patient and ask him or her to read something up close.

Blurred vision may be due to posterior capsule opacification, capsular folds, or lacrimal disturbances. Capsulotomy should be done even if there is only a very tiny fold or mild opacity, but should be avoided before explantation if the latter is inevitable.

Vision quality problems caused by the decentration of the multifocal IOL may necessitate explantation and implantation of a monofocal IOL or multifocal IOL 3-piece in the sulcus, although sulcus placement is not recommended.[6]

Intermediate vision problems with the first eye, computer, or cell phone can be solved by undercorrecting the second eye or with a Mix and Match technique. Inadequate intermediate vision is common with most multifocal IOLs. With the new FineVision trifocal refractive IOL as well as the Alcon ReSTOR +2.50 D lens, this is evidently less.[7]

Accommodative IOLs can be useful in outdoorsy patients such as golfers and computer users. The degree of accommodation is not predictable and depends on the ciliary body and the capsular bag. Near-sighted performance is not reliable, and long-term functionality is unknown. Slight overcorrection in the nondominant eye is helpful. Preoperative education of the patient is of value.

Iatrogenic monovision where the nondominant eye is undercorrected to −1.25 D is very popular and common practice. When the difference is more than −1.25 D asthenopia may be a problem. Laser vision correction is the best method to correct this.

Conclusion

It is important to spend more time with the preoperative evaluation to choose the right lens for the patient, do meticulous refractive cataract surgery, and educate patients about the advantages and disadvantages of multifocal lenses in particular.

References

1. Monetam E, Wachtmeister L. Dissatisfaction with cataract surgery in relation to visual results in a population-based study in Sweden. *J Cataract Refract Surg.* 1999;25(8):1127-1134.
2. Chatziralli IP, Kanonidou E, Papazisis L. Frequency of fundus pathology related to patients' dissatisfaction after phacoemulsification cataract surgery. *Bull Soc Belge Ophtalmol.* 2011;317:21-24.
3. de Vries NE, Webers CA, Touwslager WR, et al. Dissatisfaction after implantation of multifocal intraocular lenses. *J Cataract Refract Surg.* 2011;37(5):859-865.
4. JA Kruger. Oculentis M-Plus IOL—a South African perspective—results and patient satisfaction. Paper presented at the XXX ESCRS Congress, Milan, 2012.
5. Leccisotti A. Secondary procedures after presbyopic lens exchange. *J Cataract Refract Surg.* 2004;30:1461-1465.
6. Alio JL, Grabner G, Plaza-Puche AB, et al. Postoperative bilateral reading performance with 4 intraocular lens models: six month results. *J Cataract Refract Surg.* 2011;37:842-852.
7. Daya S. The latest generation of multifocal lenses. *Cataract and Refract Surg Today.* 2011;Nov/Dec:1-6.

Financial Disclosures

Dr. Jorge L. Alió has no financial or proprietary interest in the materials presented herein.

Dr. Domenico Boccuzzi has not disclosed any relevant financial relationships.

Dr. Stephen F. Brint has no financial or proprietary interest in the materials presented herein.

Dr. Lucio Buratto has not disclosed any relevant financial relationships.

Dr. Johann A. Kruger has not disclosed any relevant financial relationships.

Dr. Felipe Soria has no financial or proprietary interest in the materials presented herein.

Dr. Ghassan Zein has not disclosed any relevant financial relationships.

Index

Abbott Medical Optics IOLs, 29, 49
  1-piece, 30–31
aberrometry
  preoperative, 45
  for toric IOL implantation, 95, 97
accommodative IOLs, 73, 192
  binocular vision and, 115
  Crystalens, 73–76
  inside-the-bag, 178, 185–186
  sulcus-placed, 178, 186–187
  Synchrony, 76–78
Acrygel lens, 21
acrylate/methacrylate polymers, 7
acrylic IOLs
  haptics of, 13
  hydrophilic, 12–13, 18–19, 23
  hydrophobic, 12, 19
  soft, 10–13, 18–19
  3-piece, loading and insertion technique for, 137–140
acrylic-PMMA, 7
AcrySof IOLs
  evolution of, 32
  ReSTOR, 55–56
    for distance vision, 56
    general vision with, 56–57
    haloes and, 58
    for near vision, 56
    versus Oculentis lenses, 62–63
    pupil dynamics and, 64
    SN6AD3/SN6AD1, 179–180
    toric, 65–66
  toric, 46–48
AcrySof IQ, 36
age-related maculopathy, 69–71
AkkoLens, 186
Akreos AO lens, 32–33
Akreos insertion device, 145–147
Alcon IOLs. *See also* AcrySof IOLs
  1-piece, 30
  3-piece, 28–29
  toric, 51
alpha antagonists, 172, 173
anatomical-functional alterations, in reduced visual quality, 104–107
anesthetics, anterior chamber, 172–173
aniridia, 106–107
anterior chamber, anesthetics for, 172–173
antibiotics, intracameral, 173
aqueous humor, composition of, 172
Array lens, 20, 79
aspheric IOLs, 35–37
aspiration cannulas, 164
asteroid hyalosis, 110–111
astigmatism
  multifocal IOL implantation and, 63–65
  residual
    techniques to reduce, 39–44
    with toric IOLs, 43–44
  toric IOLs for, 95–97
AT LISA IOLs, 54–55
  809M, 180
  haloes and, 58
  in Mix and Match procedure, 80–81
  toric, 65
AT Shooter A2-2000 injector, 149–152
AT TORBI 709M toric IOL, 48–49
axis markers, 50–51
AZ9002 lens, 29

balanced salt solution (BSS), 171–172
balanced salt solution (BSS) Plus, 171–172

Bausch + Lomb lenses, 49–50. *See also* Crystalens
  1-piece, 32
  3-piece, 27, 29
benzalkonium chloride, 172
best-corrected visual acuity (BCVA), measurement of, 189
bimanual irrigation/aspiration technique, 163–165
binding, 8
Binkhorst, Cornelius, 4
binocular vision, 114–116
biometry, in lens power selection, 75–76
biometry errors
  correction methods for, 84–89
  IOL exchange for, 91
  with presbyopia-correcting IOLs, 83–84
bioptics
  in correcting refractive errors, 84–85
  techniques of, 43–44
blurred vision, postoperative, 191
Buratto's marker, 50

CALLISTO system, 51
capsular capture, 156–158
capsular rupture
  IOL implantation with, 155–156
  IOL power for, 156
  surgical technique for, 156–159
  visual quality and, 100–101
cataract surgery
  customization of, 63
  refractive, 83–89
  viscoelastic substances in, 123–125
CeeOn foldable lens, 20
cefuroxime, 173
cephalosporins, 173
chondroitin sulfate (CDS), 120–121
Choyce, Peter, 3–4
coatings, 8
cohesiveness, 119, 122
communication, in patient satisfaction, 190–191
contrast sensitivity
  loss of, 70
  with Synchrony lens, 78
  testing, 112, 113
contrast sensitivity function (CSF), 63, 69–70, 100
co-polymers, 7
corneal pathologies, 63
corneal relaxing incisions
  complications of, 42–43
  in IOL exchange, 91–92
  oblique, 101–102
  role of, 39–40
corneal topography
  preoperative evaluation of, 45–46
  for toric IOL implantation, 95–97
coupling effect, 40

Crystalens, 73
  characteristics of, 74–75
  in Mix and Match procedure, 80
  patient selection for, 75
  power selection for, 75–76
Crystalens HD, 185
  versus Synchrony, 185–186
Crystalens insertion device, 147–150

density, 119
diabetes
  dry eye syndrome in, 105
  maculopathy in, 111–112
diffractive IOLs
  combined with refractive lenses, 79–80
  mechanism of action of, 79
  multifocal, 53–55
  trifocal, 184–185
DisCoVisc, 120
dispersiveness, 119–120
Donnenfeld incision method, 40–42
dry eye, 104
  cause of, 105
  visual quality and, 100, 102–104
dual optic technology, 73
Dynacurve, 186

effective lens position (ELP)
  calculation of, 84
  in IOL implantation with capsular rupture, 157
  with piggyback IOLs, 89
Emerald Ease injector, 140
Emerald injector, 136
  for 3-piece acrylic IOL insertion, 137–140
emmetropia, with presbyopia-correcting IOLs, 84
endophthalmitis, postoperative, 173
endothelial decompensation, 102
enVista Toric MX60T, 49–50
epinephrine, 172, 173
excimer laser treatment
  for residual astigmatism, 43–44
  for residual refractive errors, 86
EYEVISPOD test, 99

femtosecond laser treatment, 85
FineVision diffractive trifocals, 184–185
fishmouth, 131
Five-Zero lens, 74
floaters, 109–110
floppy iris syndrome, intraoperative, 172, 173
foldable IOLs
  advantages of, 23–25
  disadvantages of, 25
  first, 5, 17, 18
  injectors for, 135–152

loading and implantation technique for, 152–153
materials for, 7
with silicone optic and PMMA haptics, 20
STAAR IOL, 22
folders
paddle-type, 132
for rigid IOLs, 125
for soft IOLs, 125–128
forceps
for rigid IOL insertion, 125
for soft IOL insertion, 126–130
for 3-piece acrylic IOL insertion, 137
Frankhauser, Franz, 5

gatifloxacin, 173
GDX test, 114
glare, with Synchrony lens, 78
glaucoma, 112
glucose, 171
glutathione, 171
gold waters of Gdansk, 111
grafting, 8
grinding, 7

haloes, 79
cause of, 55
in diffractive multifocal lenses, 54–55
light in, 58
in multifocal IOLs, 57–58
pupil diameter and, 58
with Synchrony lens, 78
tolerance to, 67
Healon 5, 123
Heidelberg Retina Tomography (HRT) test, 114
heparin-coated lenses, 8
higher-order aberrations (HOAs), 55, 57, 58, 63–65, 67
holders
for rigid IOLs, 125
for soft IOLs, 125–128
hyaluronic acid, 120, 122
hydrogel, 7, 10, 12
Hydromax lens, 29–30
hyperoptic patients, 68

iLASIK, 85–86
incisions. *See also* corneal relaxing incisions; limbal relaxing incisions; microincisional surgery (MICS); mini-incisions
closure of, 167–170
relaxing, 40–42
complications associated with, 42–44
self-sealing, 167
smaller, 17
techniques for, 167

injector cartridges, 135–136
Easy-Load, 140–141
loading, 138–139
injectors, 125
for foldable IOLs, 135–152
piston- or syringe-like, 135
screw controlled, 135, 136
types of, 135
insertion instruments, 125–133
intraocular lenses (IOLs)
exchange of, 91
reasons for, 91
surgical technique in, 91–94
folding, 126–128
history of, 3–5
implantation methods of
1-step, 133
2-step, 132
malpositioning, 101
position abnormalities with, 107–108
tear of damage of, 161–162
vision quality and, 99
iodization, 55
IOL power
for IOL implantation with capsular rupture, 156
selecting, 46
for toric IOL implantation, 95–96
iris coloboma, 107
irrigation/aspiration
bimanual, 163–165
monomanual, instruments for, 163–165
post implantation, 163–166
surgical technique for, 165–166
irrigation fluids, 171–172

K values, imprecise calculation of, 83
Kelman, Charles, 3, 5, 17
keratoconus
multifocal IOL implantation and, 63
in reduced visual quality, 104–106
keratometry, 39, 40, 95
keratotomy, astigmatic, 39, 40, 42–43
Kratz, Dick, 4

Lang's Stereo Test, 116, 117
laser surgery
refractive procedure guidelines for, 85
for residual astigmatism, 43–44
LASIK
for residual astigmatism, 43–44
for residual refractive errors, 85–86
Lenstec Tetraflex, 73
Lentis Mplus LS-312, 183–184
lidocaine, 172–173

lightning vision, 111
limbal relaxing incisions, 39, 40–42
  complications associated with, 42–44
  nomogram for, 42
loading technique, 137–140, 152–153
loops
  in the bag, 158
  for IOL insertion, 130

macula, reduced visual quality and, 111–112
macular dystrophy, 100
maculopathy
  multifocal IOLs and, 69–71
  in reduced vision quality, 111–112
  visual quality and, 100
Mainster, Martin A., 69–71
marginal pellucid degeneration, 104
materials, lens, 8–13
Mazzocco, Thomas, 5, 17, 18
Memory Lens, 18–19
Mendez ring, 50–51
MI60 lens, 33
microincisional surgery (MICS), 23–24, 27
Miller, David, 5
mini-incisions, 23–24
miodesopsias, 109–110
Mix and Match procedure, 79
  for binocular vision, 115
  choices for, 80
  combining refractive and diffractive lenses, 79–80
  current, 80
  with monofocal lenses, 81
  patient requirements for, 80
modulation transfer function (MTF), 63, 69–70, 100, 109
molding, compression and injection, 7
molecular weight, 122
Monarch III injector, 141–145
monofocal IOLs, 27
  binocular vision and, 115
  in Mix and Match procedure, 81
  1-piece, 27, 30–37
  3-piece, 27–30
monovision, iatrogenic, 192
mouches volantes, 109–110
moxifloxacin, 173
multifocal IOLs, 53, 79
  AcrySof ReSTOR, 55–57, 65–66
  astigmatism and, 64–65
  comparisons of, 62–63
  criteria for implantation of, 178
  diffractive, 53–55, 58–59, 178
  haloes and, 57–59
  ideal patients for, 68
  latest generation of, 177–185
  maculopathy and, 69–71
  optical principles for, 177
  pathologies with, 63
  patient requirements for, 63
  patient selection for, 63, 66–68
  preoperative interview for, 68–71
  pupil dynamics and, 63–64
  refractive, 53, 178
  ReZoom, 53, 54
  Tecnis toric, 53–54, 66
  toric lens technology and, 96
  Zeiss Meditec AT LISA toric, 54–55, 65
  zonal, 59–62
myopia, 81

Nd:YAG laser treatment
  damage to IOL in, 25
  for posterior capsule opacification, 109
neuroadaptation, 70–71, 81
neuroretinal visual sensitivity, 69–70
neurotransfer function (NTF), 63, 69–70, 100
Nichamin Age- and Pachymetry-Adjusted Intralimbal Arcuate Astigmatic (NAPA) nomogram, 40, 41

ocular motility, visual quality and, 115–117
Oculentis Mplus lens, 59
  design of, 62
  versus other multifocal lenses, 62–63
  structure of, 59–60
  toric version of, 60–62
1-piece IOLs
  Alcon, 30
  AMO, 30–31
  Bausch + Lomb, 32
  Hoya, 33
optic nerve abnormalities, 100
optics, 7
  capsular capture of, 156, 158
  tear of damage to, 161–162

passivated surface, 8
patient dissatisfaction
  avoiding and managing, 190–192
  causes of, 189–190
patient education, 190
patient satisfaction survey, 190
pendulum markers, 50
phacoemulsification, 3–5
phacoemulsification incisions, 23–24
PhacoFlex, 19–20
photorefractive keratectomy (PRK), 44, 85
piggyback IOLs
  calculating power of, 89
  correcting biometry errors, 88–89
  in IOL exchange, 91
  for residual refractive errors, 86–88

plasma treatment, 8–9
poly-HEMA, 7, 11–12
polyamide (Nylon), 13
polycarbonate tips, disposable, 163, 164–165
polymethylmethacrylate (PMMA), 7, 13
    surface treatment of, 8
polymethylmethacrylate (PMMA) lenses
    plasma treated, 8–9
    rigid, 15–16
    round or oval, 16
polymide, 13
polypropylene (Prolene), 13
posterior capsule
    altered transparency of, 108–112
    opacification of, 109
povidone iodine, 173
preoperative evaluation
    for toric IOL implantation, 44–46
preoperative interview, for multifocal IOLs, 68–71
presbyopia-correcting IOLs, 178–187
    objectives of, 84–85
    problems causing poor results in, 83–84
pseudophakic eyes, laser refractive procedure in, 85
pseudoplasticity, 119, 120
pupil dilation, drugs for, 172
pupil dynamics, 63–64
pupil kinetics, 36–37

red-green test, 116
refraction, preoperative, 66–67
refractive errors
    residual
        bioptics for, 84–85
        in patient dissatisfaction, 191
        piggyback IOLs for, 86–89
    risk of, 84
refractive IOLs
    combined with diffractive lenses, 79–80
    mechanism of action of, 79
    multifocal, 53, 54
ReSTOR IOLs, 79
    haloes with, 78
    in Mix and Match procedure, 80, 81
retina
    abnormalities of in visual quality, 100
    degeneration of, 63
retinal nerve fiber layer thickness, reduced, 114
ReZoom IOLs, 53, 54, 79, 181
    haloes with, 78
    in Mix and Match procedure, 81
rhexis, anterior
    capturing optic in, 156, 158
    continuous circular, 77
rhodopsin photoreceptors, sensitivity of, 70
Ridley, Sir Harold, 3, 5
rigid IOLs
    holders and folders for, 125
    of past, 15–16
Rosa, Daniele Aron, 5

scintillating synchysis, 111
SeeLens MF, 182–183
Sensar AR40 lenses, 29
Shearing Steven, 4–5
silicone, 9
silicone elastomers, 7
silicone IOLs, 17–18, 26
    disadvantages of, 25
    hydrophilic, 23–25
    production of, 9–10
Sinskey Buratto hook, 125
sodium bicarbonate, 171
SofPort Easy-Load Lens Delivery System, 147
SofPort lenses, 29, 147
soft IOLs
    holders and folders for, 125–128
    of past, 17–22
soft shell technique, 122–123
spherical aberration, 36–37
spinteropia, 111
STAAR IOL foldable lens, 22
Stegmann, Robert, 5
Storz Hydroview Lens, 20–21
strabismus, evaluation of, 116
Sulcoflex lens, 88
sunset syndrome, 107–108
surface treatments, 8
surgical compartmentalization, 122
suture placement, incorrect, 102
Synchrony lens, 74, 76, 185
    biocompatibility of, 76
    contrast sensitivity of, 78
    versus Crystalens HD, 185–186
    haloes and glare with, 78
    patient choice for, 77
    surgical suggestions for, 77
    technical features of, 76–77
    visual acuity with, 77–78

tamsulosin, 172, 173
Tecnis IOLs
    aspheric toric, 49
    MF, haloes with, 78
    in Mix and Match procedure, 80
    multifocal toric, 66
    1-piece, injection of, 140–141
    Z9000, 36
    ZMA00, 3-piece, 181–182

ZMB00, 53–54
in Mix and Match procedure, 81
1-piece, 181–182
pupil dynamics and, 64
Terry-Schanzlin knife, 43
3-piece IOLs
Alcon, 28–29
Bausch + Lomb, 29
Hoya, 29
implanting in capsular bag, 156–157
loading and insertion of, 137–140
for residual refractive errors, 86, 88
toric IOLs, 39
AcrySof, 46–48
Alcon, correct positioning of, 51
AMO, 46
for astigmatism correction, 95–97
complications of, 42–44
contraindications to, 43
corneal incision and, 39–40
correct positioning of, 51
enVista MX60T, 49–50
Oculentis Mplus, 60–62
preoperative evaluations for, 44–46
relaxing incisions and, 40–42
surgical technique for, 50–51
Tecnis aspheric, 49
Zeiss, 46, 48–49, 51
trephine, in keratoplasty, 42–43
Turner, Patricia L., 69–71

vancomycin, 173
Viscoat, 119, 120, 122
viscoelastic substance (VES), 41, 171
adaptive, 123
aspiration of, 165–166
in cataract surgery, 123–124
characteristics of, 119–123
chondroitin sulfate, 102
development of, 5
in IOL exchange, 92, 94
in IOL implantation with capsular rupture, 157
in lens loading and implantation, 152
in toric IOL implantation, 51
viscodispersive, 123
viscoelasticity, 119
viscosity, 119, 120
viscosurgical devices, chemical and physical characteristics of, 120–121
vision quality, 99
factors influencing, 100
ocular motility and, 115–117
optic nerve and, 112–117
problems with, 191–192
reduced, 102–112
surgical reasons for, 100–102
visual acuity, 78
Vitrax, 119, 122
vitreous abnormalities, 109–111
vitreous bodies, mobile, 109–110
vitreous transition temperature (VTT), 10–11

WIOL-CF, 187
Worth's light test, 116
wound burns, 102

ZA9003 IOL, 29
Zeiss IOLs
1-piece, 34–35
3-piece, 29–30
toric, 46, 51
Zernike's polynomials, 35
zonal multifocal lenses, 59–62

For Product Safety Concerns and Information please contact our EU
representative GPSR@taylorandfrancis.com
Taylor & Francis Verlag GmbH, Kaufingerstraße 24, 80331 München, Germany

www.ingramcontent.com/pod-product-compliance
Lightning Source LLC
Chambersburg PA
CBHW080013140226
39335CB00032B/3224